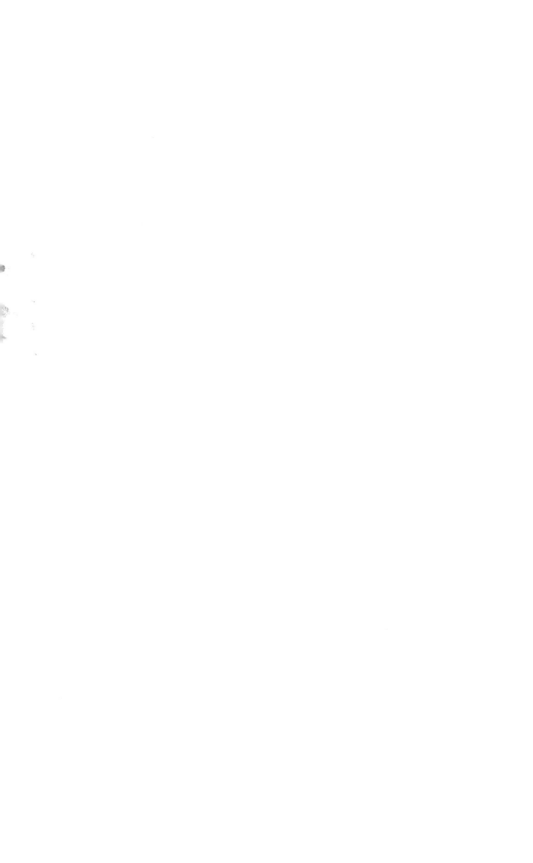

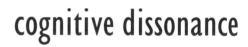

cognitive dissonance

cognitive dissonance

progress on a pivotal theory in social psychology

EDITED BY EDDIE HARMON-JONES & JUDSON MILLS

AMERICAN PSYCHOLOGICAL ASSOCIATION, WASHINGTON, DC

First printing March 1999
Second printing August 1999

Published by
American Psychological Association
750 First Street, NE
Washington, DC 20002

Copies may be ordered from
APA Order Department
P.O. Box 92984
Washington, DC 20090-2984

In the U.K., Europe, Africa, and the Middle East, copies may be ordered from
American Psychological Association
3 Henrietta Street
Covent Garden, London
WC2E 8LU England

Typeset in Minion by EPS Group Inc., Easton, MD
Printer: Sheridan Books, Inc., Ann Arbor, MI
Cover Designer: Anne Masters, Washington, DC
Technical/Production Editor: Catherine R. W. Hudson

Library of Congress Cataloging-in-Publication Data
Cognitive dissonance : progress on a pivotal theory in social psychology / edited by
    Eddie Harmon-Jones and Judson Mills.—1st ed.
        p.   cm.—(Science conference series)
    Papers presented at a two-day conference at the University of Texas at Arlington, winter of 1997.
    Includes bibliographical references and index.
    ISBN 1-55798-565-0 (acid-free paper)
    1. Cognitive dissonance—Congresses.   I. Mills, Judson, 1931–   .
II. Harmon-Jones, Eddie.   III. Series.
BF337.C63C64   1999
153.4—dc21   98-49316
                                                                                                      CIP

British Library Cataloguing-in-Publication Data
A CIP record is available from the British Library.

Printed in the United States of America

APA Science Volumes

Measuring Patient Changes in Mood, Anxiety, and Personality Disorders: Toward a Core Battery

Occasion Setting: Associative Learning and Cognition in Animals

Organ Donation and Transplantation: Psychological and Behavioral Factors

Origins and Development of Schizophrenia: Advances in Experimental Psychopathology

The Perception of Structure

Perspectives on Socially Shared Cognition

Psychological Testing of Hispanics

Psychology of Women's Health: Progress and Challenges in Research and Application

Researching Community Psychology: Issues of Theory and Methods

The Rising Curve: Long-Term Gains in IQ and Related Measures

Sexism and Stereotypes in Modern Society: The Gender Science of Janet Taylor Spence

Sleep and Cognition

Sleep Onset: Normal and Abnormal Processes

Stereotype Accuracy: Toward Appreciating Group Differences

Stereotyped Movements: Brain and Behavior Relationships

Studying Lives Through Time: Personality and Development

The Suggestibility of Children's Recollections: Implications for Eyewitness Testimony

Taste, Experience, and Feeding: Development and Learning

Temperament: Individual Differences at the Interface of Biology and Behavior

Through the Looking Glass: Issues of Psychological Well-Being in Captive Nonhuman Primates

Uniting Psychology and Biology: Integrative Perspectives on Human Development

Viewing Psychology as a Whole: The Integrative Science of William N. Dember

The Science Directorate of the American Psychological Association established its Scientific Conferences Program in 1988. Since that time,

47 conferences have received funding through this program and, to date, 42 edited volumes have been published through a collaboration with the APA Office of Communications. The scientific conference program has showcased some of the most important topics in psychological science, and the conference participants have included many leading figures in the field. This program is a source of pride for APA and for all of those who have served as conference organizers. The Science Directorate looks forward to continuing this superb program. Judging from the proposals that are submitted each year, there is no shortage of great ideas for conferences and talented scientists to implement them.

This most recent volume continues the tradition of presenting the best that psychological science has to offer. Professors Eddie Harmon-Jones and Judson Mills have taken a fresh look at one of the venerable theories in social psychology, cognitive dissonance. More than forty years ago, Leon Festinger published his landmark book, *A Theory of Cognitive Dissonance*. Since then, hundreds of studies have been conducted, and the theory has undergone changes and refinements. Harmon-Jones and Mills assembled a talented group of lecturers and discussants for their conference to capture the continuing vitality of research in this area as well as to highlight emerging controversies. The edited volume resulting from their conference captures the current views of the most important contributors to this field of inquiry. In addition, the reader is treated to a free and open exchange of ideas relating to dissonance theory. Finally, suggestions for future research directions are presented in a clear and compelling fashion.

We are very pleased that this important contribution to the literature was supported in part by the Scientific Conferences Program.

RICHARD MCCARTY, PHD
Executive Director for Science

VIRGINIA E. HOLT
Assistant Executive Director
for Science

In memory of Leon Festinger

Contents

ix

Contributors

Elliot Aronson, University of California, Santa Cruz

Joshua Aronson, University of Texas at Austin

Kenneth E. Barron, University of Wisconsin—Madison

Jean-Léon Beauvois, Université de Nice, Sophia Antipolis, France

Geoffrey Cohen, Stanford University

Joel Cooper, Princeton University

Patricia G. Devine, University of Wisconsin—Madison

Donna Eisenstadt, Saint Louis University

Andrew J. Elliot, University of Rochester

Eddie Harmon-Jones, University of Wisconsin—Madison

Robert-Vincent Joule, Université de Provence, France

Michael R. Leippe, Saint Louis University

Mark R. Lepper, Stanford University

Ian McGregor, University of Waterloo, Waterloo, Ontario, Canada

Judson Mills, University of Maryland, College Park

Paul R. Nail, Southwest Oklahoma State University

Ian R. Newby-Clark, University of Waterloo, Waterloo, Ontario, Canada

Haruki Sakai, Sapporo University, Sapporo, Japan

Thomas R. Shultz, McGill University, Montreal, Quebec, Canada

Jeff Stone, Princeton University

John M. Tauer, University of Wisconsin—Madison

Kristen M. Vance, University of Wisconsin—Madison

Mark P. Zanna, University of Waterloo, Waterloo, Ontario, Canada

Foreword

"This is more like what I had in mind" could easily be what Leon Festinger would have said about this volume had he lived to see it. He would not have been referring to the two appendices that report his own words—the first being his early, unpublished formulation of dissonance theory, the second, his comments on the state of dissonance theory 30 years after its publication. In earlier comments about the state of social psychology, after having been away from the field for several years, he had said, in effect, "it's not exactly what I had in mind."

This is a volume that Leon Festinger surely would have loved to see. It presents a variety of ideas and clever research from a collection of investigators located in Canada, France, and Japan as well as in the United States, and almost all intended to produce a better understanding of the phenomena of cognitive dissonance. Whereas the common thread is dissonance theory as first stated by Festinger, the common concern starts with the assumption that the theory must be taken seriously. From that point, these chapters fan out into a diverse array of suggestions, propositions, qualifications, and additions for the original theory.

This book contains the medication required for all those people who, quite rightly, became bored with dissonance theory in the later 1960s or early 1970s. The present collection demonstrates clearly and convincingly that the problem was not with the theory but rather with the research that was largely confined to conceptual replications of some of the major implications of the theory. Although the issues addressed in some of the chapters have been around for several years (e.g., the role of the self in the instigation of dissonance and the role of aversive consequences), even in those cases there are new and revealing programs of research reported.

What we also find in this new volume are attempts to make the theory more precise in certain respects, a summary of an ambitious research program centered on the justification of behavior, and a report of carefully crafted research to reveal dissonance arousal due to discrepancy between perception and behavior in the absence of negative consequences. There is as well a contribution that takes up the issue of multiple modes of dissonance reduction and how they are determined and interact, and then, for more formal and general points of view, there are two contributions on mathematical formulations that help to place dissonance processes in a larger conceptual context.

Finally, there are contributions that address dissonance as an affective state; one emphasizes the advantage of measuring the feeling of dissonance in pinning down how dissonance processes work, whereas the other attempts to demonstrate the connection between dissonance and ambivalence and how that connection promises to give us a much broader understanding of dissonance effects. All of these reports are preceded by a concise history of the early supporting research as well as of the theoretical and methodological controversies stirred up by the original publication of the theory.

In 1976, in his Foreword to the Wicklund and Brehm *Perspectives on Cognitive Dissonance*, Edward E. Jones wrote, "We may now have reached a less flamboyant stage of tidying of loose ends and charting out relations between dissonance theory and other psychological conceptions. . . ." Twenty years later, what this volume demonstrates is not a neat, tidy, theoretical and empirical package to which the practitioner can turn for help, but rather a remarkably exciting and growing set of research questions about how the human mind works. It is a most enticing invitation to behavioral scientists of all kinds to explore the expanding frontiers of cognitive dissonance.

Jack W. Brehm
University of Kansas

Preface

Over 40 years after the publication of Leon Festinger's (1957) book, *A Theory of Cognitive Dissonance*, research on the theory is receiving renewed attention, and revisions to the original theory have been proposed. Consequently, we felt that an assessment of the current status of the theory would be of value and that there was a need for a book to present and discuss the theoretical controversies and the recent research on important questions about the dissonance process. For this book, we are fortunate to have contributions from the prominent scientists who have made major contributions to research and theory on cognitive dissonance.

We feel honored to be able include in the book unpublished material by Leon Festinger, presenting his earliest version of the theory and his final public comment on the theory. Festinger's first paper on the theory, "Social Communication and Cognition: A Very Preliminary and Highly Tentative Draft," was distributed to students in his graduate seminar at the University of Minnesota in the winter quarter of 1954, which included Jack Brehm and Judson Mills. Festinger's last words on dissonance theory were transcribed from a tape recording of comments he made as a discussant in *Reflections on Cognitive Dissonance: 30 Years Later*, a symposium conducted at the 95th Annual Convention of the American Psychological Association in 1987. We would like to thank Trudy Festinger, for giving us permission to publish these important materials in the present volume.

To discuss the current status of cognitive dissonance theory and research, an international group of researchers met at the University of Texas at Arlington (UTA) in the winter of 1997. The 2-day meeting was attended by approximately 70 faculty, graduate students, and undergraduate students. This book does not represent the proceedings of the conference but was an outgrowth of the conference.

This book and the conference were aided immensely by UTA and the Science Directorate of the American Psychological Association (APA). We would like to thank Virginia Holt, Ed Meidenbauer, Catherine Hudson, and Maggie Nelson at APA. We would like to thank UTA Dean Vern Cox and Psychology Department Chair Roger Mellgren, for financial support and assistance with the logistics of organizing the conference. We received assistance with the conference from UTA staff members Pauline Gregory, Susan Sterling, and Karen Twohey; UTA students Bruce Frankel, Victoria Swanson, and Tracy West; and Professor Bob Schatz from Texas A & M University–Corpus Christi. We received assistance with the book from Todor Gerdjikov. We are most grateful for their generous help. Cindy Harmon-Jones also provided assistance in numerous ways, and Eddie Harmon-Jones would like to thank her. Others were invaluable and contributed to the success of the conference, and their efforts are greatly appreciated. Finally, we would like to express our appreciation to the conference participants, who made the conference an intellectually stimulating and enjoyable experience.

cognitive dissonance

An Introduction to Cognitive Dissonance Theory and an Overview of Current Perspectives on the Theory

Eddie Harmon-Jones and Judson Mills

A little more than 40 years ago, Leon Festinger published *A Theory of Cognitive Dissonance* (1957). Festinger's theory of cognitive dissonance has been one of the most influential theories in social psychology (Jones, 1985). It has generated hundreds and hundreds of studies, from which much has been learned about the determinants of attitudes and beliefs, the internalization of values, the consequences of decisions, the effects of disagreement among persons, and other important psychological processes.

As presented by Festinger in 1957, dissonance theory began by postulating that pairs of cognitions (elements of knowledge) can be relevant or irrelevant to one another. If two cognitions are relevant to one another, they are either consonant or dissonant. Two cognitions are consonant if one follows from the other, and they are dissonant if the obverse (opposite) of one cognition follows from the other. The existence of dissonance, being psychologically uncomfortable, motivates the person to reduce the dissonance and leads to avoidance of information likely to increase the dissonance. The greater the magnitude of the dissonance, the greater is the pressure to reduce dissonance.

The magnitude of dissonance between one cognitive element and the remainder of the person's cognitions depends on the number and importance of cognitions that are consonant and dissonant with the one in question. Formally speaking, the magnitude of dissonance equals the number of dissonant cognitions divided by the number of consonant cognitions plus the number of dissonant cognitions. This is referred to as the *dissonance ratio*. Holding the number and importance of consonant cognitions constant, as the number or importance of dissonant cognitions increases, the magnitude of dissonance increases. Holding the number and importance of dissonant cognitions constant, as the number or importance of consonant cognitions increases, the magnitude of dissonance decreases.

Dissonance can be reduced by removing dissonant cognitions, adding new consonant cognitions, reducing the importance of dissonant cognitions, or increasing the importance of consonant cognitions.[1] The likelihood that a particular cognition will change to reduce dissonance is determined by the resistance to change of the cognition. Cognitions that are less resistant to change will change more readily than cognitions that are more resistant to change. Resistance to change is based on the responsiveness of the cognition to reality and on the extent to which the cognition is consonant with many other cognitions. Resistance to change of a behavioral cognitive element depends on the extent of pain or loss that must be endured and the satisfaction obtained from the behavior.

An example used by Festinger (1957) may assist in elucidating the theory. A habitual smoker who learns that smoking is bad for health will experience dissonance, because the knowledge that smoking is bad for health is dissonant with the cognition that he continues to smoke. He can reduce the dissonance by changing his behavior, that is, he could stop smoking, which would be consonant with the cognition that smoking is bad for health. Alternatively, the smoker could reduce dissonance

---

[1] Increasing the importance of consonant cognitions was not specified by Festinger as a way to reduce dissonance, although it follows logically from consideration of the dissonance ratio that is used to calculate the magnitude of dissonance and Festinger's (1957) statement that "the magnitude of dissonance (and consonance) increases as the importance or value of the elements increases" (p. 18).

by changing his cognition about the effect of smoking on health and believe that smoking does not have a harmful effect on health (eliminating the dissonant cognition). He might look for positive effects of smoking and believe that smoking reduces tension and keeps him from gaining weight (adding consonant cognitions). Or he might believe that the risk to health from smoking is negligible compared with the danger of automobile accidents (reducing the importance of the dissonant cognition). In addition, he might consider the enjoyment he gets from smoking to be a very important part of his life (increasing the importance of consonant cognitions).

Since it was presented by Festinger over 40 years ago, cognitive dissonance theory has continued to generate research, revision, and controversy. Part of the reason it has been so generative is that the theory was stated in very general, highly abstract terms. As a consequence, it can be applied to a wide variety of psychological topics involving the interplay of cognition, motivation, and emotion. A person can have cognitions about behaviors, perceptions, attitudes, beliefs, and feelings. Cognitions can be about oneself, another person or group, or about things in the environment. Rather than being relevant to a single topic, the theory is relevant to many different topics.

RESEARCH PARADIGMS IN DISSONANCE RESEARCH

We now review briefly the common paradigms used in dissonance research. Important research generated by the theory has been concerned with what happens after individuals make decisions, the consequences of exposure to information inconsistent with a prior belief, the effects of effort expenditure, and what happens after persons act in ways that are discrepant with their beliefs and attitudes.

The Free-Choice Paradigm

Once a decision is made, dissonance is likely to be aroused. After the person makes a decision, each of the negative aspects of the chosen alternative and positive aspects of the rejected alternative is dissonant with the decision. On the other hand, each of the positive aspects of the chosen alternative and negative aspects of the rejected alternative is consonant with the decision. Difficult decisions should arouse more dissonance than easy decisions, because there will be a greater proportion of dissonant cognitions after a difficult decision than there will be after an easy one. Because of this, there will be greater motivation to reduce the dissonance after a difficult decision. Dissonance following a decision can be reduced by removing negative aspects of the chosen alternative or positive aspects of the rejected alternative, and it can also be reduced by adding positive aspects to the chosen alternative or negative aspects to the rejected alternative. Altering the aspects of the decision alternatives to reduce dissonance will lead to viewing the chosen alternative as more desirable and the rejected alternative as less desirable. This effect has been termed *spreading of alternatives*, and the experimental paradigm has been termed the *free-choice paradigm*.

J. W. Brehm (1956) conducted the first experiment using the free-choice paradigm to test predictions derived from dissonance theory. In his experiment, which was presented as market research, he had women rate how desirable they found eight different products (e.g., toaster or coffeemaker) and then gave each of them a choice between two products that were close in desirability (difficult decision) or between two products that were not close in desirability (easy decision). After choosing which of the two products they would keep, the women rerated the desirability of the products. Results indicated that the women who made a difficult decision changed their evaluations of the products to be more positive about the chosen product and less positive about the rejected product. Spreading of alternatives was less for the women who made an easy decision. The free-choice paradigm continues to be used to gain insights into dissonance processes (e.g., Shultz & Lepper, 1996; Stone, chap. 8, this volume).

The Belief-Disconfirmation Paradigm

Dissonance is aroused when people are exposed to information inconsistent with their beliefs. If the dissonance is not reduced by changing one's belief, the dissonance can lead to misperception or misinterpretation of the information, rejection or refutation of the information, seeking support from those who agree with one's belief, and attempting to persuade others to accept one's belief. In a study of the effect of belief disconfirmation on proselytizing, Festinger, Riecken, and Schachter (1956) acted as participant observers in a group that had become committed to an important belief that was specific enough to be capable of unequivocal disconfirmation. The group believed a prophecy that a flood would engulf the continent. The prophecy was supposedly transmitted by beings from outer space to a woman in the group. The group members also believed that they had been chosen to be saved from the flood and would be evacuated in a flying saucer.

Festinger et al. (1956) described what happened when the flood did not occur. Members of the group who were alone at that time did not maintain their beliefs. Members who were waiting with other group members maintained their faith. The woman reported receiving a message that indicated that the flood had been prevented by God because of the group's existence as a force for good. Before the disconfirmation of the belief about the flood, the group engaged in little proselytizing. After the disconfirmation, they engaged in substantial proselytizing. The group members sought to persuade others of their beliefs, which would add cognitions consonant with those beliefs. This paradigm, referred to as the *belief-disconfirmation paradigm*, continues to generate insight into dissonance processes (e.g., Burris, Harmon-Jones, & Tarpley, 1997; Harmon-Jones, chap. 4, this volume).

The Effort-Justification Paradigm

Dissonance is aroused whenever a person engages in an unpleasant activity to obtain some desirable outcome. From the cognition that the activity is unpleasant, it follows that one would not engage in the activity; the cognition that the activity is unpleasant is dissonant with engaging in the activity. Dissonance should be greater, the greater the unpleasant effort required to obtain the outcome. Dissonance can be reduced by exaggerating the desirability of the outcome, which would add consonant cognitions.

In the first experiment designed to test these theoretical ideas, E.

Aronson and Mills (1959) had women undergo a severe or mild "initiation" to become a member of a group. In the severe-initiation condition, the women engaged in an embarrassing activity to join the group, whereas in the mild-initiation condition, the women engaged in an activity that was not very embarrassing to join the group. The group turned out to be rather dull and boring. The women in the severe-initiation condition evaluated the group more favorably than the women in the mild-initiation condition. This paradigm is referred to as the *effort-justification paradigm*, and it continues to be used fruitfully in research (e.g., Beauvois & Joule, 1996).

The Induced-Compliance Paradigm

Dissonance is aroused when a person does or says something that is contrary to a prior belief or attitude. From the cognition of the prior belief or attitude, it would follow that one would not engage in such behavior. On the other hand, inducements to engage in such behavior, promises of reward or threats of punishment, provide cognitions that are consonant with the behavior. Such cognitions provide justifications for the behavior. The greater the number and importance of the cognitions justifying the behavior, the less the dissonance aroused. Dissonance can be reduced by changing the belief or attitude to correspond more closely to what was said. Instead of using Festinger's original term, *forced compliance*, this paradigm is now called the *induced-compliance paradigm*.

The first experiment using the induced-compliance paradigm was the groundbreaking study by Festinger and Carlsmith (1959). They tested the hypothesis derived from dissonance theory that the smaller the reward for saying something that one does not believe, the greater the opinion changes to agree with what one has said. In their experiment, men performed boring tasks for 1 hr. Then each was told by the experimenter that there were two groups in the experiment: the one the participant was in, which received no introduction, and a second group, which was told the tasks were enjoyable by a person who had supposedly just completed them. The experimenter asked the participant to substitute for the person who usually said the tasks were enjoyable, and the participant was given $1 or $20 to tell the next person (actually a female accomplice of the experimenter) that the tasks were enjoyable and to remain on call in the future. The participants were then asked to evaluate the tasks by an interviewer from the psychology department, who ostensibly had nothing to do with the experiment. Results indicated that those paid $1 rated the tasks as more enjoyable than did those paid $20 or those who merely performed the tasks and were not asked to describe them to another person.

The participants in the experiment by Festinger and Carlsmith (1959) engaged in what is referred to as *counterattitudinal behavior*. The finding that the less money received for engaging in the counteratti- tudinal behavior, the more positive the attitude has been labeled the *negative-incentive effect*. The reason that term is used is that there is a negative relationship between the amount of incentive (money) and the amount of attitude change in the direction of the counterattitudinal behavior.[2] Later research by Linder, Cooper, and Jones (1967) showed that the negative-incentive effect occurs when the person feels free to decide about engaging in the counterattitudinal behavior, but when there is no perceived freedom to engage in the counterattitudinal be- havior, the opposite effect occurs, that is, the more incentive, the more positive the attitude. When there is no choice about engaging in the behavior, dissonance is minimal, because there is sufficient justification for the behavior (see Festinger, Appendix B, this volume).[3]

A variant of the induced-compliance paradigm that involves threat of punishment rather than promise of reward is known as the *forbid- den-toy paradigm*. In the forbidden-toy paradigm (E. Aronson & Carl- smith, 1963), young children were given the opportunity to play with toys and were threatened with severe or mild punishment if they played

---

[2] As in many attitude-change studies, there was no measure of attitude before the experimental treatment. The measure of attitude was taken only after the experimental treatment. This type of design is referred to as an *after-only* design. In an after-only design, attitude change is shown by differences between the experimental conditions on the measure of attitude taken after the ex- perimental treatment.

[3] Later dissonance theorists have given different reasons why perceived choice is a crucial factor in dissonance effects (Beauvois & Joule, 1996; J. W. Brehm & Cohen, 1962; Cooper & Fazio, 1984; Wicklund & Brehm, 1976).

with a very attractive toy. The threatened punishment was sufficient to prevent the children from playing with the attractive toy. When asked at a later time to evaluate the attractive toy, children who were threatened with mild punishment evaluated the toy less positively than children who were threatened with severe punishment. The induced-compliance paradigm and the forbidden-toy paradigm continue to be used to address questions about dissonance processes (e.g., J. Aronson, Cohen, & Nail, chap. 6, Beauvois & Joule, chap. 3, Cooper, chap. 7, Devine, Tauer, Barron, Elliot, & Vance, chap. 12, Harmon-Jones, chap. 4, Leippe & Eisenstadt, chap. 9, Sakai, chap. 11, Shultz & Lepper, chap. 10, all in this volume).

ALTERNATIVE ACCOUNTS OF DISSONANCE PHENOMENA

Over the years, various alternative theoretical accounts have been advanced to explain the effects found in dissonance experiments. The alternative accounts of dissonance have provoked considerable controversy. In some cases, the controversy has led to important empirical and theoretical advances. We briefly review the major alternative accounts and the controversy they generated.

Alternatives to Dissonance Theory

Self-Perception Theory

Self-perception theory (Bem, 1967, 1972) argued that dissonance effects were not the result of motivation to reduce the psychological discomfort produced by cognitive dissonance but were due to a nonmotivational process whereby persons merely inferred their attitudes from their behavior and the circumstances under which the behavior occurred. The self-perception theory explanation for the negative-incentive effect found by Festinger and Carlsmith (1959) assumes that persons use their overt behavior to judge their attitudes if external cues (such as an incentive) are not seen as controlling the behavior, but they do not use their overt behavior to judge their attitudes if external cues are seen as controlling the behavior. The explanation assumes that a small incentive is not seen as controlling the behavior, whereas a large incentive is seen as controlling the behavior.

One of the consequences of the controversy generated by the self-perception account was research testing the implications of dissonance theory using the *misattribution paradigm*. In the misattribution paradigm, participants are exposed to an extraneous stimulus (e.g., a pill) that is said to have a certain effect on the person's internal state (e.g., produces tenseness). If the supposed effect of the extraneous stimulus is the same as the actual internal state the person is experiencing, the person may misattribute the internal state to the extraneous stimulus rather than attribute it to the actual cause. If this misattribution occurs, the person may not respond to the internal state in the same way (e.g., will not change cognitions to reduce dissonance, to eliminate the negative affect or arousal).

Zanna and Cooper (1974) were the first to use the misattribution paradigm to show that the attitude change found in the induced-compliance paradigm is motivated by the need to reduce negative affect or arousal, as assumed in the dissonance interpretation. In their experiment, under the guise of a study of the effects of a drug on memory, participants were given a pill to ingest that was actually a placebo with no real effect. The pill was said to cause tenseness, to cause relaxation, or to have no side effects. The participants then took part in a supposedly unrelated experiment in which they wrote a counterattitudinal message under high or low choice. If the pill was said to have no side effects, participants changed their attitudes to be more consistent with the counterattitudinal essay when choice was high but not when choice was low, in keeping with the results of other dissonance research. However, if the pill was said to cause tenseness, participants did not change their attitudes in either the low- or high-choice condition.

Zanna and Cooper (1974) reasoned that the feeling of tenseness that was experienced due to the dissonance created by writing the counterattitudinal message under high choice was misattributed to the pill when the pill was said to cause tenseness. With the tenseness misattributed to the pill, there was no need to reduce the dissonance that was the true cause of the feeling and thus no need for attitude change to reduce the dissonance.[4] Bem's self-perception account of dissonance phenomena is unable to explain the findings of the study by Zanna and Cooper. If, as assumed by the self-perception account, attitude change was not the result of motivation to reduce the discomfort produced by cognitive dissonance, then the extraneous stimulus to which the discomfort could be misattributed would have no influence on attitude change.

Prompted in part by the controversy engendered by the self-perception account, additional research has been carried out to assess the motivational and emotional nature of dissonance. By showing that dissonance is associated with physiological arousal and psychological discomfort and that the cognitive changes that occur are motivated by this discomfort, research has demonstrated that self-perception processes cannot account for all effects produced in dissonance experiments (Elliot & Devine, 1994; Fazio, Zanna, & Cooper, 1977; Gerard, 1967; Harmon-Jones, Brehm, Greenberg, Simon, & Nelson, 1996; Losch & Cacioppo, 1990; Zanna & Cooper, 1974). Beauvois and Joule (chap. 3), Devine et al. (chap. 12), and Harmon-Jones (chap. 4; all from this volume) present further experimental evidence that is consistent with dissonance theory but cannot be explained by self-perception theory.

Impression-Management Theory

Another alternative theoretical account that has been offered for the effects obtained in dissonance experiments is impression-management theory (Tedeschi, Schlenker, & Bonoma, 1971). According to this interpretation, attitudes appear to change because persons want to manage the impressions others have of them. They try to create a favorable impression or avoid an unfavorable impression by appearing to have attitudes that are consistent with their behavior. This alternative theoretical account assumes that the attitude change that occurs in disso-

---

[4]High-choice participants given the pill that was said to cause relaxation changed their attitudes more than did high-choice participants given the pill said to cause no side effects. Zanna and Cooper (1974) reasoned that when the pill was said to cause relaxation, the participants deduced the amount of their tenseness by combining the amount of tenseness actually experienced and the amount of tenseness the pill supposedly reduced.

nance experiments is not genuine and that participants in experiments only appear to change their attitudes after counterattitudinal behavior to avoid being viewed unfavorably by the experimenter.

In contrast to the assumption of the impression-management account, dissonance processes do produce genuine cognitive changes. Results supporting the dissonance interpretation have been obtained in experiments in which the attitude measure was taken by someone who did not appear connected with the experimenter that observed the participant's behavior (Festinger & Carlsmith, 1959; Linder et al., 1967) and in experiments using extremely private situations (Harmon-Jones et al., 1996). Impression-management theory has difficulty accounting for findings that show that dissonance processes that justify recent behavior can produce physiological changes (M. L. Brehm, Back, & Bogdonoff, 1964), and it has problems explaining results obtained in paradigms other than the induced-compliance paradigm, for example, the free-choice paradigm (Wicklund & Brehm, 1976).

Revisions of Dissonance Theory

Currently, there are several versions of dissonance theory that assume, along with the original version, that situations evoking dissonance produce a motivation that results in genuine cognitive changes. However, these revisions offer somewhat different theoretical interpretations for the phenomena observed in dissonance experiments. The revisions differ in what they posit to be the underlying motivation for dissonance effects. Those differences are a major source of the current controversy about dissonance. The different theoretical positions are covered extensively in the present volume by authors who have been intimately involved in the development of the revisions and the controversy they have generated.

Self-Consistency

One of the first revisions proposed was the *self-consistency* interpretation of dissonance (E. Aronson, 1968, 1992). It is based on the idea that situations that evoke dissonance do so because they create inconsistency between the self-concept and a behavior. Because most persons have a positive self-concept, persons are likely to experience dissonance when they behave in a way that they view as incompetent, immoral, or irrational. This revision interprets the effects observed in the Festinger and Carlsmith (1959) experiment as resulting from an inconsistency between the person's self-concept as a moral person and the person's behavior of telling a lie to another person. This revision has led to an examination of the way in which variables related to the self, such as self-esteem, are involved in dissonance processes and to the generation of new research paradigms (see E. Aronson, chap. 5, and Stone, chap. 8, both this volume).

The New Look

Another revision has proposed that the effects observed in dissonance studies are the result of feeling personally responsible for producing foreseeable aversive consequences (Cooper & Fazio, 1984; Scher & Cooper, 1989). This revision, often referred to the *new look* version of dissonance, proposes that the attitude change observed in the Festinger and Carlsmith (1959) experiment resulted from the desire to avoid feeling personally responsible for producing the aversive consequence of having harmed the other participant by leading them to believe that a boring task was enjoyable. This revision has generated research concerned with identifying necessary and sufficient conditions for the production of dissonance and with the role of arousal and its interpretation in dissonance processes. Controversy about this revision has spurred empirical and theoretical advances (see E. Aronson, chap. 5, Beauvois & Joule, chap. 3; Harmon-Jones, chap. 4; Sakai, chap. 11, all this volume).

Self-Affirmation

Self-affirmation theory proposes that dissonance effects are not the result of cognitive inconsistency, self-inconsistency, or feeling personally responsible for producing aversive consequences, but of behaving in a manner that threatens one's sense of moral and adaptive integrity (Steele, 1988; Steele, Spencer, & Lynch, 1993). This revision interprets the Festinger and Carlsmith (1959) results by assuming that the participants in that experiment changed their attitudes about the task because saying that the tasks were enjoyable when they knew they were boring

14

made them feel foolish and threatened their sense of self-worth. The self-affirmation revision also has generated much controversy that has led to empirical and theoretical advances (see J. Aronson et al., chap. 6; Cooper, chap. 7; Stone, chap. 8, all this volume).

The Original Version Reaffirmed

Although the revisions of dissonance theory have produced serious challenges to the original version of the theory, other theorists maintain that the original version continues to be viable and that it can explain the evidence generated by the revisions (Beauvois & Joule, 1996, chap. 3; Harmon-Jones, chap. 4; McGregor, Newby-Clark, & Zanna, chap. 13; Mills, chap. 2, all this volume). The resurgence of the original version has generated new experimental paradigms and conceptual advances.

Areas of Agreement and Disagreement

Although there is controversy about the underlying motivation for dissonance effects, there is also much agreement about important issues. Dissonance theorists currently agree that genuine cognitive changes occur in dissonance studies, for example, studies of the induced-compliance paradigm, the free-choice paradigm, and the effort-justification paradigm. Moreover, it is agreed that these cognitive changes are motivated in nature and that the source of this motivation is a form of psychological discomfort.

Currently, the major area of disagreement is the nature of the motivation underlying the cognitive and other changes that result from dissonance. Just as the earlier controversies in the history of dissonance research have led to important empirical and theoretical advances, the controversy regarding the nature of the motivation underlying dissonance effects has been, and promises to continue to be, the source of new research findings. Understanding the nature of the motivation underlying dissonance effects should assist in developing a better understanding of the interplay of cognition, motivation, emotion, and behavior. By advancing knowledge about the determinants of cognitive, emotional, motivational, and behavioral change, dissonance research has the potential to produce significant practical applications to problems of society.

OVERVIEW OF THE PRESENT VOLUME

The chapters written for this volume by dissonance researchers and scholars have been grouped into four parts, organized on the basis of themes shared by the chapters. The placement of the chapters into different parts should not be taken to mean that what is included in the chapters in one part is not relevant to the material contained in the chapters in a different part. Each of the chapters shares the common theme of dealing with issues of importance for the continued development of theory and research on dissonance processes.

Part One, "Perspectives Employing the Original Version of the Theory," consists of chapters discussing work that uses the original version of dissonance theory. In chapter 2, Judson Mills presents suggestions for improving the original version. He contends that the magnitude of avoidance of new dissonance is not influenced by the amount of existing dissonance and that spreading of alternatives occurs before a choice. He proposes changing the definition of dissonance to include the degree to which a behavior will lead to a consequence and the desirability of the consequence.

Jean-Léon Beauvois and Robert-Vincent Joule present their radical dissonance theory in chapter 3. They suggest that dissonance theory is a theory concerned with rationalization of behavior and that as such, it is not a theory of cognitive consistency, the management of personal responsibility, or the management of one's moral worth. They review experiments supporting their viewpoint and describe two new paradigms for dissonance research.

In chapter 4, Eddie Harmon-Jones presents arguments suggesting, in contrast to the new look version of dissonance, that feeling personally responsible for the production of aversive consequences is not necessary to create cognitive dissonance and that dissonance will occur even when aversive consequences are not produced. He presents recent empirical evidence supporting this view and offers a new theoretical interpretation for dissonance theory.

Part Two, "The Role of the Self in Dissonance," comprises chapters that discuss the revisions of cognitive dissonance theory that use the self as a crucial factor in dissonance processes. In chapter 5, Elliot Aronson presents his self-consistency interpretation of dissonance and describes a new paradigm for dissonance theory, the *hypocrisy paradigm*, that makes persons mindful of the fact that they are not practicing what they are preaching. He argues that evidence obtained in this paradigm indicates that the production of aversive consequences is not essential for the creation of dissonance.

Joshua Aronson, Geoffry Cohen, and Paul R. Nail present the self-affirmation reformulation of dissonance theory in chapter 6. They describe research derived from self-affirmation theory that was used to challenge the original version of dissonance theory and discuss recent evidence that poses challenges for a self-affirmation theory account of dissonance research.

In chapter 7, Joel Cooper presents the new look version of dissonance theory and discusses recent research on how the self is implicated in dissonance processes. Proposing an interpretation different from self-consistency and self-affirmation theories, he reviews evidence showing that the self is multiply involved in dissonance processes.

Jeff Stone presents an analysis of the conditions under which the self plays a role in dissonance in chapter 8. He considers when the self operates as a standard determining dissonance and when the self operates as a resource for dissonance reduction. He describes research on self-focused attention aimed at determining when effects occur that are predicted by self-consistency theory, self-affirmation theory, or neither theory.

In chapter 9, the final chapter of Part Two, Michael Leippe and Donna Eisenstadt present their self-accountability model of dissonance reduction, which deals with the conditions under which various modes of dissonance reduction are used. They review evidence showing that in addition to attitude change, dissonance can be reduced by forgetting the dissonant cognitions, by elaborate cognitive restructuring, or by changing related beliefs.

Part Three, "Mathematical Models of Dissonance," comprises chapters that present novel mathematical models of dissonance processes. In chapter 10, Thomas R. Shultz and Mark R. Lepper present a computational model of cognitive dissonance, which they refer to as the *consonance* model, because it assumes that the motivation underlying dissonance phenomena is to increase cognitive consonance. The model is based on principles of constraint satisfaction. They describe simulations of the results of dissonance experiments using an artificial neural network model.

Haruki Sakai presents a mathematical formulation of dissonance, termed the *multiplicative power-function model* in chapter 11. He discusses implications of the model for important theoretical issues, such as the calculation of magnitude of dissonance and specifying the key element around which dissonance is calculated. He also describes research on shared responsibility for negative consequences that casts doubt on the new look version of dissonance.

Part Four, "Dissonance and Affect," comprises chapters that present recent work on the role of emotion in dissonance processes. Patricia G. Devine, John M. Tauer, Kenneth E. Barron, Andrew J. Elliot, and Kristen M. Vance argue in chapter 12 that attitude change, the most commonly used dependent variable in dissonance research, is limited in what it can reveal about the nature of dissonance motivation and dissonance reduction. They describe research demonstrating the value of measures of self-reported affect in dissonance studies.

In the final chapter, chapter 13, Ian McGregor, Ian R. Newby-Clark, and Mark P. Zanna present an account of dissonance in terms of the simultaneous accessibility of inconsistent cognitions. They describe research on attitudinal ambivalence indicating that felt ambivalence arising from the existence of inconsistent cognitions is moderated by the extent to which both cognitions are readily and easily accessible.

As editors of the book, we encouraged the authors to present their own personal views on the important issues in cognitive dissonance research and theory. We hoped to encourage a free and open exchange of ideas relevant to the theory. As expected, differing viewpoints about dissonance are expressed in the different chapters. Also as expected, the differences are not resolved within the book. We hope that the debate about the differences and the controversy about the nature of dissonance will stimulate theoretical development and lead to new insights and findings. We believe that the future of dissonance research promises to be as exciting and valuable as the past 40 years of work on the theory.

REFERENCES

Aronson, E. (1968). Dissonance theory: Progress and problems. In R. P. Abelson, E. Aronson, W. J. McGuire, T. M. Newcomb, M. J. Rosenberg, & P. H. Tannenbaum (Eds.), *Theories of cognitive consistency: A sourcebook* (pp. 5–27). Chicago: Rand McNally.

Aronson, E. (1992). The return of the repressed: Dissonance theory makes a comeback. *Psychological Inquiry, 3,* 303–311.

Aronson, E., & Carlsmith, J. M. (1963). Effect of severity of threat on the valuation of forbidden behavior. *Journal of Abnormal and Social Psychology, 66,* 584–588.

Aronson, E., & Mills, J. (1959). The effect of severity of initiation on liking for a group. *Journal of Abnormal and Social Psychology, 59,* 177–181.

Beauvois, J.-L., & Joule, R.-V. (1996). *A radical dissonance theory.* London: Taylor & Francis.

Bem, D. J. (1967). Self-perception: An alternative interpretation of cognitive dissonance phenomena. *Psychological Review, 74,* 183–200.

Bem, D. J. (1972). Self-perception theory. In L. Berkowitz (Ed.), *Advances in experimental social psychology* (Vol. 6, pp. 1–62). New York: Academic Press.

Brehm, J. W. (1956). Postdecision changes in the desirability of alternatives. *Journal of Abnormal and Social Psychology, 52,* 384–389.

Brehm, J. W., & Cohen, A. R. (1962). *Explorations in cognitive dissonance.* New York: Wiley.

Brehm, M. L., Back, K. W., & Bogdonoff, M. D. (1964). A physiological effect of cognitive dissonance under stress and deprivation. *Journal of Abnormal and Social Psychology, 69,* 303–310.

Burris, C. T., Harmon-Jones, E., & Tarpley, W. R. (1997). "By faith alone": Religious agitation and cognitive dissonance. *Basic and Applied Social Psychology, 19,* 17–31.

Cooper, J., & Fazio, R. H. (1984). A new look at dissonance theory. In L. Berkowitz (Ed.), *Advances in experimental social psychology* (Vol. 17, pp. 229–264). Orlando, FL: Academic Press.

Elliot, A. J., & Devine, P. G. (1994). On the motivational nature of cognitive dissonance: Dissonance as psychological discomfort. *Journal of Personality and Social Psychology, 67*, 382–394.

Fazio, R. H., Zanna, M. P., & Cooper, J. (1977). Dissonance and self-perception: An integrative view of each theory's proper domain of application. *Journal of Experimental Social Psychology, 13*, 464–479.

Festinger, L. (1957). *A theory of cognitive dissonance.* Evanston, IL: Row, Peterson.

Festinger, L., & Carlsmith, J. M. (1959). Cognitive consequences of forced compliance. *Journal of Abnormal and Social Psychology, 58*, 203–210.

Festinger, L., Riecken, H. W., & Schachter, S. (1956). *When prophecy fails.* Minneapolis: University of Minnesota Press.

Gerard, H. B. (1967). Choice difficulty, dissonance and the decision sequence. *Journal of Personality, 35*, 91–108.

Harmon-Jones, E., Brehm, J. W., Greenberg, J., Simon, L., & Nelson, D. E. (1996). Evidence that the production of aversive consequences is not necessary to create cognitive dissonance. *Journal of Personality and Social Psychology, 70*, 5–16.

Jones, E. E. (1985). Major developments in social psychology during the past five decades. In G. Lindzey & E. Aronson (Eds.), *The handbook of social psychology* (3rd ed., pp. 47–108). New York: Random House.

Linder, D. E., Cooper, J., & Jones, E. E. (1967). Decision freedom as a determinant of the role of incentive magnitude in attitude change. *Journal of Personality and Social Psychology, 6*, 245–254.

Losch, M. E., & Cacioppo, J. T. (1990). Cognitive dissonance may enhance sympathetic tonus, but attitudes are changed to reduce negative affect rather than arousal. *Journal of Experimental Social Psychology, 26*, 289–304.

Scher, S. J., & Cooper, J. (1989). Motivational basis of dissonance: The singular role of behavioral consequences. *Journal of Personality and Social Psychology, 56*, 899–906.

Shultz, T. R., & Lepper, M. R. (1996). Cognitive dissonance reduction as constraint satisfaction. *Psychological Review, 103*, 219–240.

Steele, C. M. (1988). The psychology of self-affirmation: Sustaining the integrity of the self. In L. Berkowitz (Ed.), *Advances in experimental social psychology* (Vol. 21, pp. 261–302). San Diego, CA: Academic Press.

Steele, C. M., Spencer, S. J., & Lynch, M. (1993). Self-image resilience and dissonance: The role of affirmational resources. *Journal of Personality and Social Psychology, 64,* 885–896.

Tedeschi, J. T., Schlenker, B. R., & Bonoma, T. V. (1971). Cognitive dissonance: Private ratiocination or public spectacle? *American Psychologist, 26,* 685–695.

Wicklund, R. A., & Brehm, J. W. (1976). *Perspectives on cognitive dissonance.* Hillsdale, NJ: Erlbaum.

Zanna, M. P., & Cooper, J. (1974). Dissonance and the pill: An attribution approach to studying the arousal properties of dissonance. *Journal of Personality and Social Psychology, 29,* 703–709.

PART ONE

Perspectives Employing the Original Version of the Theory

2

Improving the 1957 Version of Dissonance Theory

Judson Mills

In this chapter, I am going to do something audacious. I am going to propose some improvements in Leon Festinger's most important contribution to psychology, his 1957 theory of cognitive dissonance. Some of the proposed changes have to do with Festinger's assumptions about the magnitude of avoidance of dissonance and about what occurs before a choice. A major proposed change is concerned with how dissonance is determined by desired consequences and importance of cognitions.

In Festinger's last public reflections on dissonance theory made at the symposium, *Reflections on Cognitive Dissonance: 30 Years Later*, conducted at the 95th Annual Convention of the American Psychological Association (1987; see Appendix B), he described why he left social psychology: "I left and stopped doing research on the theory of dissonance because I was in a total rut. The only thing I could think about was how correct the original statement had been" (Appendix B, this volume, p. 383). If Festinger, the master theoretician, could not improve dissonance theory, what hope is there?

However, in his remarks, Festinger also said, "If a theory is at all testable it will not remain unchanged. It has to change. All theories are wrong. One doesn't ask about theories, can I show they are wrong or can I show they are right, but rather one asks, how much of the empirical realm can it handle and how must it be modified and changed as it matures?" (Appendix B, this volume, p. 383). Referring to dissonance theory, Festinger said, "I am quite sure that there is enough validity to the theory, and as changes are made, emendations are made, there will be even more validity to the theory, that research on it will continue, and a lot will get clarified" (Appendix B, this volume, p. 384). So although Festinger felt unable to improve the theory and left dissonance research and social psychology in 1964, his retrospection gives us hope and encouragement to develop and improve the theory.

As is well known, dissonance theory has been extremely fruitful and has stimulated an enormous amount of research. Beyond that, as I noted when moderating the 1987 symposium on dissonance, Festinger's theorizing about dissonance has had repercussions far outside the field of social psychology. It has changed the meaning of the word *dissonance*. No longer do educated people immediately think of music when the word dissonance is mentioned. *Cognitive dissonance* has become a part of the language. For example, the term has appeared in articles on the op-ed page of the *Washington Post*.

Why was dissonance theory, and specifically the 1957 version, so fruitful and important? One answer to that question emphasizes Festinger's unique research style. In the obituary for Festinger in the *American Psychologist*, Zajonc (1990) likened Festinger to Dostoyevski and Picasso. Zajonc wrote, "Like Dostoyevski and like Picasso, Festinger set in motion a *style* of research and theory in the social sciences that is now the common property of all creative workers in the field," (p. 661). Zajonc said about Festinger, "Leon is to social psychology what Freud is to clinical psychology and Piaget to developmental psychology," (p. 661). Such a statement made by a Festinger advisee such as myself would be viewed as biased and possibly self-serving, but Zajonc, who is a very distinguished psychologist, was not a Festinger advisee.

I prefer to answer the question about why the theory became so important in terms of the content of the theory. I believe that it has been so important because it has uncovered a large number of new and interesting phenomena, phenomena dealing primarily with the effect of actions on beliefs and attitudes. The theory went far beyond the simple idea that saying is believing. It specified the conditions under which saying is believing and doing is valuing. The concern with the effect of behavior on cognition that is the hallmark of dissonance theory can be seen in the earliest version of the theory, in an unpublished paper Festinger distributed in his seminar in 1954 (see Appendix A, this volume). In that first version of dissonance theory, Festinger hypothesized that there exists a tendency to make one's cognition and one's behavior consonant, to reduce dissonance between behavior and cognition.

I am going to concentrate on the 1957 version of dissonance theory, which has been, and I believe continues to be, a very useful theoretical statement. The 1957 version started with a (seemingly) simple definition of dissonance. "Two elements are in dissonant relationship if, considering these two alone, the obverse of one element would follow from the other. To state it a bit more formally, x and y are dissonant if not-x follows from y" (Festinger, 1957, p. 13). I prefer to focus on the second sentence of the definition because it avoids the obscure term *obverse*.[1]

The key element of dissonance theory that made the theory so useful was, I believe, the assumption that dissonance varies in magnitude, that the total amount of dissonance depends on the proportion of relevant elements that are dissonant with the one in question. The focal element was typically a behavior or what Festinger called a *behavioral element*. The assumption concerning the magnitude of the dissonance, with the assumptions that dissonance was uncomfortable and that the pressure to reduce dissonance was a function of the magnitude of the dissonance, allowed the derivation of many interesting predictions, for example, the prediction that the less money one receives for convincing someone that a boring task is enjoyable, the more positive one's attitude toward the boring task will be (Festinger & Carlsmith, 1959).

Festinger's assumption about the magnitude of dissonance was very

---

[1] The term *obverse* does not seem to have been used in accord with the dictionary definition of *obverse* as a proposition inferred immediately from another by denying the opposite of that which the given proposition affirms, for example, the obverse of "all *a* is *b*" is "no *a* is not *b*."

different than what was assumed in the other theories of cognitive consistency common in the 1950s and 1960s. It allowed not only derivations about when dissonance would be more likely to be created and thus when tendencies to reduce dissonance would be stronger but predictions about how dissonance would be reduced. The assumption that dissonance was a function of the proportion of dissonant elements enabled predictions concerning the reduction of dissonance by adding consonant cognitions as well as by removing dissonant cognitions. Those predictions were not made by the other cognitive consistency theories, which did not make assumptions about degrees of inconsistency or alleviating an inconsistency by adding a different consistency.

THE MAGNITUDE OF AVOIDANCE OF DISSONANCE

There are some assumptions in the 1957 version of dissonance theory that have received insufficient attention and are in need of revision. One is Festinger's assumption that the greater the magnitude of existing dissonance, the greater will be the magnitude of avoidance of new information expected to increase dissonance (up to an extreme point; p. 130).

Some of the earliest research on dissonance theory examined the implications of the theory for selectivity in exposure to information. It was known in the 1950s that the mass media were generally ineffective in changing socially significant attitudes and that one prominent reason for this was self-selection of mass media audiences (Hovland, 1959). Dissonance theory was particularly useful in understanding bias in voluntary exposure to information because it specified conditions under which persons will seek out or avoid information. It predicted that persons will seek out information expected to increase consonance (*consonant* information) and avoid information expected to increase dissonance (*dissonant* information). It also predicted that the greater the existing dissonance, the stronger will be the tendencies to seek out consonant information and to avoid dissonant information.

The early dissonance studies of selective exposure to information showed that there was a preference for consonant information (Ehrlich, Guttman, Schonbach, & Mills, 1957; Mills, Aronson, & Robinson, 1959). However, the fact that people prefer consonant information does not provide evidence of avoidance of dissonant information, because such a preference can be due solely to the seeking of consonant information. To show actual avoidance of dissonant information, it is necessary to make comparisons against a neutral baseline.

Later experiments on interest in consonant and dissonant information had a neutral baseline, and evidence of avoidance of dissonant information was found (Mills, 1965a). The effect of amount of existing dissonance on interest in consonant and dissonant information was tested (Mills, 1965b). Evidence was found that the greater the postdecision dissonance, the greater the interest in consonant information. Interest in information favoring the chosen alternative was stronger when the chosen and rejected alternatives were closer in attractiveness. However, it was not found that avoidance of dissonant information was greater, the greater the postdecision dissonance. Avoidance of information favoring the rejected alternative was not stronger when the chosen and rejected alternatives were closer in attractiveness.

The failure to find that the magnitude of avoidance of dissonance was influenced by the amount of existing dissonance in the experiment by Mills (1965b) cannot be explained away on the basis of inadequate procedures. It cannot be attributed to inadequate manipulation of amount of dissonance or inadequate measurement of interest in information. The reason is that, in the same experimental situation using the same manipulation of amount of dissonance and the same measure of interest in information, it was found that interest in consonant information was greater, the greater the amount of existing dissonance. The positive result for interest in consonant information would not have occurred unless the manipulation of amount of dissonance and the measurement of interest in information had been adequate in that experiment. That positive result provides evidence that the negative result for the effect of amount of existing dissonance on the magnitude of avoidance of dissonance was not due to inadequate procedures.

The experiment on the effect of amount of existing dissonance on interest in consonant and dissonant information (Mills, 1965b) is the only one I am aware of that has tested Festinger's assumption about the effect of existing dissonance on the magnitude of avoidance of new dissonance. There is no evidence that I know of that supports the assumption that avoidance of new dissonance is greater, the greater the amount of existing dissonance. On the basis of what little research there is on the topic, I conclude that the assumption in the 1957 version that the magnitude of avoidance of dissonance is influenced by the amount of existing dissonance is in need of revision.

WHAT HAPPENS BEFORE A CHOICE

Another aspect of the 1957 version that is in need of revision is Festinger's assumption about what happens before a choice. Festinger assumed that there is no cognitive bias in the prechoice situation. Festinger took the position, which, strictly speaking, was not integral to the theory, that "the preaction or predecision situation will be characterized by nonselective seeking of relevant information" and "there will be a lack of resistance to accepting and cognizing any relevant information" (p. 126).

Contrary to what Festinger assumed, research on the topic of exposure to information before a choice has found evidence of selective exposure to information. When people are not committed to a position, the more certain they are that their position is the best one, the more they prefer information supporting their position (Mills & Ross, 1964), whereas the opposite occurs when commitment is high. Before a choice, people who are certain that an alternative is not the best are less interested in information favoring that alternative than people uncertain about which alternative is best (Mills, 1965c). People certain that an alternative is not the best before a choice show evidence of avoidance of information favoring that alternative by displaying less interest in it than people who can not even choose that alternative (Mills & Jellison, 1968).

The research on selective exposure before commitment has been based on the assumption that people want to be certain when they take an action that it is better than the alternatives. That conception was termed *choice certainty theory* (Mills, 1968). Another line of research based on choice certainty theory found evidence of cognitive bias before a choice. The anticipation of making a choice about other people increases the halo effect in the impressions of those other people on positive traits, reflecting a greater difference in evaluations of those other people (Mills & O'Neal, 1971; O'Neal, 1971; O'Neal & Mills, 1969). When a prospective choice is nearer in time, there is greater difference in private evaluations of the alternatives (Brounstein, Ostrove, & Mills, 1979) but smaller difference in public evaluations of the alternatives.

The effects of importance of a prospective choice on private and public evaluations of the alternatives were tested in a recent experiment (Mills & Ford, 1995). It found that the more important the prospective choice, the greater the difference in private evaluations of the alternatives and the less the difference in public evaluations of the alternatives. Those results can be interpreted in terms of dissonance, specifically, avoidance of dissonance expected to occur after the choice.[2]

The greater difference in private evaluations of the alternatives when the prospective choice was more important can be interpreted in terms of greater motivation to avoid the dissonance that would otherwise be expected to occur after the choice. Spreading the attractiveness of the alternatives in private before a choice will reduce dissonance that might otherwise be expected after the choice. The dissonance expected after the choice should be greater, the more important the choice, and so spreading the attractiveness of the alternatives in private to avoid dissonance after the choice should be greater, the more important the choice.[3] The finding that the more important the choice, the less the difference in public evaluations of the alternatives provides evidence

---

[2] The interpretation in terms of dissonance was relegated to a footnote in the article by Mills and Ford, in accordance with the wishes of the article's editor.

[3] The assumption that the magnitude of avoidance of dissonance is determined by the amount of dissonance otherwise expected to occur is separate and distinct from the assumption questioned earlier that the magnitude of avoidance of dissonance is determined by the amount of existing dissonance.

that the private and public evaluations were made in a prechoice situation. If the evaluations were made in a postchoice situation, opposite effects for private and public evaluations should not have occurred.

The smaller difference in public evaluations of the alternatives when the prospective choice is more important can be explained in terms of the assumption Festinger (1957) made that the fear of dissonance may lead to a reluctance to commit oneself (p. 30). The explanation involves the assumption that the public expression of a preference for one alternative before a choice is regarded as involving commitment to choose that alternative. Commitment can be avoided by minimizing the difference in public evaluations of the alternatives. The greater the importance of the prospective choice, the greater the fear of dissonance and the minimizing of the difference in public evaluations.

In *Conflict, Decision, and Dissonance,* Festinger (1964) emphasized that dissonance does not occur until after a choice. However, in discussing the consequences of the anticipation of postdecision dissonance for predecision behavior, Festinger (1964) stated, "If a person anticipates dissonance as a consequence of making a decision, he would be expected to react by attempting to minimize, or to avoid completely, the anticipated dissonance" (1964, pp. 144–145). If the need to be certain about the correctness of a prospective choice is construed in terms of the need to avoid dissonance that would otherwise be expected to occur after the choice, the research based on *choice-certainty* theory (which found bias in information seeking and evaluations before a choice) can be interpreted in terms of dissonance. As mentioned in the article by Mills and Ford (1995), choice-certainty theory can be integrated with dissonance theory.[4]

On the basis of a fair amount of research dealing with the issue, I conclude that when faced with a prospective choice, people will be motivated to avoid dissonance anticipated as a consequence of making a decision. They will avoid information expected to increase dissonance after the decision, and they will spread the attractiveness of the alternatives, in private, to avoid the dissonance that would otherwise be

---

[4]The mention occurred in a footnote about the dissonance interpretation.

expected to occur after the choice. That is contrary to what Festinger assumed. The avoidance of dissonance is an important aspect of the theory, which has been neglected in most recent work on dissonance. It needs to be addressed in any revision of the theory.

HOW DISSONANCE IS DETERMINED BY DESIRED CONSEQUENCES AND IMPORTANCE OF COGNITIONS

There are some other important aspects of the 1957 version that I feel have been ignored or have not received sufficient attention. One is that Festinger said that "motivations and desired consequences may also be factors in determining whether or not two elements are dissonant," (p. 13) Another is Festinger's assumption that if two elements are dissonant, the magnitude of dissonance will be a function of the importance of the elements (p. 16). Those neglected aspects of the theory are involved in a proposal I make for a change in the definition of *dissonance*.[5] The change I will propose also stems from some aspects of the theory that have concerned me for a long time, ever since the time I was working as Festinger's research assistant in the period 1954–1957, when he was developing the theory.

One thing about the 1957 version that has always troubled me is that the definition of dissonance disregards the existence of all the other cognitive elements that are relevant to either or both of the two under consideration and simply deals with those two alone (p. 13). For a long time, I have thought that if motivations and desired consequences determine whether there is dissonance, then one would not simply consider the two cognitive elements alone. Desired consequences would seem to constitute a third cognition that must be taken into account.

Immediately after Festinger (1957) made the statement about the role of desired consequences in determining whether cognitions are

---

[5] I was stimulated to consider the role of importance in dissonance by conversations with Haruki Sakai when he visited Maryland during the summer of 1995.

dissonant, he gave the following example: "A person in a card game might continue playing and losing money while knowing that the others in the game are professional gamblers. This latter knowledge would be dissonant with his cognition about his behavior, namely, continuing to play. But it should be clear that to specify the relation as dissonant is to assume (plausibly enough) that the person involved wants to win. If for some strange reason this person wants to lose, this relation would be consonant" (p. 13).

In the situation in Festinger's example, it would seem reasonable to assume that if the person wants to win, there would be a cognition that the person wants to win. If the person wants to win but for some strange reason does not have the cognition that he wants to win, it would seem that the playing the game would not be dissonant with the knowledge that the others in the game are professional gamblers. Taking desired consequences into account when determining the presence of dissonance seems to require considering more than just two cognitive elements alone.

Another aspect of the theory that has long bothered me has to do with the assumption that elements either follow or do not follow from one another but that there is no variation in the degree to which one element follows from another. I recall an argument with Festinger about that issue. It occurred when I was working on the study that was to be my doctoral dissertation. That study examined the effect of resistance to temptation on changes in attitudes toward cheating (Mills, 1958). One aspect of that study varied restraints against cheating by making it seem highly likely that cheating would be detected or very unlikely that cheating would be detected.

I suggested to Festinger that the cognition that there was a high likelihood of being caught was more dissonant with cheating than the cognition that there was a low likelihood of being caught and went further than that and suggested that a 95% chance of being caught was more dissonant with cheating than a 55% chance of being caught. Festinger maintained that dissonance was either/or, that there was no degree to which a behavior followed from a cognition. He took the position that there were a larger number of cognitions dissonant with cheating if there was a 95% chance of being caught than if there was a 55% chance. As with every argument I ever had with Festinger, I did not win that argument.

Festinger did make an assumption in the 1957 version about degrees of dissonance between two cognitions, when he assumed that the magnitude of the dissonance between two cognitions depends on the importance of the cognitions. Unfortunately, the variable of importance of cognitions has not been given much emphasis in research and theorizing about dissonance. One possible reason is that Festinger (1957) did not say much about what he meant by importance beyond saying that "the more these elements are important to, or valued by the person, the greater will be the magnitude of a dissonant relation between them" (p. 16). Another possible reason, perhaps more consequential, is that Festinger did not do any studies varying importance.

Festinger often made his points by giving examples, which he was a master at constructing. He gave an example of reducing dissonance by reducing importance, when a habitual cigarette smoker has the belief that smoking is bad for health. "Our smoker, for example, could find out all about accidents and death rates in automobiles. Having then added the cognition that the danger of smoking is negligible compared to the danger he runs driving a car, his dissonance would also have been somewhat reduced. Here the total dissonance is reduced by reducing the *importance* of the existing dissonance" (Festinger, 1957, p. 22). Like most of Festinger's examples, this one seems clear, but it does not provide a general conceptualization of the variable of importance.

The variable of importance seems to be involved with the consequences of the behavior for things that are valued or desired or with the consequences of the behavior for things regarded as undesirable. Now that appears similar to the idea that motivation and desired consequences determine dissonance, except that the variable of importance varies the magnitude of the dissonance. It seems reasonable to assume that a behavior follows from a cognition about a consequence of the behavior, if there is a desire for that consequence, and that the obverse (or opposite) of the behavior follows from a cognition about a consequence of the behavior, if there is a desire to avoid that consequence.

Such a formulation would incorporate desired (and undesired) consequences within the definition of dissonance.

One result of incorporating the desirability (or undesirability) of consequences of the behavior within the definition of dissonance is that the determination of dissonance would involve three cognitions: (a) a cognition about the behavior, (b) a cognition about a consequence of the behavior, and (c) a cognition about the desirability (or undesirability) of the consequence. Using three cognitions when specifying dissonance would make dissonance theory more like *balance* theory. Some years ago, Insko and collaborators (Insko, Worchel, Folger, & Kutkus 1975) proposed a balance theory interpretation of dissonance, although in somewhat different terms. In their recent constraint-satisfaction neural network model of dissonance, Shultz and Lepper (1996) made assumptions that they noted were reminiscent of cognitive balance theory.

Sticking as closely as possible to the language of the 1957 version, my suggestion for specifying dissonance is that a behavior follows from (is consonant with) a cognition about a consequence of the behavior, if the consequence is desirable, and a behavior does not follow from (is dissonant with) a cognition about a consequence of the behavior, if the consequence is undesirable. Thinking about dissonance in terms of three cognitions clarifies why dissonance is sometimes reduced by changing an attitude and sometimes by changing a belief. A smoker can reduce dissonance by believing there is no evidence smoking causes cancer or by downplaying the undesirability of having cancer, although the latter is less likely because negative attitudes toward cancer are very strong and resistant to change. Most dissonance research has focused on reducing dissonance by changing an attitude (e.g., disliking someone to whom one has made disparaging comments; Davis & Jones, 1960) and has used situations in which it was very difficult to reduce dissonance by changing a belief (e.g., by denying that one's comments were disparaging to the other).

The idea that a behavior is dissonant with a cognition about a consequence of the behavior if there is a desire to avoid the consequence sounds very similar to the assumption of Cooper and Fazio

(1984) about the necessity of aversive consequences for the arousal of dissonance. However, the similarity is not quite so clear when one looks at their definition of an aversive event as "an event that blocks one's self-interest or an event that one would rather not have occur" (Cooper & Fazio, 1984, p. 232). Their definition of an aversive event has two distinct aspects. An event may be one that one would rather not have occur, but it may not be an event that blocks one's self-interest.

It seems clear that the consequence of the behavior has to be undesirable, something the person is motivated to avoid, for dissonance to be aroused. Using ideas similar to the general version of balance proposed by Rosenberg and Abelson (1960), it is possible to state in general terms what constitutes a desirable or undesirable consequence. A consequence is desirable if it has a positive effect on or promotes something that is positively evaluated or if it has a negative effect on or negates something that is negatively evaluated. A consequence is undesirable if it promotes something that is negatively evaluated or if it negates something that is positively evaluated.

As Brehm and Cohen (1962) emphasized, dissonance trades on the frustration of other motives. But whether the self has to be involved is another matter. The recent research by Harmon-Jones, Brehm, Greenberg, Simon, and Nelson (1996), showing that a public statement of one's position is not necessary for the arousal of dissonance, indicates that blocking one's self-interest or harming another person is not required for dissonance arousal. The way in which the self is involved in dissonance is an important matter that I return to later.

Explicitly including desired (and undesired) consequences in the definition of dissonance has other advantages. It includes importance or value directly in the specification of dissonance. In addition, it makes it easy to take the next step of allowing for degrees of dissonance between cognitions, depending on the strength of the motivation to avoid the particular consequence. What determines importance is not just that a behavior has consequences for something that is desirable or undesirable but also the degree of likelihood that a behavior has the consequence and the degree to which the consequence is desirable or undesirable.

I propose that the degree to which the obverse (or opposite) of a behavior follows from a cognition about a consequence depends on the amount of the desire to avoid the consequence. Dissonance should depend on the degree of certainty that a behavior will lead to a consequence and on the degree to which the consequence is desirable or undesirable. To give some examples, there should be more dissonance if a smoker thinks there is a 100% probability that smoking causes cancer than if she or he thinks the chance that smoking causes cancer is only 1%. There should be more dissonance if a smoker believes that smoking will cause cancer within 5 years than if she or he believes smoking will cause cancer within 50 years. There should be more dissonance if a smoker believes smoking will cause large inoperable tumors than if she or he thinks it will cause only very small tumors that are easily removed. And, of course, there should be more dissonance for a smoker to believe that smoking causes cancer than to believe that smoking causes something less undesirable, such as discolored teeth.

This formulation of dissonance in terms of the degree to which a behavior follows from a consequence and the desirability of the consequence has another advantage. It avoids the awkwardness of the original version that requires that degrees of dissonance always be described in terms of the number of consonant and dissonant cognitions. In some cases, such as the amount of money received for convincing someone a boring task is enjoyable (Festinger & Carlsmith, 1959), it is not unreasonable to talk about a person receiving $20 as having a larger number of consonant cognitions than a person receiving $1. But in other cases, such as the amount of effort involved in engaging in an action, it is rather awkward to talk in terms of number of cognitions. It is strained to say that a highly effortful action involves more cognitions than one involving moderate effort. That kind of awkward usage can be avoided if one thinks of dissonance in terms of the strength of the relationship between the cognitive elements as opposed to simply counting the number of consonant versus dissonant elements.

The formulation which I propose which explicitly takes into account the desirability of consequences and thus, in effect, the importance of the elements, has another potential advantage. It could help to reconcile the current theories that place emphasis on the role of the self in dissonance processes (Thibodeau & Aronson, 1992) with the formulation of dissonance in the original 1957 version. When considering the role of the self, I am going to assume that there is a distinction between the motivation of the person and the role of the self. If lower animals such as rats have dissonance and reduce dissonance as Festinger believed (Lawrence & Festinger, 1962), then the self does not have to be involved for dissonance to occur. We do not assume that rats have self-concepts. But, of course, rats do have motivations. For rats, there are desired and undesired consequences, such as the presence of food or electric shock.

In the case of humans, in addition to motives that do not require invoking the concept of the self, there are, of course, self-concepts, self-esteem, self-beliefs, and self-attitudes. All of these self-aspects have important implications for motivation. In my interpretation of dissonance, the engagement of the self may increase desired consequences or undesired consequences. If we use the definition of dissonance that allows for degrees of dissonance depending on the degree of the consequences and the degree of the desirability or undesirability of the consequences, we can unify the current thinking about the role of the self in dissonance with the general framework of the original version of the theory.

In some cases, self-relevance may increase dissonance by increasing the motivation to avoid certain consequences, and in other cases, a focus on the self may reduce dissonance by reducing the motivation to avoid the consequences. Some important work recently by Simon, Greenberg, and Brehm (1995) has provided evidence that the self-affirmation manipulation of Steele and Liu (1983), which has been shown to reduce dissonance, can be explained in terms of the lowering of the importance of the dissonant action. The present formulation, which explicitly includes importance in the definition of dissonance, can explain why sometimes dissonance is greater when the self is involved and also why it is less under other circumstances when the self is involved.

Obviously, my proposal (that the degree of dissonance depends on the degree to which the opposite of the behavior follows from the cognitions about the degree of the consequences of the behavior and the degree of desirability or undesirability of the consequences) is something that goes beyond Festinger's original definition of dissonance. However, I feel it is within the spirit of Festinger's original 1957 version and fits with many of the examples that he gave. There are many complexities in this formulation that need to be addressed, which could pose formidable problems. How does one measure the degree to which a behavior follows from a consequence? How does one measure the degree of desirability or undesirability of a consequence? A number of important issues need to be considered.

CONCLUSION

I am frequently reminded of the statement attributed to Einstein that everything should be made as simple as possible, but no simpler. This formulation of dissonance is not as simple as the 1957 version, which I believe was deceptively simple. However, I believe it provides a more precise and accurate account of the domain of dissonance research. If that is true, it should prove useful in providing new insights. Hopefully, it will promote the continued development of dissonance theory. I believe we honor Festinger's contribution by continuing to develop the theory.

REFERENCES

Brehm, J. W., & Cohen, A. R. (1962). *Explorations in cognitive dissonance.* New York: Wiley.

Brounstein, P. J., Ostrove, N., & Mills, J. (1979). Divergence of private evaluations of alternatives prior to a choice. *Journal of Personality and Social Psychology, 37,* 1957–1965.

Cooper, J., & Fazio, R. H. (1984). A new look at dissonance theory. In L. Berkowitz (Ed.), *Advances in experimental social psychology* (Vol. 17, pp. 220–262). New York: Academic Press.

Davis, K., & Jones, E. E. (1960). Changes in interpersonal perception as a means of reducing cognitive dissonance. *Journal of Abnormal and Social Psychology, 61,* 402–410.

Ehrlich, D., Guttman, I., Schonbach, P., & Mills, J. (1957). Post-decision exposure to relevant information. *Journal of Abnormal and Social Psychology, 54*, 98–102.

Festinger, L. (1957). *A theory of cognitive dissonance*. Evanston, IL: Row, Peterson.

Festinger, L. (1964). *Conflict, decision, and dissonance*. Stanford, CA: Stanford University Press.

Festinger, L., & Carlsmith, J. M. (1959). Cognitive consequences of forced compliance. *Journal of Abnormal and Social Psychology, 58*, 203–210.

Harmon-Jones, E., Brehm, J., Greenberg, J., Simon, L., & Nelson, D. E. (1996). Evidence that the production of aversive consequences is not necessary to create cognitive dissonance. *Journal of Personality and Social Psychology, 70*, 5–16.

Hovland, C. I. (1959). Reconciling conflicting results derived from experimental and survey studies of attitude change. *American Psychologist, 14*, 8–17.

Insko, C. A., Worchel, S., Folger, R., & Kutkus, A. (1975). A balance theory interpretation of dissonance. *Psychological Review, 82*, 169–183.

Lawrence, D. H., & Festinger, L. (1962). *Deterrents and reinforcement*. Stanford, CA: Stanford University Press.

Mills, J. (1958). Changes in moral attitudes following temptation. *Journal of Personality, 26*, 517–531.

Mills, J. (1965a). Avoidance of dissonant information. *Journal of Personality and Social Psychology, 2*, 589–593.

Mills, J. (1965b). Effect of certainty about a decision upon postdecision exposure to consonant and dissonant information. *Journal of Personality and Social Psychology, 2*, 749–752.

Mills, J. (1965c). The effect of certainty on exposure to information prior to commitment. *Journal of Experimental Social Psychology, 1*, 348–355.

Mills, J. (1968). Interest in supporting and discrepant information. In R. P. Abelson, E. Aronson, W. J. McGuire, T. M. Newcomb, M. J. Rosenberg, & P. H. Tannenbaum (Eds.), *Theories of cognitive consistency: A source book*. Skokie, IL: Rand McNally.

Mills, J., Aronson, E., & Robinson, H. (1959). Selectivity in exposure to information. *Journal of Abnormal and Social Psychology, 59*, 250–253.

Mills, J., & Ford, T. E. (1995). Effects of importance of a prospective choice upon private and public evaluations of the alternatives. *Personality and Social Psychology Bulletin, 21*, 256–266.

Mills, J., & Jellison, J. (1968). Avoidance of discrepant information prior to commitment. *Journal of Personality and Social Psychology, 8*, 59–62.

Mills, J., & O'Neal, E. (1971). Anticipated choice, attention, and the halo effect. *Psychonomic Science, 22*, 231–233.

Mills, J., & Ross, A. (1964). Effects of commitment and certainty on interest in supporting information. *Journal of Abnormal and Social Psychology, 68*, 552–555.

O'Neal, E. (1971). Influence of future choice, importance, and arousal on the halo effect. *Journal of Personality and Social Psychology, 19*, 334–340.

O'Neal, E., & Mills, J. (1969). The influence of anticipated choice on the halo effect. *Journal of Experimental Social Psychology, 5*, 347–351.

Rosenberg, M. J., & Abelson, R. P. (1960). An analysis of cognitive balancing. In C. I. Hovland & M. J. Rosenberg (Eds.), *Attitude organization and change* (112–163). New Haven, CT: Yale University Press.

Shultz, T. R., & Lepper, M. R. (1996). Cognitive dissonance reduction as constraint satisfaction. *Psychological Review, 103*, 219–240.

Simon, L., Greenberg, J., & Brehm, J. (1995). Trivialization: The forgotten mode of dissonance reduction. *Journal of Personality and Social Psychology, 68*, 247–260.

Steele, C. M., & Liu, T. J. (1983). Dissonance processes and self-affirmation. *Journal of Personality and Social Psychology, 41*, 831–846.

Thibodeau, R., & Aronson, E. (1992). Taking a closer look: Reasserting the role of the self-concept in dissonance theory. *Personality and Social Psychology Bulletin, 18*, 591–602.

Zajonc, R. B. (1990). Leon Festinger (1919–1989). *American Psychologist, 45*, 661–662.

3

A Radical Point of View on Dissonance Theory

Jean-Léon Beauvois and Robert-Vincent Joule

In 1957, Leon Festinger put forth the theory of cognitive dissonance (Festinger, 1957b). His book described research and proposed a theory that explained the experimental results presented. It also contained a metatheory that borrowed from the zeitgeist of the period and incited Festinger to make various generalizations, including one that made a connection between his theory and cognitive-consistency theories. In fact, extracted from the metatheory, the central element of Festinger's theory boils down to this: A person can experience an unpleasant state of arousal (state of dissonance) that can be quantified by a ratio (the *dissonance* ratio; see chapter 2, this volume, for further explanation) and is reduced when this ratio decreases. Cognitions are relevant and taken into consideration only to the degree that they allow for composing this ratio. Further, in 1962, Brehm and Cohen stated that everything nontrivial that this theory offers relates to the dissonance ratio. When we speak below of the "theory of '57," we are referring to this central element of Festinger's presentation.

After functioning on this basis for about 10 years and producing the experimental results and classical paradigms that made its reputation, the theory was revised. These revisions consisted of the introduction of new propositions (assumptions?) that were supposed to explain why the state of dissonance existed. These propositions pulled the theory of dissonance toward a theory of the ego, and in fact, researchers neglected the rate of dissonance ratio and its theoretical implications,[1] to deal with a new kind of cognition that Festinger had not foreseen (e.g., I was free to accept or to refuse). In spite of the interest of these revisions and the experimental work that they inspired, we believe that in abandoning the dissonance ratio, these revisions broke with the theory of '57. The conception that we propose rests, on the contrary, on the idea that we must stick as close as possible to the theory of '57, which was never disproven and produced the most fascinating products of dissonance theory. Thus, all hypotheses must be derived from the dissonance ratio.

Does this mean that the revisions were ill timed? Of course not! They had a genuine problem as their origin: The effects of dissonance are observed only in certain conditions (e.g., free choice or weighing consequences of the performed behavior). To deal with this problem, we favored a course other than revising the theory.[2] In fact, we strove to resolve this problem without altering the theory of '57 but rather by adding to it a single proposition, which was faithful, moreover, to Brehm and Cohen (1962): An act induces a state of dissonance only when there is commitment. Accepting this proposition amounts to making an important theoretical decision. It actually amounts to inserting dissonance theory into a more general theoretical framework, that of the psychology of commitment (Kiesler, 1971). However, this framework does not have affinities with that of ego theories. In fact, the same situation applies to Kiesler's book as to Festinger's. It contains a theory packaged within a metatheory. When one takes it out of the metatheory, Kiesler's theory looks like a theory of *external* commitment (rather than the person commiting to the act, the situation commits

---

[1] For example, in establishing a dissonance ratio and putting the relevant, considered perceptions in the numerator or denominator, one can consider only the psychological implications of two perceptions at a time.

[2] Further, this course was more or less suggested by Brehm and Cohen (1962), who were the first to introduce the idea of commitment. Similar to Kiesler (1971), we think that the concept of commitment was a throwaway construct for dissonance theorists.

the person to the act), and this external commitment is rather incompatible with an ego theory.

This option, which implies the careful distinction between theory and metatheory,[3] led us to propose a *radical dissonance theory* (Beauvois & Joule, 1996), which conserves only the central element of Festinger's (1957b) work, and a *theory of external commitment* (Joule & Beauvois, 1998), which conserves only the central element of Kiesler's (1971) book. It goes without saying that returning to the central element of a theory does not mean that one is sticking to a theoretical status quo. It also goes without saying that giving up the metatheories of Festinger and Kiesler can result in new theoretical developments likely to astonish Festinger and Kiesler themselves.

The goal of the chapter is twofold. On the one hand, we want to show how our theoretical developments result in original hypotheses and even in new experimental paradigms. On the other hand, we want to present the particularities of the radical view relative to other versions of dissonance theory. For this, we select from the experimental work on which this radical view is based, and we describe several experimental results that, although compatible with the theory of '57, seem quite incompatible with the other versions of the theory. Thus, we show that, within the experimental framework of forced compliance, (a) dissonance theory is not a theory of consistency, (b) the reduction of dissonance is not to serve a morally good ego, and (c) dissonance arousal does not necessarily imply personal responsibility for the act. Finally, we show that this radical view allows for the proposal of new experimental paradigms.

DISSONANCE REDUCTION VERSUS INCONSISTENCIES REDUCTION

Two basic features of the theory of '57 are important here:
  1. The dissonance ratio, the reduction of which corresponds to the

---

[3] Experimental practice is a good criterion. One needs a theory to explain experimental practice and experimental results.

dissonance-reduction process, is defined with reference to one and only one cognition. This cognition appears in neither the numerator nor the denominator of the ratio. It represents the participant's behavior.

Shortly before Festinger decided to quantify the state of dissonance, structural balance theorists had proposed a measure of structure imbalance (Cartwright & Harary, 1956), which derived from a fundamentally different conception. This measure was the ratio of the unbalanced triads to the total number of triads implied by the structure. It was therefore a measure relating to the whole structure under consideration and accorded no particular status to any of the cognitions involved. This type of measure was in perfect conformity with Heider's premises, which viewed the cognitive universe as a scene contemplated by the perceiver and that satisfied, to a greater or lesser degree, his or her preference for balance (Heider, 1958).

Festinger chose a different approach. In effect, for him, the evaluation of the total amount of dissonance requires that one define a special element that makes it possible to assign the status of consonant or dissonant to the other cognitions. Therefore, this measure is oriented by a special cognition. We call it the *generative* cognition (Mills, chap. 2, this vol., calls it the *focal* element). Formal and experimental arguments do at least suggest that this cognition is behavioral in nature. Several experiments (see Beauvois & Joule, 1996) allowed us to develop two types of hypotheses: one in which the behavioral cognition was generative and one in which it was attitudinal. All the results indicate that the generative cognition is provided by the representation of behavior. This is the case of Experiment 1, which we report below.

2. Decreasing the dissonance ratio is compatible with the emergence of inconsistent relations between certain cognitions implicated by the dissonance ratio. The reason for this is that cognitions in the ratio are determined solely by their relation with the generative cognition. So if the generative cognition is behavioral, the goal of the dissonance-reduction process is not the production of cognitive consistency, but rather the rationalization of the behavior that produced the generative cognition. That is why the dissonance-reduction process may result in greater inconsistency among other cognitions. Therefore, the reduction

of the ratio, which for us remains the unconditional objective of the dissonance-reduction process, in no way implies that there is consistency among the cognitions that it contains. These two basic features come into play in the following experiment (Experiment 1).

Festinger and Carlsmith (1959) realized that the condition that produced the greatest attitude change also produced less argumentation about the position being defended. Rabbie, Brehm, and Cohen (1959) observed incidentally that in a counterattitudinal role-playing situation, participants who had produced the greatest number of arguments in favor of the position being defended were also the ones whose attitudes changed the least. These observations suggested an inverse relationship between the elaborateness of argumentation and attitude change. In fact, these findings were never formalized by dissonance theorists, who, on the contrary, mentioned them as mere curiosities. Yet they clearly fit quite well into the strict (let us say "radical") view of the theory of '57: The counterattitudinal arguments that participants produce furnish cognitions that are consistent with the counterattitudinal behavior precisely because it consists of defending the argued viewpoint. There is nothing shocking about this statement to a dissonance theorist, who "naturally" recognizes that arguments consistent with the initial private attitude imply defending it by writing an attitudinal essay. As such, every argument that psychologically implies the viewpoint being defended must be regarded as a consonant cognition and, as such, is a dissonance-reducing cognition. It is thus easy to see why, in a counterattitudinal role-playing situation, the more arguments participants find supporting the attitude that they defend and against their initial attitude, the less dissonance they experience, and consequently, the less they change their mind to reduce dissonance. We would therefore expect an inverse relation between argumentation and attitude change. Beauvois, Ghiglione, and Joule (1976) obtained results supporting this hypothesis. For participants who were free to choose, as opposed to those with no choice, the more time allotted to supporting the counterattitudinal position, the less the participants' attitudes changed. Joule and Lévèque (1993) tested this hypothesis more recently with a 2 × 3 factorial design, with participants in a classical counterattitudinal role-playing situation (individual training).

In the Joule and Lévèque (1993) experiment, 120 participants (literature students at the University of Provence) had to write a persuasive essay favoring the counterattitudinal position that "leisure activities are a waste of time for students." All participants had volunteered to participate in what was said to be a study on persuasion. Half were told that they were free to accept or refuse to write the essay (free-choice instructions), whereas the other half heard no such statement (Independent Variable 1). A third of the participants were given 20 min to write the advocacy essay before assessing their attitude. Another third were given 5 min before assessing their attitude, and the final third expressed their attitudes immediately, before beginning to write (Independent Variable 2). The postexperimental attitude was measured on a 21-point scale where the participants rated their degree of agreement with the position they were asked to defend (Dependent Variable 1). Of course, the arguments produced by the participants in the 20-min condition significantly outnumbered those generated in the 5-min condition (Dependent Variable 2). The results are given in Table 1. As for the postexperimental attitude, the expected interaction between the two

Table 1

Effects of Counterattitudinal Advocacy on Attitude

Assessment	Free-choice condition			No-choice condition		
	0 min	5 min	20 min	0 min	5 min	20 min
Arguments	0.00	2.85	5.05	0.00	2.80	5.40
Attitude	6.20	3.40	2.50	1.30	2.90	8.00

Note. For attitude, the higher the figure, the more closely the measured attitude conforms to the counterattitudinal act. In a control group ($n = 20$), the mean attitude was 2.60. Judges who were unaware of conditions were asked to assess the arguments furnished by the participants. The arguments given in the 5-min conditions were found also in the 20-min conditions, along with new arguments deemed acceptable by the judges. From Joule and Lévèque (1993).

independent variables was significant and did indeed exhibit the predicted pattern: In the free-choice condition, the more time the participants had to find arguments, the further away their postexperimental attitudes were from the position being defended (i.e., less attitude change). The opposite pattern was obtained in the no-choice condition.

As in the Beauvois et al. (1976) study, the results observed in the free-choice condition support the hypothesis that producing more arguments reduces the dissonance generated by the behavior executed during the counterattitudinal role-playing. Note that these results are incompatible with self-perception theory: No self-perception view could possibly be used to derive the idea that participants are less likely to adhere to the position they are defending as the number of arguments they produce increases.

These results fit fully with the theory of '57, with the arguments found being cognitions that implicate psychologically the counterattitudinal behavior and that therefore increase the denominator of the dissonance ratio (i.e., add consonant cognitions). They support the view that the behavioral cognition functions as the generative cognition in the evaluation of the total amount of dissonance. It is self-evident that taking the private attitude as the generative cognition would force us to the opposite expectation, with participants experiencing more dissonance, the more time they had to find arguments opposed to their private attitude. Results do not support this expectation. Moreover, results go against the widely accepted idea (see the classical presentations of dissonance theory: Feldman, 1966; and especially Zajonc, 1968) that dissonance theory is a theory of consistency. It is indeed difficult to see how there could be a consistency effect in the fact that participants change their attitude even less when they come up with numerous arguments against it. Brehm and Cohen (1962) even judged dissonance theory to be ambiguous in this respect, claiming that another hypothesis opposing the one we have just set forth was just as compatible with the theory and, needless to say, more compatible with the consistency axiom ("the higher the quality of the participant's arguments, the more dissonance there should be, assuming an initial disagreement with the advocated position," p. 34). But as we have already seen, the inverse relationship between argument quantity and attitude change is not ambiguous from the standpoint of dissonance theory.

THE DISSONANCE IN TELLING THE TRUTH

The principal reformulations of dissonance theory (Aronson, 1968, 1969; Cooper & Fazio, 1984; Wicklund & Brehm, 1976) have gradually turned the original theory into a cognitive-defense theory, describing the mechanisms used by responsible participants concerned about their own morality. These reformulations date back, as we noted previously, to the discovery in the sixties of factors that Kiesler (1971) considered to be the conditions for commitment (e.g., free choice, irrevocability, and consequences). We would now like to demonstrate that even if one agrees that commitment is necessary, it does not have to be interpreted in terms of the morally good self. Let us begin by showing that we can derive hypotheses from dissonance theory that are incompatible with this interpretation. Contrary to what the versions based on the morally good self and centered around the idea of lying would lead us to expect, dissonance can be increased by a perfectly moral act: telling the truth.

But first, let us analyze this situation used in Festinger and Carlsmith's (1959) classic experiment. Participants were induced to perform two consecutive behaviors likely to generate dissonance. The first behavior consisted of accomplishing a particularly boring and mindless task. Thus, the cognition, "This task is boring" would imply the opposite psychologically of the cognition "I will do this work," just as the cognition "I'm thirsty" implied the opposite psychologically of "I do not drink." The second behavior consisted of telling a peer that the task was interesting (counterattitudinal advocacy). Joule and Girandola (1995) demonstrated that this situation would be regarded as one of *double compliance* (Joule, 1991), making it necessary to consider the relationship between the two behavioral cognitions. This relationship would be obviously consonant if we confined ourselves to dual relationships involving two cognitions only, as required by the 1957 definition of psychological implication and dissonance relations. Dissonance theory treats relationships two at a time, and psychological implication indeed only looks at relationships between two cognitions. Saying that a task is interesting goes quite well (is consonant) with having carried out that task. This is true regardless of one's attitude toward the task, and the attitude constitutes a third cognition. In short, the actual accomplishment of the task provided Festinger and Carlsmith's participants who said the task was interesting with a consonant cognition. They would thus experience less dissonance than participants who said the same thing but had not been required to carry out the task.

What happens when participants are led to tell the truth, namely, to say that the task is uninteresting? This time, the two acts are inconsistent with each other. The requested statement, which involves telling the truth, should thus increase the dissonance induced by task execution. In short, once they have executed the tedious task, participants having "lied" should experience less dissonance than participants having told the truth. These conjectures have been confirmed by the experiment conducted by Joule and Girandola (1995), described next (Experiment 2).

The participants, all volunteers, were 80 female literature students at the University of Provence, assigned to the four cells of a 2 × 2 design. They were asked to take part in unpaid research ostensibly concerning the effects of concentration on performance. Half had to accomplish a tedious task (turning knobs on a board for 13 min). The other half simply had the task described to them and were clearly told that they would not have to perform it (Independent Variable 1). Then all participants described the task to a peer, either positively (counterattitudinal role playing) or negatively (attitudinal role playing; Independent Variable 2), using arguments supplied by the experimenter (e.g., "It was very enjoyable" or "I had a lot of fun" vs. "It was tedious" or "I got bored"). Finally, the participants rated their attitude toward the task on an 11-point scale (dependent variable). This scale was strictly identical to the one used by Festinger and Carlsmith (1959; the scale that produced the most significant findings). The results are given in Table 2.

Festinger and Carlsmith's (1959) main finding was replicated: Par-

Table 2		
Attitude Toward a Tedious Task		
Condition	Positive presentation	Negative presentation
With task	−0.5	1.5
Without task	1.4	−1.3

Note. Entries are participant ratings of the task on a 11-point scale ranging from −5 (not at all interesting) to 5 (very interesting). In Control Situation 1 of simple compliance (task execution only), the participants' mean rating of the task was −0.2. In Control Situation 2 of simple task assessment, the mean rating by the participants who neither executed nor presented the task was −2.1. From "Tâche fastidieuse et jeu de rôle dans le paradigme de la double soumission" [Tedious task and role-playing in the double compliance paradigm], by R. V. Joule and F. Girandola, 1995, *Revue Internationale de Psychologie Sociale, 8,* 101–116. Copyright 1995 by Presses Universitaires de Grenoble. Reprinted with permission.

ticipants who had to accomplish and positively present the task had a better attitude toward it than Control Group 2 participants, who only had to rate the task (−0.5 vs. −2.1). But what these results showed above all was that participants who performed the tedious task found it more interesting after telling a peer it was boring than after telling a peer it was interesting (1.5 vs. −0.5). In addition, participants who performed the task and negatively described it found it more interesting than Control Condition 1 participants, who only had to perform the task (1.5 vs. −0.2). This last result was absolutely incompatible with a self-perception view of dissonance phenomena.

Thus, the immorality of the "lie" was not behind the dissonance experienced by the Festinger and Carlsmith (1959) participants, nor was the fact that they had tricked their peer. Joule and Girandola's (1995) results showed that participants would have felt even more dissonance, had the researchers asked them to tell the truth. Thus, counterattitudinal advocacy does not evoke dissonance because it is immoral, but, from a theoretical perspective, because there are some cognitions that would have implied doing the opposite. From this same theoretical perspective, it is possible that the same would apply to proattitudinal advocacy. We have just seen, for example, that having previously performed the task sufficed for the participant to experience more dissonance for telling the truth than for telling a lie.

This conclusion prompts us to think about the role played by the consequences of the act. Indeed, it is probably because they shared this somewhat moral interpretation of dissonance that certain researchers (in particular, Cooper & Fazio, 1984) insisted so strongly on the importance of what they called the act's *aversive* consequences (here, tricking a peer), to the point of making it the core of their "new look." Granted, we are not questioning the necessity of the commitment, and even less so the importance of the act's consequences as a commitment factor. Nevertheless, having shown in this situation that telling the truth to a peer (and in doing so, suggesting that he or she not agree to perform the tedious task) leads to an increase in dissonance compels us to reconsider the theoretical role sometimes ascribed to these consequences. As we have just seen (see also Harmon-Jones, Brehm, Greenberg, Simon, & Nelson, 1996), they need not be morally aversive at all for dissonance to be generated. Note once again that we have adhered strictly to the stipulations of the theory of '57.

COMMITMENT TO COMPLIANCE

Since Brehm and Cohen (1962), dissonance theorists accepted the idea that the simple presence of relations of inconsistency among cognitions is not a sufficient condition for the arousal of dissonance. In fact, the 1960s were to prove a rich source of experiments showing that the primary reward effect of dissonance in forced-compliance situations is observed only if the participants are allowed to choose whether to perform the requested act. When participants do not have this choice, the dissonance effect is replaced by a reinforcement effect (Holmes & Strickland, 1970; Linder, Cooper, & Jones, 1967). At the same time that the critical importance of free choice was being demonstrated, researchers revealed the significance of other cognitions relating to the public or anonymous nature of the problematic behavior (Carlsmith, Collins, & Helmreich, 1966), the irrevocable or reversible nature of the act (Helmreich & Collins, 1968), and, above all, the role of cognitions concerning its consequences (Calder, Ross, & Insko, 1973; Cooper & Worchel, 1970). Like free choice, such cognitions seem to function as more or less necessary conditions for dissonance arousal. In our view, the idea of commitment, in the form proposed by Kiesler (1971), provides the best conceptual synthesis of this rich research tradition and allows us to hypothesize that the induction of a state of dissonance in a forced-compliance situation requires the participant's commitment to the problematic behavior. In fact, Kiesler treated all the cognitions that have been studied as preconditions for dissonance effects (e.g., free choice, public nature of the behavior, irrevocability, and consequences) as variables affecting a person's level of commitment. Since 1971, a number of dissonance theorists have placed at least two of the conditions of commitment (free choice and consequences) at the heart of their formulations. To the extent that they thought they had discovered the psychological reason for the arousal of dissonance in these conditions of commitment, they were led to revise Festinger's original theory, turning it into a theory of personal responsibility (Wicklund & Brehm, 1976) or a theory of the cognitive management of the consequences of behavior (Cooper & Fazio, 1984).

It is clear that for these researchers commitment to one's behavior is a key element of the revised theory. Was it really necessary to change the basic assumptions of the original theory to introduce commitment? Before addressing this question, we clarify the meaning of the most important factor of commitment: free choice.

Indeed, the traditional way to manipulate free choice (i.e., "You are entirely free to do or not to do what I ask you. It's up to you") authorizes two interpretations with very different theoretical implications. Free choice can mean that the participant agrees (or, in a few cases, refuses) to execute the particular act requested of him or her, such as writing an essay in favor of police intervention, refraining from eating or drinking, stopping smoking temporarily, or saying that a task is interesting. No one would deny that this is the traditional interpretation. In fact, this is the interpretation that allows for understanding the effects of dissonance in terms of self-perception. Yet manipulating free choice can be interpreted to mean something else, namely, that the participant agrees (or, in a few cases, refuses) to comply with the obedience relationship proposed by an experimenter in a research framework. It is obvious that this is not the same choice as above. Replying "No, I don't want to do that particular thing, but you can ask me to do some other thing" (first interpretation) is not the same as replying "I have no reason to comply with your demands" (second interpretation). In the first case, accepting means agreeing to perform a specific act (and, thus, to be held responsible for that act), as several post-Festinger theorists assume. In the second case, which is closer to our idea of what a forced compliance contract is (Beauvois & Joule, 1996, pp. 146–154), accepting means being willing to comply with the experimenter, in which case the experimenter can be held responsible for whatever happens. The following description of Experiment 3 (Beauvois, Bungert, & Mariette, 1995) shows that the commitment necessary to induce a state of dissonance corresponds to the second interpretation of free choice.

Three independent variables were manipulated in a 2 × 2 × 2 design. In every case, participants were asked in the end to write a counterattitudinal essay, for which they did or did not choose the topic (Independent Variable 1: commitment to act). Before writing the essay, they either chose to or were assigned to (Independent Variable 2: compliance commitment) an experimental situation in which they had to perform problematic behaviors. The third independent variable dealt with the problematic behaviors announced to participants before the manipulation of the second independent variable. For the first half of the participants, the stated problematic behavior was writing counterattitudinal essays, like that which they would genuinely have to write (paradigmatic-sequence condition). For the second half of the participants, these problematic behaviors consisted of doing tedious tasks (which they would never be asked to perform in reality: nonparadigmatic-sequence condition). Further details with regard to this third independent variable are described in the following paragraphs.

In the *paradigmatic-sequence condition*, the participants were either given the choice or not (Independent Variable 2) to take part in a counterattitudinal role-playing situation. Before they made their decision or, in the no-choice condition, before they were told to do the behavior, Beauvois et al. (1995) presented the participants with the topics (all counterattitudinal) that they might be asked to write about (i.e., drivers under 16 years old no longer allowed to drive when accompanied by an adult, shorter holidays, or scholarships to be limited to students achieving an average grade of 14/20, approximately a "B" in the American system, in the preceding year). In the commitment-to-compliance condition, the experimenter said that the participants were entirely free to agree or to refuse to take part in the research and asked them to make their own decision. However, they were not told which of these essays they would ultimately have to produce but that this would be decided later. In contrast, in the other condition (no commitment to compliance), the experimenter stated that the research had been requested by the government and made no mention of the possibility of refusing to take part. Independent Variable 1, commitment to the counterattitudinal act, was then manipulated. In the commitment condition, the experimenter reformulated the three topics and asked the participant which one he or she would like to write about. In the no-committment condition, the experimenter told the participant to write about "today's topic," which were topics that matched those chosen by the participants in the commitment to the counterattitudinal act condition.

In the no-paradigmatic-sequence condition (Independent Variable 3), the participants were either given the choice or not, to take part in a tedious task experiment. Before manipulating the commitment to compliance (statement of participant's free choice to participate in the experiment), the experimenter gave examples of problematic behaviors that were very different from the ones the participants would actually have to accomplish (e.g., glue a piece of confetti on every occurrence of the letter *a* in a long text, copy three pages of the telephone book, or take a lengthy test involving crossing out symbols). The commitment-to-compliance manipulation was the same as the paradigmatic-sequence condition. In the commitment-to-compliance condition, the experimenter told the participants that they were entirely free to agree or to refuse to take part in the research. Then, once commitment to compliance was manipulated, the experimenter claimed she had made a mistake and told the participants that the task would be something completely different from what had just been said. Without repeating the statement that participants were free to participate, she went on to the counterattitudinal essays paradigm and manipulated the chosen or nonchosen topic variable. In summary, all participants wrote a counterattitudinal essay for which they had chosen or not chosen the topic (commitment to act vs. no commitment to act). Before this, they either could choose to accept or were assigned to a situation (commitment to compliance vs. no commitment to compliance), with or without the knowledge of what problematic act this situation really involved (paradigmatic sequence vs. nonparadigmatic sequence). Finally, after the completion of the essays, a postexperimental questionnaire was used to assess three attitudes (vacations, driving, and scholarships).

Let us consider first the paradigmatic-sequence condition. As shown in Table 3, participants who changed attitudes the most, and thereby reduced dissonance the most, were the ones who had been given the choice to enter or not, into the situation (commitment to compliance) but who were required to write about the topic of the day. This result has important theoretical implications. If the traditional free choice were indeed the choice to execute or not to execute the specific behavior

Table 3

Commitment to Compliance and Free Choice of the Problematic Act in a Forced-Compliance Situation

Commitment to compliance	Paradigmatic sequence		Nonparadigmatic sequence	
	Choice	No choice	Choice	No choice
Choice	5.36	6.63	4.72	4.82
No choice	3.36	2.59	2.77	2.05

Note. The higher the number, the more closely the participant's attitude conforms to the position defended in the selected essay (dissonance effect).

requested, then the choice of one particular act among three in Experiment 3 would indeed be the best approximation of this type of free choice. Yet being able to choose one of three acts did not generate dissonance in this case. On the contrary, it seemed to have reduced it when the participant was committed to compliance, and this is what we expected.[4] Imagine a participant who has just agreed to comply with the experimenter, knowing that he or she will have to execute a counterattitudinal behavior but not knowing which. Once this commitment to compliance is obtained, the participant is given the choice between various obviously counterattitudinal behaviors. In such a decision-making situation, being able to choose must reduce the dissonance ratio, compared with a classical forced-compliance situation, in which the participant is proposed one and only one act. Indeed, insofar as the chosen alternative is the least discomforting for the participant (the lesser of three evils), it must reduce the total amount of dissonance by creating consistent cognitions (the higher cost of the nonselected alternatives psychologically implies choosing the selected one). The fact that having chosen one out of three acts in Experiment 3 reduced dissonance is thus perfectly compatible with the theory of '57.

The most important point in this experiment is that commitment to compliance must be considered as the factor that aroused the dissonance in the commitment-to-compliance–nonchosen-issue situation. These results were confirmed in the nonparadigmatic-sequence condition. We discovered that participants who committed to compliance by agreeing to perform boring tasks modified their attitude in favor of the essay topic when it was imposed. Here again, the choice of one of three counterattitudinal acts did not induce dissonance per se. However, in the commitment-to-compliance condition, being able to choose a topic does not seem to have reduced the dissonance (as in the paradigmatic condition). This is probably because in the nonparadigmatic condition, the participants had been told nothing about the two nonchosen topics when they had to pick one of three, so they had not already implicitly

---

[4]The interaction between these two independent variables was statistically significant in the paradigmatic-sequence condition.

agreed to write about them (during the commitment-to-compliance manipulation). In effect, avoiding two topics one has never heard about and therefore never agreed to write about does not provide any consonant cognitions, unlike the case in which participants could choose to write about the least problematic of three topics.

In opposition to the traditional understanding of free choice, it is indeed commitment to compliance, not commitment to a particular counterattitudinal act, that is the condition needed to induce a state of dissonance. The results of Experiment 3 point out the limitations of a view of the dissonance-reduction process that reduces it to the management of responsibility. In our minds, revisions based on responsibility, the anticipation of aversive consequences, and other similar concepts stem from a faulty interpretation of what free choice really is in classic forced-compliance experiments. Of course it is quite understandable that participants who experience the feelings involved in having chosen to perform the particular counterattitudinal act just performed have some problems about their own values and have trouble accepting that the act has aversive consequences. But these feelings have nothing to do with the state of dissonance. Note first of all, against this view, that dissonance is induced in a number of situations void of moral implications. Such is the case in situations of abstinence from smoking, for example, or in situations involving eating an unappetizing dish. Note also, and still opposing this view, that the traditional free-choice effects are not incompatible with very slight although real differences in the feeling of freedom between participants who had free choice and those given no choice: Either they all globally experience a strong feeling of constraint (Steiner, 1980), or on the contrary, they all experience a strong feeling of freedom (Beauvois, Michel, Py, Rainis, & Somat, 1996). In the studies mentioned by Steiner (1980), as well as in those described by Beauvois et al. (1996), dissonance effects are observed only in participants assigned to a free choice condition, whether they experience a strong feeling of freedom (as in Beauvois et al.) or, on the contrary, a strong feeling of obligation (as reported by Steiner).

Furthermore, for us, the key element for dissonance arousal is not the feeling of freedom, but rather whether the participant is said to have choice. In any case, the results of Experiment 3, described here, and those of another experiment described by Beauvois et al. (1995), more clearly pinpoint the limits of personal responsibility in a "morally good self" and the ideological confusion this view implies: Are participants morally responsible when they accept a condition of obedience and perform an imposed, unexpected act, which they do (no refusals observed) simply because they accept their state of compliance with the experimenter? Even if we obviously have to answer no to this question, the results show that participants nevertheless experience cognitive dissonance right from the very moment they are told they are free to comply or not to comply.

A RADICAL VIEW

In our minds, no theory other than dissonance theory can make sense out of all of the effects presented here. This also applies to the theories devised by Festinger's critics (e.g., self-perception and impression management) and even to the revised versions proposed by his followers. Yet if dissonance theory indeed remains the only theory that can make sense out of these effects, then it is not just one of many theories of dissonance. Does the radical theory really diverge that far from the theory of '57? The answer to this question is no to the extent that the radical theory conserves the key element of this theory of '57. In the remainder of this section, we discuss what is necessary for it to do so.

Strictly calculating the dissonance ratio and accepting its implications. The use of this ratio has several repercussions: Insofar as the state of dissonance is calculated from relationships (both dissonant and consonant) between cognitions, the calculation requires making the important theoretical distinction between the state of dissonance and the presence (vs. absence) of dissonant relationships between cognitions. The fact that Festinger used the word *dissonance* to refer to both of these instances may have led to the assumption that a state of dissonance exists whenever dissonant relationships between cognitions exist.

Radically calculating the total amount of dissonance means recognizing that all cognitions do not have the same status. To calculate, one of the cognitions must be designated as the generative cognition. This cognition allows us to say that the other cognitions (the ones we put in the numerator or denominator of the dissonance ratio) are consistent (whenever there is psychological implication) or inconsistent (whenever there is implication of the obverse of the generating cognition). The other cognitions enter into play only as a result of potential psychological implications that link them to the generating cognition or to its obverse.

Radically calculating the dissonance ratio also means only considering those relationships involving the generative cognition. Indeed, relationships are included in this calculation only to the extent that they link the generative cognition (or its obverse) to other cognitions. This implies that certain relationships, and in particular those between the cognitions in the numerator or denominator of the dissonance ratio, are not part of the calculation of the total amount of dissonance. For instance, anyone would agree that Festinger and Carlsmith (1959) were correct in ignoring the potential relationship between personal attitude and reward, that is, between two cognitions included in the dissonance ratio because of the relationships (inconsistency for the former and consistency for the latter) they had with the generative cognition (the counterattitudinal behavior). Note that in the present case, the relationship between these two cognitions is irrelevant. There may exist cases however, in which there is a relevant relationship between two cognitions in the dissonance ratio. If so, should it also be ignored in the calculation of total dissonance? The answer is yes. We have even seen that total dissonance could be decreased by the generation of new inconsistencies between the cognitions in the dissonance ratio. In Experiment 1, for instance, the counterattitudinal advocacy that led to the production of cognitions that were inconsistent with the participant's personal attitude was accompanied by less overall dissonance, because the total amount of dissonance was reduced by those cognitions.

Finally, radically calculating the total dissonance calculation implies considering only those relationships that link two cognitions (two-term relationships). Coming back to the role of the reward in the Festinger and Carlsmith (1959) experiment we can agree once again—because the findings support their reasoning—that Festinger and Carlsmith (1959) were quite right to call the relationship between the reward and the counterattitudinal behavior consistent. Yet it would suffice to bring a third cognition into the picture, personal attitude, for the relationship between the reward and the behavior to change in nature, because the participants might think that they were being bribed by the experimenter. In this case, the reward would become outright immoral, even aversive, and would generate dissonance. This type of reasoning is invalid, because the findings clearly show that rewards reduce dissonance. So why, then, would this reasoning become valid when we looked at other possible cases of relationships among three cognitions, in particular, when the consequences of the act were at stake? Indeed, the very idea of aversive consequences (Cooper & Fazio, 1984), presumably responsible for dissonance, relies on the consideration of three-term relationships (the relationship between one's act and its consequences being modified by one's personal attitude).

Granting a particular status to commitment cognitions. Discovery of commitment factors had a strong impact on the evolution of dissonance theory. Was it really necessary to change it? First of all, if we limit ourselves to two-term relationships, which are the only ones defined in the theory, then *commitment* cognitions (e.g., "I was told I was free to accept or refuse," "What I do will have such and such a consequence," and "I will not be able to go back on my word") do not really fall within the scope of the theory of '57. Such cognitions are obviously relevant, because they condition the dissonance-reduction process. They are definitely consistent with the act. Indeed, it makes no sense to contend that knowing one is free to do something (psychologically) implies that one does not do it. Commitment cognitions thus pose a real theoretical problem: Although relevant, they are not inconsistent with the act, even though their presence is necessary to induce a state of dissonance. This is the reason why theorists quickly veered away from the theoretical constraints of the 1957 version of dissonance theory, especially those involving the calculation of the dissonance ratio. They began to reason in a very flexible fashion by intuitively ascertaining a state of dissonance that participants experience as they engage in a sort of reasoning based on three, if not four, cognitions ("I say x, but I am against x, and yet I was free not to say x" or "I say x, but I am against x, and it is even worse because my act is going to have such and such a consequence").

We think there is an alternative, one that is in keeping with the experimental practices and data. This alternative fits into one proposition: Commitment to an act is a necessary condition (but insufficient, because the act must also be discomforting, i.e., counterattitudinal or countermotivational) for the induction of a state of dissonance. This proposition has three implications. The first goes without saying: The theory of '57 can remain unchanged. The second is that it forces us to carefully examine this mandatory dissonance-inducing commitment. Reflection about this problem should give rise to a second branch of a more complete theory (see Experiment 3 above). The third is that dissonance theory is a local theory of the psychology of commitment; more precisely, it is a theory of the effects of commitment to a problematic act. From an experimental point of view, one can imagine that there is no arousal below a certain threshold of commitment and that experimental operationalizations (declaration of free choice or the salience of consequences) ordinarily allow us to attain this threshold. This proposition allows us to distinguish two types of cognitions: cognitions generating arousal (commitment cognitions) and cognitions composing the total amount of dissonance (specific cognitions). This perspective is justified first because commitment cognitions are not consistent or inconsistent cognitions and so cannot be located in the dissonance ratio (e.g., "I was free to accept or to refuse"). It is justified also by the fact that some cognitions facilitate commitment, therefore arousal, even though they reduce the total amount of dissonance. This is the case of internal explanations. These explanations increase commitment because they reinforce the link between the individual and the behavioral act. But because they psychologically imply the act, they are consistent cognitions, which reduce the total amount of dissonance (see Beauvois et al., 1996, for experimental support).

Thus, on a formal level we can distinguish commitment cognitions, which define the committing character of the generative cognition, from specific cognitions. Both types of cognitions are represented in the dissonance ratio on either the right or the left side of the equal sign in the formula:

$$D_g - b(F, C, \ldots) = A/A + R + \ldots$$

where D is the total amount of dissonance induced by the generative cognition g relative to the behavior b and F (free choice) and C (consequences) are commitment cognitions without which there would be no dissonance arousal. Their status comes from the theory of commitment. A (attitude) and R (reward) are specific cognitions that appear in the numerator and denominator of the dissonance ratio. These cognitions allow for the quantification of the state of dissonance.

TWO NEW PARADIGMS

By focusing on the generative cognition as a behavior-related cognition and on the rationalization of behavior, the radical theory has made it possible to explore two new paradigms (for a review, see Beauvois & Joule, 1996): *double forced compliance* (see Experiment 2 above) and *act rationalization.*

In the double forced compliance paradigm, we are interested in the dissonance-reduction process after the execution of two behaviors, at least one of which is discomforting. Let us consider a participant who has produced two behaviors, B_1 and B_2. Naturally, if this participant is to experience a state of dissonance, it is necessary and sufficient for one of these behaviors to contradict the participant's attitudes or motivations A. Let us suppose that the discrepant behavior is B_1. If we reason on the basis of behavior B_1 alone, then we will consider the participant to be in a classic forced-compliance situation. However, if we also consider behavior B_2, we must take account not only the relations between this new behavior and the attitudes or motivations A of the participant (inconsistent, consistent, or neutral relations) but also the relations that exist between behavior B_2 and behavior B_1 (inconsistent, consistent, or neutral relations).

First of all, let us consider only the relevant relations that may exist

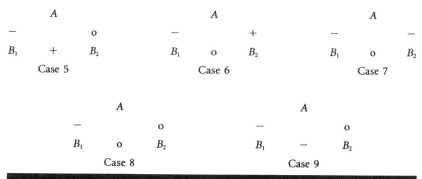

	A			A			A			A	
$-$		$-$	$-$		$+$	$-$		$+$	$-$		$-$
B_1	$+$	B_2	B_1	$-$	B_2	B_1	$+$	B_2	B_1	$-$	B_2
	Case 1			Case 2			Case 3			Case 4	

Figure 1

Double compliance situations: Relevant relationships.

Note. $-$ = inconsistent relationship. $+$ = consistent relationship.

among B_1, B_2 and A. If we assume the inconsistent relation between B_1 and A to be constant, then logic indicates the presence of four possible cases, as shown in Figure 1.

Let us now consider both the relevant and irrelevant relations among B_1, B_2 and A. If we once again assume the relation of inconsistency between B_1 and A to be constant, then logic this time presents us with 9 possible cases, namely, the 4 cases presented in Figure 1 and the 5 cases presented in Figure 2.

Of these theoretically possible cases, two have been studied in particular detail: Cases 1 and 2. These are easier to imagine than the others, possibly because they correspond to balanced triads. Festinger and

	A			A			A	
$-$		o	$-$		$+$	$-$		$-$
B_1	$+$	B_2	B_1	o	B_2	B_1	o	B_2
	Case 5			Case 6			Case 7	

	A			A	
$-$		o	$-$		o
B_1	o	B_2	B_1	$-$	B_2
	Case 8			Case 9	

Figure 2

Double compliance situations: Relevant and irrelevant relationships.

Note. $-$ = inconsistent relationship. $+$ = consistent relationship. 0 = irrelevant relationship.

Carlsmith's (1959) situation implemented Case 1 (B_1: perform a boring task; B_2: lie). Joule and Girandola's (1995) "truth situation" (Experiment 2) implemented Case 2. In a study by Joule (1991), the first behavior (B_1), produced by smokers, consisted of refraining from smoking for an evening (B_1). The second behavior consisted of writing an essay either against (B_2: Case 1) or in favor (B_2: Case 2) of smoking. As expected on the bases of radical considerations, the participants who had to write an essay against tobacco after being induced to refrain from smoking found it most difficult to go without tobacco and felt the greatest need for tobacco.

In the act rationalization paradigm, we are interested in the conditions that are likely to lead a participant who has just carried out a discomforting act to rationalize that act by carrying out another discomforting act. The dissonance state is one of tension, which as such must be reduced. One can imagine that the participant will adopt the most convenient route or the first one available. But whatever the case may be, the arousal can only be reduced by two principal kinds of processes. These processes serve to make the act less problematic. Some processes affect the commitment to the act and reduce this commitment, and other processes reduce the total amount of dissonance by changing one or several existing cognitions or by producing new ones.

In ordinary circumstances, the behavior cannot be denied, and the easiest route available is the change of the private attitude that would have implied the contrary. This is most likely what happens in daily life, and it is natural that it was the first studied and remains the most traditional route of study. But if the participant is given the chance to trivialize his behavior and therefore make it less or even not at all problematic (to the point of no longer having commitment: a great distance between the participant and his act), it is probable that he or she will resort to this route (Simon, Greenberg, & Brehm, 1995). This route is probably less spontaneous than the preceding one (except in the case of a very polarized or salient initial attitude) because in daily life people are reluctant to say to themselves or others that they engage in trivial behaviors. But the participant can also reduce this tension by any other route that becomes available.

We have more specifically studied act rationalization. In fact, along-side the classic forms of rationalization (attitude change and triviali-zation), which we might term *cognitive* rationalization, we have been persuaded of the possibility of another form of rationalization. We have given the name *act* rationalization to this new type of rationalization because the problematic behavior that underlies the generative cogni-tion is rationalized (and thereby rendered less problematic) by the pro-duction of a new, more problematic behavior rather than by cognitive realignment, which has been the classic object of investigation by dis-sonance theorists.

The hypothesis of the alternative nature of the cognitive path and behavioral path of dissonance reduction has received substantial sup-port (Beauvois, Joule, & Brunetti, 1993; Joule, 1996): Act rationalization is hindered when cognitive rationalization is promoted, and in contrast, it is promoted when cognitive rationalization is blocked. For example (Beauvois et al., 1993, Experiment 1), smokers who had just accepted a first period of abstinence (18 hr without smoking) were proposed a second, much longer abstinence period (6 days without smoking), which was the final request. Before making this final request, the ex-perimenter asked half of the participants to write down the reasons that led them to accept the first abstinence period; nothing of this sort was asked of the other half. Thus, we gave the first group, but not the second, the chance to cognitively rationalize their first abstinence. Fewer of the participants who had the chance to rationalize the first abstinence (26.1%) accepted the final request than of those who did not have this rationalization opportunity (82.6%).

Since the discovery of the conditions necessary for inducing a state of dissonance, dissonance theory has greatly evolved, to the point where previously rival theories are now considered as ways of thinking about dissonance reduction. We do not want to imply here that this evolution has been infertile or that it has not produced substantial data. It remains the case, however, that this evolution has led to the neglect of essential points of Festinger's theory and that this theory can still teach us a lot. And who knows, what it still has to teach us may contain many new surprises.

REFERENCES

Aronson, E. (1968). Dissonance theory: Progress and problems. In R. P. Abelson, E. Aronson, W. J. McGuire, T. M. Newcomb, M. J. Rosenberg, & P. H. Tannenbaum (Eds.). *Theories of cognitive consistency: A sourcebook.* Chicago: Rand McNally.

Aronson, E. (1969). The theory of cognitive dissonance: A current perspective. In L. Berkowitz (Ed.), *Advances in experimental social psychology,* (Vol. 4). New York: Academic Press.

Aronson, E. (1992). *The social animal.* San Francisco: Freeman.

Beauvois, J. L., Bungert, M., & Mariette, P. (1995). Forced compliance: Commitment to compliance and commitment to activity. *European Journal of Social Psychology, 25,* 17–26.

Beauvois, J.-L., Ghiglione, R., & Joule, R.-V. (1976). Quelques limites des réinterprétations commodes des effets de dissonance [some limitations of convenient reinterpretations of dissonance affects]. *Bulletin de Psychologie, 29,* 758–765.

Beauvois, J.-L., & Joule, R.-V. (1996). *A radical dissonance theory.* London: Taylor & Francis.

Beauvois, J.-L., Joule, R.-V., & Brunetti, F. (1993). Cognitive rationalization and act rationalization in an escalation of commitment. *Basic and Applied Social Psychology, 14,* 1–17.

Beauvois, J.-L., Michel, S., Py, J., Rainis, N., & Somat, A. (1996). Activation d'explications internes et externes du comportement problématique dans une situation de soumission forcée [Activation of internal and external explanations of problematic behavior in a forced compliance situation]. In J.-L. Beauvois, R.-V. Joule, & J. M. Monteil (Eds.), *Perspectives cognitives et conduites sociales: 5. Contextes et contextes sociaux.* Neuchâtel, Switzerland: Delachaux et Niestlé.

Brehm, J. W., & Cohen, A. R. (1962). *Explorations in cognitive dissonance.* New York: Wiley.

Calder, B. J., Ross, M., & Insko, C. A. (1973). Attitude change and attribution: Effect of incentive, choice and consequences. *Journal of Personality and Social Psychology, 25,* 95–99.

Carlsmith, J. M., Collins, B. E., & Helmreich, R. I. (1966). Studies in forced compliance: 1. The effect of pressure for compliance on attitude change produced by face to face role playing and anonymous essay writing. *Journal of Personality and Social Psychology, 4,* 1–13.

Cartwright, D., & Harary, F. (1956). Structural balance: A generalization of Heider's theory. *Psychological Review, 63,* 277–293.

Cooper, J., & Fazio, R. H. (1984). A new look at dissonance theory. In L. Berkowitz (Ed.), *Advances in experimental social psychology,* (Vol. 17, pp. 229–266). New York: Academic Press.

Cooper, J., & Worschel, S. (1970). Role of undesired consequences in arousing cognitive dissonance. *Journal of Personality and Social Psychology, 16,* 199–206.

Feldman, S. (1966). Motivational aspects of attitudinal elements and their place in cognitive interaction. In S. Feldman (Ed.), *Cognitive consistency* (pp. 75–108). New York: Academic Press.

Festinger, L. (1957a). The relation between behavior and cognition. In J. S. Bruner, E. Brunswik, L. Festinger, F. Heider, K. F. Muenzinger, C. E. Osgood, D. Rapaport (Eds.). *Contemporary approaches to cognition* (pp. 127–150). Cambridge, England: Oxford University Press.

Festinger, L. (1957b). *A theory of cognitive dissonance.* Stanford, CA: Stanford University Press.

Festinger, L., & Carlsmith, J. M. (1959). Cognitive consequences of forced compliance. *Journal of Abnormal and Social Psychology, 58,* 203–210.

Harmon-Jones, E., Brehm, J. W., Greenberg, J., Simon, L., & Nelson, D. E. (1996). Evidence that the production of aversive consequences is not necessary to create cognitive dissonance. *Journal of Personality and Social Psychology, 70,* 5–16.

Heider, F. (1958). *The psychology of interpersonal relations.* New York: Wiley.

Helmreich, R. I., & Collins, B. E. (1968). Studies in forced compliance: Commitment and magnitude of inducement to comply as determinants of opinion change. *Journal of Personality and Social Psychology, 10,* 75–81.

Holmes, J. G., & Strickland, L. H. (1970). Choice freedom and confirmation of incentive expectancy as determinants of attitude change. *Journal of Personality and Social Psychology, 14,* 39–45.

Joule, R.-V. (1991). Practicing and arguing for abstinence from smoking: A test of the double forced compliance paradigm. *European Journal of Social Psychology, 21,* 119–129.

Joule, R.-V. (1996). Une nouvelle voie de réduction de la dissonance: La rationalisation en acte [A new model for dissonance reduction: Act rationalization]. In J.-L. Beauvois, R.-V. Joule, & J. M. Monteil (Eds.), *Perspectives cognitives et conduites sociales: 5. Contextes et contextes sociaux* (pp. 293–307). Neuchâtel, Switzerland: Delachaux et Niestlé.

Joule, R.-V. & Beauvois, J. L. (1998). *La soumission librement consentie*. Paris, Presses Universitaires de France.

Joule, R.-V., & Girandola, F. (1995). Tâche fastidieuse et jeu de rôle dans le paradigme de la double soumission [Tedious task and role-playing in the double compliance paradigm]. *Revue Internationale de Psychologie Sociale, 8*, 101–116.

Joule, R.-V., & Lévèque, L. (1993). *Le changement d'attitude comme fonction du temps d'argumentation* [Attitude change as a function of argumentation length]. Unpublished manuscript, Provence University, Aix-en-Provence, France.

Kiesler, C. A. (1971). *The psychology of commitment: Experiments linking behavior to belief.* New York: Academic Press.

Leippe, M. R., & Eisenstadt, D. (1994). Generalization of dissonance reduction: Decreasing prejudice through induced compliance. *Journal of Personality and Social Psychology, 67*, 395–413.

Linder, D. E., Cooper, J., & Jones, E. E. (1967). Decision freedom as determinant of the role of incentive magnitude in attitude change. *Journal of Personality and Social Psychology, 6*, 245–254.

Rabbie, J. M., Brehm, J. W., & Cohen, A. R. (1959). Verbalization and relations to cognitive dissonance. *Journal of Personality, 27*, 407–417.

Simon, L., Greenberg, J., & Brehm, J. (1995). Trivialization: The forgotten mode of dissonance reduction. *Journal of Personality and Social Psychology, 68*, 247–260.

Steiner, I. D. (1980). Attribution of choice. In M. Fishbein (Ed.), *Progress in social psychology* (pp. 1–47). Hillsdale, NJ: Erlbaum.

Wicklund, R. A., & Brehm, J. W. (1976). *Perspectives on cognitive dissonance.* New York: Wiley.

Zajonc, R. K. (1968). Cognitive theories in social psychology. In G. Lindzey & E. Aronson (Eds.), *Handbook of social psychology* (Vol. 1, pp. 320–411). Reading, MA: Addison-Wesley.

4

Toward an Understanding of the Motivation Underlying Dissonance Effects: Is the Production of Aversive Consequences Necessary?

Eddie Harmon-Jones

In the 1960s, researchers began to challenge the original theory of cognitive dissonance and proposed that *cognitive discrepancy* (as defined by the original version of the theory; see Harmon-Jones & Mills, chap. 1, this volume) was not the cause of the cognitive and behavioral changes that were observed in experiments testing dissonance theory. Several revisions to the original theory emerged (Aronson, 1969; Collins, 1969; Cooper & Worchel, 1970). One of the most prevalent revisions posited, in contrast to the original theory of dissonance, that cognitive discrepancy was not necessary or sufficient to generate the cognitive and behavioral changes. This revision, which I refer to as the *aversive-consequences* revision, posited that feeling personally responsible for the production of foreseeable aversive consequences was necessary and sufficient to cause these effects (Cooper & Fazio, 1984). Addressing whether the production of aversive consequences is necessary to create dissonance is one of the most fundamental and important questions for dissonance theory and research—it concerns the under-

Thanks to Jack Brehm, Trish Devine, Cindy Harmon-Jones, and Judson Mills for providing helpful comments on a draft of this chapter.

lying motivational force driving dissonance effects. In the present chapter, I provide a brief overview of the original version of the theory of cognitive dissonance (see Festinger, 1957, and Harmon-Jones & Mills, chap. 1, this volume, for more complete descriptions) and the aversive-consequences revision. I then review evidence obtained in a variety of experimental paradigms that indicates that the production of aversive consequences is not necessary to create dissonance effects and that cognitive discrepancy, as defined by the original theory, is sufficient to cause dissonance effects. I conclude by proposing an extension of the original theory that assists in understanding the function of dissonance processes.

THE ORIGINAL VERSION

The original statement of cognitive dissonance theory (Festinger, 1957) proposed that discrepancy between cognitions creates a negative affective state that motivates individuals to attempt to reduce or eliminate the discrepancy between cognitions (see Devine, Tauer, Barron, Elliot, & Vance, chap. 12, this volume, and Harmon-Jones, in press, for a more complete description of this process). Several paradigms have been used to test predictions derived from dissonance theory. In each of these paradigms, the availability of the cognitions that serve to make the entire set of relevant cognitions more or less discrepant is manipulated. In the induced-compliance paradigm, participants are induced to act contrary to an attitude, and if they are provided few consonant cognitions (few reasons or little justification) for doing so, they are hypothesized to experience dissonance and reduce it, usually by changing their attitude to be more consistent with their behavior. In one of the first induced-compliance experiments, Festinger and Carlsmith (1959) paid participants either $1 (low justification) or $20 (high justification) to tell a fellow participant (confederate) that dull and boring tasks were very interesting and to remain on call to do it again in the future. After participants told this to the confederate, they were asked how interesting and enjoyable the tasks were. As predicted, participants given little justification for performing the counterattitudinal behavior rated the tasks as more interesting than did participants given much justification. Festinger and Carlsmith posited that participants provided low justification (just enough justification to say the counterattitudinal statement) experienced dissonance and changed their attitudes because of the inconsistency between their original attitude (they believed that the task was boring) and their behavior (they had said that the task was interesting). Participants provided with high justification, on the other hand, experienced little dissonance, because receiving $20 to perform the behavior justified the behavior or was consonant with the behavior.

In later research (Brehm & Cohen, 1962), dissonance was manipulated by means of perceived choice. Having low choice to behave counterattitudinally is consonant with that behavior whereas having high choice is not. Experiments found that participants who were given high choice, as opposed to low choice, to write counterattitudinal essays changed their attitudes to be more consistent with their behavior.

AVERSIVE-CONSEQUENCES REVISION

Within the decade after the publication of the provocative Festinger and Carlsmith (1959) experiment, researchers offered alternative theoretical and experimental accounts for their results. One alternative account suggested that low-justification participants in the Festinger and Carlsmith experiment changed their attitudes not because of cognitive discrepancy, but because their actions brought about an aversive event (convincing another person to expect boring tasks to be interesting). In one of the first experiments testing this explanation, Cooper and Worchel (1970) replicated and extended the Festinger and Carlsmith study. Cooper and Worchel found that low-justification participants changed their attitudes to be consistent with their behavior when the confederate believed their statement but not when the confederate did not believe their statement.

Using a slightly different procedure, other research has suggested that when the counterattitudinal actions do not cause aversive consequences, attitude change does not occur (e.g., Collins & Hoyt, 1972; Goethals & Cooper, 1975; Hoyt, Henley, & Collins, 1972). In these experiments, participants' counterattitudinal statements were to be shown to persons who could or could not affect a disliked policy. For example, Hoyt et al. (1972) gave participants low or high choice to write counterattitudinal essays saying that "toothbrushing is a dangerous, unhealthy habit" (p. 205). Participants were told that the essays would or would not produce the aversive consequence of influencing junior high school students to quit toothbrushing. Hoyt et al. found that only high-choice—aversive-consequences participants changed their attitudes. Other experiments have been offered as support for this revision (Cooper & Fazio, 1984; Scher & Cooper, 1989), and this revision has been widely accepted.

According to the aversive-consequences revision, a sufficient cognitive discrepancy is neither necessary nor sufficient to cause dissonance and discrepancy reduction. Instead, feeling personally responsible for the production of foreseeable aversive consequences is necessary and sufficient. Aversive consequences are events that one would not want to occur (Cooper & Fazio, 1984).

Alternative Explanations for the Evidence Produced by the Aversive-Consequences Revision

The aversive-consequences revision is supported by evidence obtained in the induced-compliance paradigm. More specifically, the support for the aversive-consequences revision comes from the absence of measurable attitude change in the conditions in which aversive consequences are not produced. Note that there are numerous explanations for the absence of this attitude-change effect in the no-aversive-consequences conditions, and these alternative explanations must prevent us from concluding that cognitive discrepancy is not necessary or sufficient to create dissonance. First, this is a null effect. It is difficult to draw clear inferences from null effects. A variety of factors could have produced the null effects. Had these past theorists and researchers drawn the conclusion that feeling personally responsible for producing an aversive outcome intensifies dissonance, I would be in complete agreement, for it is likely that feeling personally responsible for such will intensify dissonance and dissonance-produced attitude change. However, these past theorists and researchers did not draw this conclusion but instead proposed that feelings of personal responsibility for aversive outcomes were necessary to produce dissonance effects.

At least two sets of alternative explanations can be offered for the lack of attitude change in the no-aversive-consequences conditions. The first set of alternative explanations argues that the level of dissonance was not large enough to generate dissonance sufficient to produce attitude change and that the addition of the production of aversive consequences was necessary to produce dissonance sufficient to cause attitude change. Several of the past induced-compliance experiments that included a no-aversive-consequences and an aversive-consequences condition used attitudinal issues that were not extremely negative or positive, that is, control-condition participants reported moderately negative or positive attitudes (e.g., Calder, Ross, & Insko, 1973; Nel, Helmreich, & Aronson, 1969). Moreover, the lack of extremity might have reflected ambivalence or a mix of positive and negative attitudes toward the issues. Because the attitudes used in past experiments were not extremely positive or negative and might have been held with ambivalence, they were likely not to arouse much dissonance when behavior counter to them occurred. In essence, the magnitude of dissonance aroused may have been too small to generate attitude change.

In the past experiments, the researchers often encouraged participants to generate lengthy counterattitudinal statements. This may increase the likelihood of finding no attitude change in the no-aversive-consequences conditions. Research has shown that the length of the counterattitudinal statement relates inversely with the amount of attitude change that occurs (e.g., Beauvois & Joule, chap. 3, this volume; Rabbie, Brehm, & Cohen, 1959), that is, longer essays are likely to produce less attitude change. This inverse relationship between essay length and attitude change may occur because participants may provide their own justifications and hence more cognitions consonant with the behavior in these lengthy essays. As the number of consonant cognitions increases, the magnitude of dissonance decreases.

In addition, because of the salience of the audiences in these experiments, the participants' attention may have been focused more on the audience and whether they were convinced or could affect a disliked policy than on the nature of their own counterattitudinal actions or their own attitudes. As a result of this, the magnitude of dissonance may have been determined in large part by what the audience did or would do as a result of the counterattitudinal advocacy. Thus, the unconvinced audience, in contrast to the convinced audience, may have reduced the importance of the dissonant cognitions, to the point of making the counterattitudinal action seem trivial. If the perceived importance of dissonant cognitions is low, dissonance may not reach a magnitude that requires reduction.

Another possible explanation is that participants in these past experiments may have been provided too much justification (too many consonant cognitions) for producing the counterattitudinal statement, and the production of aversive consequences may have been necessary to elicit enough dissonance to produce measurable attitude change. This explanation seems very reasonable when one considers the high compliance rates observed in most if not all of this past research.[1] Typically, 100% of the participants have complied with the experimenter's request to write the counterattitudinal statement. As Festinger (1957) has explained, for attitude change to result from dissonance, the person should be offered *"just enough reward or punishment to elicit the overt compliance"* (p. 95, italics in original). Thus, the past experiments on the necessity of aversive consequences may have had inducing forces (the friendliness of the experimenter, the benefits to science) that were so great that little or no dissonance was produced, and the addition of feeling personally responsible for producing aversive consequences may have been necessary to produce sufficient dissonance to cause measurable discrepancy reduction (e.g., attitude change).

Another set of alternative explanations for the lack of attitude

---

[1]An examination of the past experiments that manipulated whether participants produced an aversive consequence revealed extremely high compliance rates in the high-choice and low-justification conditions. These experiments are listed with the number of noncompliers indicated in parentheses after the date of publication: Nel et al., 1969 (1); Cooper & Worchel, 1970 (1); Collins & Hoyt, 1972 (0); Goethals & Cooper, 1972 (2 experiments; 0); Hoyt et al., 1972 (1); Calder et al., 1973 (1); Cooper, Zanna, & Goethals, 1974 (0); Goethals & Cooper, 1975 (1); Scher & Cooper, 1989 (1); Johnson, Kelly, & LeBlanc, 1995 (0).

change in the no-aversive-consequences conditions argues that dissonance may have been aroused in participants in the no-aversive-consequences conditions of the past experiments but was not detected. The sole method of detecting dissonance in the experiments testing the aversive-consequences model against the original version of the theory has been assessment of attitude change. Because no assessments of dissonance were obtained in experiments testing the aversive consequences model, it is impossible to know whether dissonance was aroused in the no-aversive-consequences conditions. The only conclusion that can safely be drawn is that measurable attitude change did not occur. On the other hand, attitude change may have occurred in the no-aversive-consequences conditions but may have been small, and it would not have been detected if one had only 10–12 persons per condition, as was done in much of the past research (e.g., Calder et al., 1973; Cooper & Worchel, 1970). In addition, the dissonance may have been reduced in a route other than attitude change. Persons whose counterattitudinal actions had no undesired effects may have reduced dissonance by reducing the importance (Simon, Greenberg, & Brehm, 1995) or the perceived effectiveness (Scheier & Carver, 1980) of the counterattitudinal behavior.

It is unlikely that one of these possible alternative explanations accounts for all of the nonsignificant effects that have been found in the past no-aversive-consequences conditions. However, given the number of plausible alternative explanations for the null effects produced in the past experiments that had been used to support the aversive-consequences revision, my colleagues and I thought it was premature to abandon the original version of the theory.

Induced-Compliance Experimental Results Inconsistent With the Aversive-Consequences Revision

All of the research on the aversive-consequences revision has been conducted using the *induced-compliance* paradigm, which is the focal paradigm in which predictions derived from dissonance theory and its revisions have been tested. My colleagues and I have conducted several induced-compliance experiments to test the hypothesis that feeling personally responsible for producing aversive consequences is not necessary to produce dissonance and that cognitive discrepancy is sufficient to produce dissonance even in the induced-compliance paradigm. In conducting these experiments, we created a situation in which participants would write counterattitudinal statements but not produce aversive consequences. We designed the experiments so that conditions present in previous induced-compliance experiments that might have prevented attitude change from occurring were not present. We took special care to ensure that the inducing force was "just barely sufficient to induce the person" to behave counterattitudinally (Festinger & Carlsmith, 1959, p. 204), to reduce the number of consonant cognitions to a bare minimum, so that the dissonance aroused after the action would be at high levels. In addition, we had participants write short counterattitudinal statements about objects toward which they held attitudes that were highly salient, strongly negative (or positive), simple, and not ambivalent. Also, in some of the experiments, we assessed negative affect and arousal, to provide measures of dissonance.

In each experiment, under the guise of an experiment on recall, participants were exposed to a stimulus, were given low or high choice to write a counterattitudinal statement about that stimulus, threw away the statement they wrote, and then completed questionnaires that assessed their attitudes toward the stimulus. We assured participants that their counterattitudinal statements and their responses to the questionnaires would be made in private and would be anonymous. We did so to create a situation in which the counterattitudinal behavior would not lead to aversive consequences, because, as Cooper and Fazio (1984) argued, "making a statement contrary to one's attitude while in solitude does not have the potential for bringing about an aversive event" (p. 232). We predicted that participants provided high choice for engaging in the counterattitudinal behavior would change their attitudes to be more consistent with their behavior, whereas participants provided low choice would not.

Dissonance and a Bitter Beverage

In Experiment 1 (Harmon-Jones, Brehm, Greenberg, Simon, & Nelson, 1996), the experimenter told participants that he was interested in factors that affect the recall of characteristics of products and that at this point in his research, he was seeing how writing a sentence evaluating a product would affect recall of the characteristics of the product. He told participants that he would have them drink a beverage and that they would be asked to recall characteristics of it. He also informed participants that he was using a variety of drinks, that he would not know what type of drink they would receive, and that they should not let him know what type of drink they received. He also explained that all of their responses would be anonymous and that he would not see their responses to questionnaires but that an assistant would enter them into a computer.

Then the experimenter gave the participant a cup covered with a lid. The cup contained 4 oz of fruit-punch-flavored Kool-Aid. The Kool-Aid was mixed either with the amount of sugar suggested on the package (1 cup per two qt), to create a pleasant-tasting drink, or with 2 teaspoons of white vinegar (no sugar), to create an unpleasant-tasting drink. Because the experimenter was unaware of whether participants were given a pleasant- or an unpleasant-tasting drink, he was unaware of whether participants experienced dissonance.

After the participant drank some of the beverage, the experimenter returned to the participant's cubicle and induced the choice manipulation. He told participants in the low-choice condition that they were randomly assigned to write a statement saying they liked the beverage. He told participants in the high-choice condition that they could write a statement saying they liked or disliked the beverage and that it was their choice. The experimenter explained that he needed some more persons to write that they liked the beverage, and he asked the participant if she or he would write that she or he liked the beverage. Once the experimenter gained compliance from the participant, he reminded her or him that it was her or his choice.

The experimenter then asked both low-choice and high-choice participants to write one sentence saying they liked the beverage. He also told participants that he did not "need the sheet of paper you will write your sentence on; we just need for you to go through the process of writing the sentence. So when you are done, just wad it up and throw it in the wastebasket." He did this to ensure that the participants perceived that they had anonymity and that there would be no consequences to their behavior. The experimenter then left the participants alone to write the sentence.

After the participant discarded the sentence, the experimenter gave the participant an envelope and said that previous research had indicated that the characteristics a person recalls about a product may be affected by whether they liked the product and that to take this into account, he needed them to answer a questionnaire that assessed their thoughts about the drink. The questionnaire assessed how much the drink was liked. The experimenter left the participant alone to answer this questionnaire. After the participant finished with this questionnaire, the experimenter had the participant complete a questionnaire that assessed the effectiveness of the manipulation of choice. After assessing suspicion, ensuring that participants perceived their questionnaires and statements to be anonymous, and debriefing, the experimenter collected the participants' statements from the trash can, to assess whether participants complied with the request to write the counterattitudinal statement, and placed the statement with the participants' questionnaires.

Approximately 15% of the participants did not write counterattitudinal statements. This effect suggests that we had designed a situation in which there was just enough but not too much external justification to write the counterattitudinal statement. Results indicated that unpleasant-tasting drink–high-choice participants reported more positive attitudes toward the drink than did unpleasant-tasting drink–low-choice participants. This effect was significant when both compliers and noncompliers were included in the analysis. Thus, the results of the first experiment suggested that dissonance can be created in induced-compliance situations void of aversive consequences.

Dissonance, Boring Passages, and Electrodermal Activity

To increase confidence that the results obtained in Experiment 1 were valid, my colleagues and I attempted to conceptually replicate the effects by means of a different manipulation of choice and a different attitudinal object. Using the same procedures as used in the first experiment, we had participants read a boring passage and gave them low or high choice, by means of written instructions, to write a statement saying that the passage was interesting. Thus, in this experiment, we had only two conditions: low choice and high choice. Because choice was induced by means of written instructions, the experimenter was unaware of when dissonance was expected. Results from Experiment 2 replicated those of Experiment 1, showing that high-choice participants rated the boring passage as more interesting than did low-choice participants (Harmon-Jones et al., 1996).

In Experiment 3 (Harmon-Jones et al., 1996), we measured nonspecific skin conductance responses (NS-SCRs) that occurred in the 3 min after the writing of the counterattitudinal statement but before the assessment of attitude. Previous research has indicated that increased NS-SCRs are associated with increased sympathetic nervous system activity, which is increased during emotional arousal. If our experimental procedure evoked dissonance, we would observe increased NS-SCRs. Results indicated that participants given high choice to write the counterattitudinal statement evidenced more NS-SCRs and reported that the passage was more interesting than did participants given low choice to write the statement.

Dissonance and a Hershey's Kiss

The previous results demonstrate that the production of aversive consequences is not necessary to arouse dissonance and dissonance-related attitude change. However, they may be subject to an alternative explanation: Perhaps the manipulation of choice to write the statement affected individuals' reconstructive construal of the situation, so that high-choice participants felt as though they had high choice to partake of the negative stimulus, whereas low-choice participants felt as though they had low choice to partake of the negative stimulus. If this were so, then the aversive-consequences revision could explain these results as being due to feeling personally responsible for inflicting a negative event on oneself (choosing to drink the bitter Kool-Aid). To eliminate this alternative explanation, I recently conducted the following experiment (Harmon-Jones, 1998). In this experiment, instead of having persons write a counterattitudinal statement about a negative stimulus, I had them write a counterattitudinal statement about a positive stimulus.

Using the same cover story as used in the previous two experiments,

I had participants eat a Hershey's Kiss and then gave them high or low choice to write that they did not enjoy it. In keeping with the previous results, high-choice participants reported that they disliked the Hershey's Kiss more than did low-choice participants (see Figure 1).

In addition, in this experiment, I assessed state self-reported affect. It was assessed immediately after the writing of the counterattitudinal statement or after the attitude-change opportunity. Time between counter-attitudinal action and attitude assessment was controlled by having participants complete an affect questionnaire or a filler questionnaire, comparable in length. From the state affect measure, four indexes of affect were derived. Discomfort was measured with the scale developed by Elliot and Devine (1994). State social self-esteem and appearance self-esteem were measured with the subscales of the State Self-Esteem Scale (Heatherton & Polivy, 1991). Positive affect was measured with the items happy, proud, and enthusiastic.

Results indicated that participants who were given high choice and who completed the affect questionnaire before the attitude measure reported significantly more discomfort than did participants in the other conditions (see Figure 2). Positive affect, state social self-esteem, and state appearance self-esteem did not differ significantly among conditions. These results suggest that the cognitive discrepancy evoked in this situation increased discomfort. The present results also suggest that the cognitive discrepancy evoked in this situation was more likely to increase discomfort than to decrease state self-esteem or positive affect.[2]

---

[2] In the three induced-compliance experiments by Harmon-Jones et al. (1996) that are described in this chapter, compliance was approximately 85%. However, in the reported experiment by Harmon-Jones (1998), in which participants ate a piece of chocolate and then wrote that they did not enjoy it, only 1 participant did not comply. In the experiments by Harmon-Jones et al., persons were asked to write that they believed a boring passage they had just read was interesting or that an unpleasant-tasting beverage was pleasant tasting. The attitudes toward these simple stimuli were quite negative, as evidenced by low-choice-condition and control-condition participants (see Harmon-Jones et al., 1996). In contrast, in the experiment by Harmon-Jones (1998), persons' attitudes toward the chocolate were not extremely positive. Thus, although this latter experiment had compliance rates similar to the ones discussed above, it still produced dissonance. Thus, compliance rates are not an inviolable assessment of amount of justification within an experiment. Other factors, such as the size and importance of the discrepancy between attitude and behavior and number and importance of justifications for the behavior (promised rewards or punishments, which are probably largely social in nature), need to be taken into account. Attempts to measure size and importance of discrepancy and justifications would aid tremendously in specifying the magnitude of dissonance.

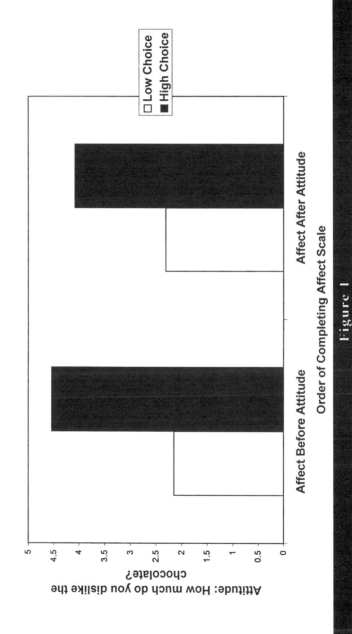

Attitudes as a Function of Choice and Order of Completing Affect Scale

Figure 1

Attitudes as a function of choice and order of completing the affect scale.

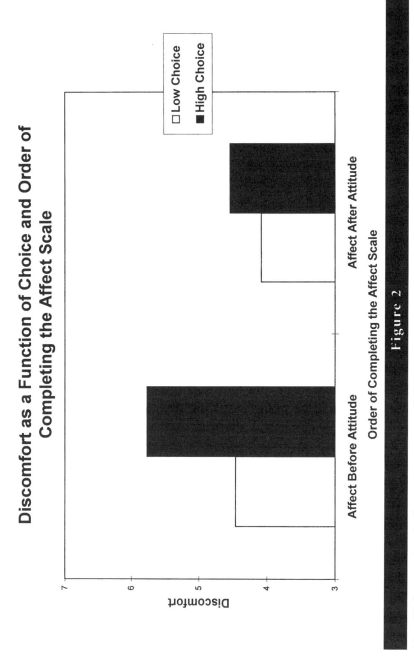

Discomfort as a Function of Choice and Order of Completing the Affect Scale

Figure 2

Note. Higher numbers indicate more reported discomfort.

Summary

The experiments presented thus far were all conducted using the induced-compliance paradigm. The results from these experiments support the original theory of dissonance and are inconsistent with the aversive-consequences revision. These experiments are important because they show that dissonance arousal, dissonance affect, and dissonance-produced attitude change can occur in situations in which a sufficient cognitive discrepancy is present but feeling personally responsible for the production of aversive consequences is not present. The present evidence convincingly demonstrates that dissonance effects can be generated by a cognitive discrepancy that does not produce aversive consequences. Indeed, these results suggest that the original version of the theory was abandoned prematurely (see also Beauvois & Joule, 1996, chap. 3, this volume).

Aversive Consequences and Attitude Change

Earlier I argued that producing aversive consequences might intensify dissonance. Why would this occur? The production of aversive consequences may intensify dissonance because aversive consequences are a cognition dissonant with one's preexisting attitude. If the attitude were the generative cognition, the cognition about the counterattitudinal behavior and the cognition of producing aversive consequences would be dissonant cognitions. Thus, the magnitude of dissonance aroused would be greater in psychological situations where counterattitudinal behavior and aversive consequences were produced than in situations where only counterattitudinal behavior was produced, because there are more dissonant cognitions in the former than in the latter situation. However, if the counterattitudinal behavior were the generative cognition, then the cognition of producing aversive consequences would be a consonant cognition (it follows from the behavior), and thus it would decrease the magnitude of dissonance aroused. Beauvois and Joule (1996) have reported results consistent with this latter interpretation, but the past research on the aversive-consequences model is consistent with the former. This inconsistency between these two sets of data can be resolved by positing that in the induced-compliance paradigm, both the attitude and the behavior can serve as generative cognitions, and there may be a potential dissonance associated with each. That is, there is a potential dissonance associated with the attitude and a potential dissonance associated with the behavior. In general, the greater dissonance would be the one reduced. The generative cognition associated with that greater dissonance would not be altered, whereas the generative cognition associated with the lesser dissonance would be altered. However, the reduction of dissonance depends also on the availability of discrepancy-reduction routes. Hence, when the potential dissonances are not very different in magnitude, the discrepancy may be reduced by means of the most available route, which has been attitude change in most previous dissonance experiments.

In contrast, the production of aversive consequences may increase the dissonance because it increases the commitment to the behavior, making the behavior more resistant to change and attitude change more likely to result. In addition, when behavior produces important consequences, it will be regarded as a more important cognition and thus has the potential to create more dissonance. Although these explanations are more elegant in their simplicity, they do not fit with the large body evidence presented by Beauvois and Joule (1996), whereas the explanation offered in the previous paragraph does.

Past Evidence From the Belief-Disconfirmation Paradigm Inconsistent With the Aversion Consequences Revision

Research on the aversive-consequences revision has focused exclusively on the induced-compliance paradigm. However, other paradigms have been used to test predictions derived from dissonance theory, and evidence obtained in these paradigms is difficult to explain with the aversive-consequences revision (see also Berkowitz & Devine, 1989).

One such paradigm is the *belief-disconfirmation* paradigm. This paradigm is based on Festinger, Riecken, and Schachter's (1956) observations of belief intensification among members of a group whose belief that a flood would destroy the continent was disconfirmed. This evidence suggests that the cognitive discrepancy that occurs when an important and highly resistant to change belief is disconfirmed produces dissonance, leading to the use of dissonance-reducing strategies such as belief intensification. Results obtained in this paradigm are not subject to an aversive-consequences alternative explanation, because individuals involuntarily exposed to belief-discrepant information have not produced an aversive consequence and thus cannot feel responsible for having done so.

In an experiment by Brock and Balloun (1967), committed churchgoers were confronted with audiotaped information that did or did not support their religious values. These individuals were less likely to press a button to eliminate white noise from the communication and thus clarify it when the information was inconsistent with their values. Other research has replicated these findings (e.g., Schwarz, Frey, & Kumpf, 1980), further suggesting that dissonance effects occur even when inconsistencies are produced by outside information, not from actions that produce aversive consequences.

In a quasi-experiment by Batson (1975), girls attending a church youth program were asked to declare publicly whether they believed in the divinity of Jesus. After completing a measure of Christian orthodoxy, the girls were then presented with belief-disconfirming information (i.e., information that indicated that Jesus was not the son of God). Orthodoxy was once again assessed. As expected, those who believed in the divinity of Jesus and accepted the truthfulness of the disconfirming information intensified their belief in Jesus' divinity, whereas those who were not believers or who believed but did not accept the truthfulness of the disconfirming information did not.

It is difficult to explain the results obtained in the belief-disconfirmation paradigm as resulting from the motivation to avoid feeling personally responsible for producing aversive consequences. That is, the person exposed to belief-inconsistent information has not acted in a manner to produce aversive consequences and thus cannot feel responsible for having done so. In this paradigm, persons are exposed to information from an external source; they have not done anything for which to feel responsible. Note that Cooper and Fazio (1989), two of the main proponents of the aversive-consequences revision, have stated that according to the aversive-consequences revision, evidence obtained in the belief-disconfirmation paradigm is not the result of dissonance. Cooper and Fazio (1989) have stated that exposure to belief-discrepant information "will not necessarily create an unwanted consequence and will not necessarily arouse dissonance" (p. 525). In my view, this is not an accurate statement, and the aversive-consequences revision has unfortunately excessively narrowed the range of application of dissonance theory. One way to demonstrate that evidence obtained in the belief-disconfirmation paradigm is the result of dissonance processes is to show that the negative affect that motivates the cognitive effects occurs as a result of belief disconfirmation and is reduced after reconciliation of the cognitive discrepancy.

Recent Evidence From the
Belief-Disconfirmation Paradigm Inconsistent With the
Aversion Consequences Revision

My colleagues and I recently conducted two belief-disconfirmation experiments, to assess whether the reactions observed in past belief-disconfirmation experiments resulted from the affective and motivational pressures presumed by dissonance theory to drive the cognitive effects (Burris, Harmon-Jones, & Tarpley, 1997). We tested Allport's (1950) idea that "the suffering of innocent persons is for most people the hardest of all facts to integrate into religious sentiment" (p. 81). In the experiments, Christian participants were exposed to a newspaper article that highlighted the discrepancy between belief in a loving, protecting, just, and omnipotent God and knowledge of the gratuitous suffering humans often experience. The newspaper article reported the drive-by shooting death of an infant boy in his grandmother's arms as she and the child's father prayed for protection because a similar incident had occurred two nights earlier. The article concluded with a quote from the infant's grandfather that expressed his continued faith in God. The cognitive discrepancy between the participants' religious beliefs (God is a good God who protects the innocent and answers prayers) and this tragic outcome (the infant dies during a prayer for protection) was highlighted by having participants read, "Some people would think that the grandfather's continued belief and trust in a good God is naive and misguided."

Belief Disconfirmation and Transcendence Experiment

In the first experiment, we tested the hypothesis, offered by Abelson (1959), that "the theosophical dilemma of God's presumed permissiveness toward evil is sometimes resolved by appeal to transcendent concepts" (p. 346). If participants exposed to this belief-discrepant story were allowed to engage in transcendence (i.e., allowed to reconcile dissonant cognitions under a superordinate principle), they would experience less negative affect. Moreover, the more they engaged in transcendence, the less their negative affect would be.

Participants were randomly assigned to one of two conditions. In the transcendence-opportunity condition, they read the newspaper article and then completed a questionnaire that allowed them to engage in transcendence. These participants were given the explicit opportunity to reconcile the cognitive discrepancy after the dissonance had been aroused, when they were most in need of reducing the dissonance brought about by exposure to the belief-inconsistent information. They then completed a measure of self-reported state negative affect. In the no-transcendent-opportunity condition, participants completed the transcendence measure, read the tragic newspaper article, and then completed the measure of negative affect. These participants were thus not given an explicit opportunity to engage in transcendence after the dissonance had been aroused, when they were most in need of reducing the dissonance. The transcendence measure included questions such as, How much does God intervene in persons' lives? and How often do things happen to persons because of God's greater purpose? The measure of negative affect included items to measure discomfort (uncomfortable, uneasy, bothered; Elliot & Devine, 1994) and agitation (angry, frustrated, distressed, and threatened).

We hypothesized that endorsement of higher levels of transcendence subsequent to reading the newspaper article would relate to lower levels of dissonance-related affect, whereas higher levels of transcendence before the reading were not expected to relate to lower levels of dissonance-related affect. To test this hypothesis, separate regression analyses were conducted, in which agitation and discomfort served as criterion variables. In each, experimental condition (effect coded) and transcendence were first entered as main effects, followed by their interaction.

For agitation, neither main effect approached significance, but in keeping with predictions, a significant two-way interaction emerged. Higher endorsement of transcendence predicted decreased agitation in the transcendence-opportunity condition, whereas it did not in the no-opportunity condition. A similar pattern emerged for discomfort. Moreover, individuals in the transcendence-opportunity condition engaged in more transcendence than did individuals in the no-transcendence-opportunity condition.

As expected, more extreme endorsement of transcendent beliefs after exposure to a belief-discrepant article was associated with reduced dissonance-related affect. In contrast, belief transcendence before exposure to the belief-discrepant article did not relate to reduced dissonance-related affect. This evidence strongly suggests that exposure to belief-discrepant information arouses dissonance that motivates persons to engage in discrepancy reduction, which then reduces the dissonance. Because persons in the belief-disconfirmation paradigm do not produce aversive consequences for which to feel responsible, this evidence suggests that the production of aversive consequences is not necessary to create dissonance.

Belief Disconfirmation and Belief Affirmation Experiment

In the previous experiment, time and transcendence opportunity were confounded, making it difficult to infer what caused the observed effects. That is, those who completed the transcendence scale after reading the article and before responding to the affect measures may have been distracted by this intervening task compared with those who completed the transcendence scale before the article. This explanation does not seem plausible, given that there was no main effect of transcendence-opportunity condition on dissonance-related affect but only an interaction with level of transcendence endorsement. However, to eliminate this explanation, we conducted a second study that conceptually replicated the first. In addition, instead of assessing transcendence in response to belief disconfirmation, we assessed belief affirmation, much like Batson (1975) and Festinger et al. (1956) did, to test the hypothesis that religious individuals would "rigidly maintain or even intensify" (Batson, 1975, p. 178) their beliefs when faced with disconfirming evidence. Religiously interested participants completed religious belief measures either after (belief-affirmation condition) or before (no-affirmation condition) reading the belief-discrepant article or completed comparable-length nonreligious belief measures after the article (distraction condition). All then completed affect measures (e.g., agitation). Results revealed that, as predicted, agitation was lower in the religious-affirmation condition than in either the no-affirmation or the distraction condition; agitation levels in the latter two conditions did not differ.

Past results from the belief-disconfirmation paradigm cannot be interpreted in terms of the aversive-consequences revision. This past research, however, suffers from an important limitation because no measures of dissonance-related affect were obtained either during the experience of dissonance or after discrepancy reduction, rendering it difficult to know whether the effects generated in this belief-disconfirmation paradigm were indeed caused by the mechanisms proposed by dissonance theory. The recent research by Burris et al. (1997) demonstrates quite convincingly that the effects produced in the belief-disconfirmation paradigm are due to dissonance processes.

Other Experimental Results Inconsistent With the Aversive-Consequences Revision

Other experiments provide evidence of dissonance in situations void of the production of aversive consequences. For instance, Aronson and Carlsmith (1962) found that individuals with experimentally created expectancies for failure reacted with dissonance to behaving successfully. In the experiment, after individuals had repeatedly failed at a task, they were given feedback indicating that they were succeeding at the task. Then the individuals were given an opportunity to change their responses. Results indicated that these individuals changed their responses from being correct to being incorrect. Because failure is regarded as negative and success as positive, the behavior of these individuals would be difficult to interpret in the aversive-consequences formulation. In addition, Aronson, Stone, and colleagues (Aronson, chap. 5, this volume; Aronson, Fried, & Stone, 1991; Fried & Aronson, 1995; Stone, Aronson, Crain, Winslow, & Fried, 1994) have demonstrated that dissonance can occur even when participants engage in proattitudinal behavior that has positive consequences. Beauvois and Joule (1996, chap. 3, this volume) and McGregor, Newby-Clark, and Zanna (chap. 13, this volume) also have reported recent experimental evidence indicating that dissonance can occur in the absence of the production of aversive consequences.

SUMMARY OF EVIDENCE

Results from experiments using several methodologies suggest that a cognitive discrepancy in the absence of feeling personally responsible for the production of aversive consequences can cause increased dissonance-related negative affect and discrepancy reduction. The results of these experiments suggest that a cognitive discrepancy is enough to generate dissonance and discrepancy reduction. Feeling personally responsible for producing aversive consequences is not necessary to generate dissonance and discrepancy reduction, but it may enhance the magnitude of dissonance effects because producing aversive consequences is an important cognition that is dissonant with one's preexisting attitude or because the aversive consequences increase the commitment to behavior.

A cognitive discrepancy, however, will produce an aversive state, in keeping with Festinger's speculations and the data presented in this chapter. This aversive state is not equivalent to the aversive consequences that dissonance theory revisionists discussed. Further research is necessary to understand why cognitive discrepancy creates a negative affective state and motivates discrepancy reduction.

WHAT IS THE MOTIVATION UNDERLYING DISSONANCE EFFECTS?

The reviewed research cogently demonstrates that the motivation to avoid the production of aversive consequences is not the motivation underlying dissonance effects. According to the original version of the theory, a sufficient cognitive discrepancy is the source of the motivation underlying dissonance and its effects. But why would a cognitive discrepancy evoke such a motivation? What function does the capacity to experience negative affect in response to a sufficient cognitive discrepancy and then be motivated to reduce it have for the organism? Is this set of psychological mechanisms adaptively beneficial? That is, is the dissonance mechanism functional or beneficial for the organism?

Understanding of dissonance processes could be improved and extended with an explanation of why cognitive inconsistency arouses negative affect and how and why this negative affect motivates the cognitive and behavior adjustments. The present model begins with the assumption that cognitions (broadly defined) can serve as action tendencies. The idea that cognition is for action is seen not only in the writings of William James (1890/1950) but also in ecological approaches to perception (Gibson, 1979; McArthur & Baron, 1983) and in the study of attitudes, both historically (Bain, 1868; Spencer, 1865) and currently (Cacioppo & Berntson, 1994). In this sense, the cognitions that are of primary concern for this approach are those that provide useful information, and usefulness of information is defined by its relevance to actions and goals. When information inconsistent with cognitions that guide action is encountered, negative emotion (dissonance) is aroused because the dissonant information has the potential to interfere with effective and unconflicted action. For the present model, effective behavior can occur in the absence of consciousness; in other words, effective behavior can be produced automatically. Thus, the present model does not propose that cognitive consistency is necessary for effective behavior. It only proposes that cognitive inconsistency interferes with effective behavior.

Thus, cognitive discrepancy may create negative affect because discrepancy among cognitions undermines the requirement for effective and unconflicted action (Beckmann & Irle, 1985; Harmon-Jones, in press; Jones & Gerard, 1967). Research on the theory of dissonance has identified commitment as an important, if not necessary, condition for the arousal of dissonance (Beauvois & Joule, 1996; Brehm & Cohen,

1962; Festinger, 1964). For most dissonance theorists, the notion of commitment implies that the person has engaged in a behavior for which he or she feels responsibility and that he or she has a definite understanding of the consequences of the behavior. However, persons can regard cognitions that may not involve a behavioral commitment as true or certain (Mills, 1968) and would experience dissonance if information were presented that was inconsistent with these cognitions. A good example of this type of cognition is a person's knowledge of the law of gravity. Information that violates the law of gravity would probably arouse dissonance in most persons. Therefore, a commitment occurs when a person regards a behavior, belief, attitude, or value as a meaningful truth. Defining commitment in this way allows for viewing commitment as a continuous variable. When commitment is defined as overt behavior, as with previous dissonance theorists, commitment is reduced to a categorical variable, which then may present problems. The psychological commitment to the cognition guides information processing, which serves the ultimate function of producing and guiding behavior.

If dissonant information is encountered, negative emotion may result and cause the person to engage in cognitive work to support the commitment. However, if dissonant information continues to mount, the negative emotion that results may motivate the person to discontinue supporting the commitment and give in to the dissonant information. Whether the person's cognitive work is aimed toward supporting the commitment or discontinuing the commitment would be determined by the resistance to change of each cognition. If the commitment is more resistant to change than the dissonant information, then cognitive work would be aimed at supporting the commitment. If, however, the dissonant information is more resistant to change than the commitment, then the cognitive work would be aimed at discontinuing the commitment. Resistance to change of cognitions is determined by the responsiveness of the cognitions to reality (e.g., the grass is green), the extent to which the cognitions are in relations of consonance to other cognitions, the difficulty of changing the cognition, and so on. From the present view, resistance to change is ultimately determined by the degree to which individuals believe the information assists them in controlling and predicting outcomes and thus behaving effectively. When knowledge about the environment, about oneself, or about one's actions, beliefs, or attitudes is in a dissonant relation, the sense of being able to control and predict outcomes may be threatened, and ultimately, the need to act effectively would be undermined.

From the current perspective, the proximal motivation to reduce cognitive discrepancy stems from the need to reduce negative emotion, whereas the distal motivation to reduce discrepancy stems from the requirement for effective action. When the maintenance of true and certain knowledge and thus the potential for effective action are threatened by information that is sufficiently discrepant from the psychological commitment, negative emotion results, which prompts attempts at the restoration of cognitions supportive of the commitment (i.e., discrepancy reduction). Thus, negative emotion works much like pain in that it provides the information and motivation that prompts the person to engage in cognitive action aimed at resolving the discrepancy. These speculations about the adaptive function of dissonance processes suggest interesting avenues of research.

REFERENCES

Abelson, R. P. (1959). Modes or resolution of belief dilemmas. *Journal of Conflict Resolution, 3,* 343–352.

Allport, G. W. (1950). *The individual and his religion.* New York: Macmillan.

Aronson, E. (1969). The theory of cognitive dissonance: A current perspective. In L. Berkowitz (Ed.), *Advances in experimental social psychology* (Vol. 4, pp. 1–34). New York: Academic Press.

Aronson, E., & Carlsmith, J. M. (1962). Performance expectancy as a determinant of actual performance. *Journal of Abnormal and Social Psychology, 65,* 178–183.

Aronson, E., Fried, C., & Stone, J. (1991). Overcoming denial and increasing the intention to use condoms through the induction of hypocrisy. *American Journal of Public Health, 81,* 1636–1638.

Bain, A. (1868). *Mental science: A compendium of psychology, and the history of philosophy.* New York: Appleton-Century-Crofts.

Batson, C. D. (1975). Rational processing or rationalization?: The effect of disconfirming information on a stated religious belief. *Journal of Personality and Social Psychology, 32*, 176–184.

Beauvois, J.-L., & Joule, R.-V. (1996). *A radical dissonance theory.* London: Taylor & Francis.

Beckmann, J., & Irle, M. (1985). Dissonance and action control. In J. Kuhl & J. Beckmann (Eds.), *Action control: From cognition to behavior* (pp. 129–150). Berlin: Springer-Verlag.

Berkowitz, L., & Devine, P. G. (1989). Research traditions, analysis, and synthesis in social psychological theories: The case of dissonance theory. *Personality and Social Psychology Bulletin, 15*, 493–507.

Brehm, J. W., & Cohen, A. R. (1962). *Explorations in cognitive dissonance.* New York: Wiley.

Brock, T. C., & Balloun, J. C. (1967). Behavioral receptivity to dissonant information. *Journal of Personality and Social Psychology, 6*, 413–428.

Burris, C. T., Harmon-Jones, E., & Tarpley, W. R. (1997). "By faith alone": Religious agitation and cognitive dissonance. *Basic and Applied Social Psychology, 19*, 17–31.

Cacioppo, J. T., & Berntson, G. G. (1994). Relationship between attitudes and evaluative space: A critical review, with emphasis on the separability of positive and negative substrates. *Psychological Bulletin, 115*, 401–423.

Calder, B. J., Ross, M., & Insko, C. A. (1973). Attitude change and attitude attribution: Effects of incentive, choice, and consequences. *Journal of Personality and Social Psychology, 25*, 84–99.

Collins, B. E. (1969). The effect of monetary inducements on the amount of attitude change produced by forced compliance. In A. C. Elms (Ed.), *Role playing, reward, and attitude change* (pp. 209–223). New York: Van Nostrand Reinhold.

Collins, B. E., & Hoyt, M. F. (1972). Personal responsibility-for-consequences: An integration and extension of the "forced compliance" literature. *Journal of Experimental Social Psychology, 8*, 558–593.

Cooper, J., & Fazio, R. H. (1984). A new look at dissonance theory. In L. Berkowitz (Ed.), *Advances in experimental social psychology* (Vol. 17, pp. 229–264). Orlando, FL: Academic Press.

Cooper, J., & Fazio, R. H. (1989). Research traditions, analysis, and synthesis:

Building a faulty case around misinterpreted theory. *Personality and Social Psychology Bulletin, 15*, 519–529.

Cooper, J., & Worchel, S. (1970). Role of undesired consequences in arousing cognitive dissonance. *Journal of Personality and Social Psychology, 16*, 199–206.

Cooper, J., Zanna, M. P., & Goethals, G. R. (1974). Mistreatment of an esteemed other as a consequence affecting dissonance reduction. *Journal of Experimental Social Psychology, 10*, 224–233.

Elliot, A. J., & Devine, P. G. (1994). On the motivational nature of cognitive dissonance: Dissonance as psychological discomfort. *Journal of Personality and Social Psychology, 67*, 382–394.

Festinger, L. (1957). *A theory of cognitive dissonance.* Evanston, IL: Row, Peterson.

Festinger, L. (1964). *Conflict, decision, and dissonance.* Stanford, CA: Stanford University Press.

Festinger, L., & Carlsmith, J. M. (1959). Cognitive consequences of forced compliance. *Journal of Abnormal and Social Psychology, 58*, 203–210.

Festinger, L., Riecken, H. W., & Schachter, S. (1956). *When prophecy fails.* Minneapolis: University of Minnesota Press.

Fried, C. B., & Aronson, E. (1995). Hypocrisy, misattribution, and dissonance reduction. *Personality and Social Psychology Bulletin, 21*, 925–933.

Gibson, J. J. (1979). *The ecological approach to visual perception.* Boston: Houghton Mifflin.

Goethals, G. R., & Cooper, J. (1972). Role of intention and postbehavioral consequence in the arousal of cognitive dissonance. *Journal of Personality and Social Psychology, 23*, 293–301.

Goethals, G. R., & Cooper, J. (1975). When dissonance is reduced: The timing of self-justificatory attitude change. *Journal of Personality and Social Psychology, 32*, 361–367.

Harmon-Jones, E. (1998). *Dissonance and affect: Evidence that dissonance-related negative affect occurs in the absence of aversive consequences.* Manuscript in preparation.

Harmon-Jones, E. (in press). *A cognitive dissonance theory perspective on the role of emotion in the maintenance and change of beliefs and attitudes.* In

N. Frijda, A. R. S. Manstead, & S. Bem (Eds.), *Emotions and beliefs*. Cambridge, England: Cambridge University Press.

Harmon-Jones, E., Brehm, J. W., Greenberg, J., Simon, L., & Nelson, D. E. (1996). Evidence that the production of aversive consequences is not necessary to create cognitive dissonance. *Journal of Personality and Social Psychology, 70,* 5–16.

Heatherton, T. F., & Polivy, J. (1991). Development and validation of a scale for measuring state self-esteem. *Journal of Personality and Social Psychology, 60,* 895–910.

Hoyt, M. F., Henley, M. D., & Collins, B. E. (1972). Studies in forced compliance: Confluence of choice and consequence on attitude change. *Journal of Personality and Social Psychology, 23,* 205–210.

James, W. (1950). *The principles of psychology*. New York: Dover. (Original work published 1890)

Johnson, R. W., Kelly, R. J., & LeBlanc, B. A. (1995). Motivational basis of dissonance: Aversive consequences or inconsistency. *Personality and Social Psychology Bulletin, 21,* 850–855.

Jones, E. E., & Gerard, H. B. (1967). *Foundations of social psychology*. New York: Wiley.

McArthur, L. Z., & Baron, R. M. (1983). Toward an ecological theory of social perception. *Psychological Review, 90,* 215–238.

Mills, J. (1968). Interest in supporting and discrepant information. In R. P. Abelson, E. Aronson, W. J. McGuire, T. M. Newcomb, M. J. Rosenberg, & P. H. Tannenbaum (Eds.), *Theories of cognitive consistency: A source book* (pp. 771–776). Skokie, IL: Rand McNally.

Nel, E., Helmreich, R., & Aronson, E. (1969). Opinion change in the advocate as a function of the persuasibility of his audience: A clarification of the meaning of dissonance. *Journal of Personality and Social Psychology, 12,* 117–124.

Rabbie, J. M., Brehm, J. W., & Cohen, A. R. (1959). Verbalization and reactions to cognitive dissonance. *Journal of Personality, 27,* 407–417.

Scheier, M. F., & Carver, C. S. (1980). Private and public self-attention, resistance to change, and dissonance reduction. *Journal of Personality and Social Psychology, 39,* 390–405.

Scher, S. J., & Cooper, J. (1989). Motivational basis of dissonance: The singular role of behavioral consequences. *Journal of Personality and Social Psychology, 56,* 899–906.

Schwarz, N., Frey, D., & Kumpf, M. (1980). Interactive effects of writing and reading a persuasive essay on attitude change and selective exposure. *Journal of Experimental Social Psychology, 16,* 1–17.

Simon, L., Greenberg, J., & Brehm, J. W. (1995). Trivialization: The forgotten mode of dissonance reduction. *Journal of Personality and Social Psychology, 68,* 247–260.

Spencer, H. (1865). *First principles.* New York: Appleton.

Stone, J., Aronson, E., Crain, A. L., Winslow, M. P., & Fried, C. B. (1994). Inducing hypocrisy as a means for encouraging young adults to use condoms. *Personality and Social Psychology Bulletin, 20,* 116–128.

Thibodeau, R., & Aronson, E. (1992). Taking a closer look: Reasserting the role of self-concept in dissonance theory. *Personality and Social Psychology Bulletin, 18,* 591–602.

PART TWO

The Role of the Self in Dissonance

5

Dissonance, Hypocrisy, and the Self-Concept

Elliot Aronson

This chapter focuses primarily on the relationship between cognitive dissonance and the self-concept. At the outset, however, note that when Leon Festinger invented the theory of cognitive dissonance, he conceived of dissonance arousal and reduction as a much more universal phenomenon—not as tied to a person's self-concept. Accordingly, before getting to the heart of this chapter, I trace the evolution of the theory from its exciting universalistic beginnings, in 1957, when it revolutionized the way social psychologists think about human behavior, through its "doldrums" period (roughly, 1975–1990), when it was largely ignored by most researchers, to its reemergence in the 1990s as a powerful means of predicting and changing human behavior in a variety of areas, including those that have abiding societal importance (such as condom use and water conservation).

Because dissonance theory arrived on the social psychological scene at virtually the same moment I started graduate school, my involvement with the theory is a personal one as well as an intellectual one. Accordingly, it might be useful to tell the story of the dissonance "revolution" through my own rather fortuitous experience with the theory —almost from its inception.

As a 1st-year graduate student at Stanford, in 1956, I had very little interest in social psychology, and what little I knew about that discipline seemed both boring and pedestrian. Central to social psychology was the issue of social influence, which is certainly an important topic, but in the mid-1950s, the existing knowledge of social influence seemed fairly cut and dried and rather obvious. What did social psychologists know for sure about social influence at that time?

1. If you want people to go along with your position, offer tangible rewards for compliance and clear punishments for noncompliance.
2. Present an audience with a reasonable communication, attributing it to a highly credible communicator.
3. Present the individual with the illusion that everyone else in sight agrees with one another.
4. If a member of your discussion group disagrees with you, you will send him more messages (in attempt to get him to see the light) than if he agrees with you. If he persists in being stubborn, you will try to eject him from the group.

In those days, the overwhelming trend in all of American empirical psychology was "Let's find the reinforcer." If a person (or a rat) does something, there must be a reason, and that reason has to be the gaining of an identifiable reward, such as food, money, or praise, or the removing of a noxious state of affairs, such as pain, fear, or anxiety. If food will induce a hungry rat to press the lever of a Skinner box or turn left in a Y maze, surely conceptually similar rewards can induce a person to adopt a given opinion. The classic experiment that seemed to epitomize experimental social psychology in the mid-1950s was the still-classic Asch (1951) experiment, in which a unanimous majority apparently disagreed with an individual on a simple, unambiguous perceptual judgment. Why do most people conform to this kind of group pressure? Perhaps it makes them anxious to be alone against a unanimous majority; they fear being considered crazy, being held in low esteem, and so on. It's comforting to be in agreement with others. That's the reward for conformity.

Or take the equally classic experiment done by Hovland and Weiss (1951). Why do people tend to believe a statement attributed to a credible source (such as Oppenheimer) rather than a noncredible one (such as Pravda)? Perhaps it increases the probability of being right, and being right reduces anxiety and makes one feel good, smart, and esteemed. That is the reward for changing one's belief.

These data are true enough, but hardly worth getting excited about. My old bobbeh (grandmother), a fountainhead of folk wisdom, could have told me those things without having done an elaborate experiment to demonstrate the obvious. Then, in 1957, Leon Festinger invented the theory of cognitive dissonance, deftly combining cognition and motivation, and produced a revolution that revitalized social psychology and changed it forever. I first read Festinger's book in the form of a pre-publication carbon copy that he thrust into my hands (rather disdainfully!) after I told him I was trying to decide whether to enroll in his graduate seminar. Reading that manuscript was something of an epiphany for me. It was (and still is) the single most exciting book I have ever read in all of psychology.

The core proposition of the theory is a very simple one: If a person were to hold two cognitions that were psychologically inconsistent, she or he would experience dissonance. Because dissonance is an unpleasant drive state (like hunger, thirst, or pain), the person will attempt to reduce it—much like she or he would try to reduce hunger, thirst, or pain. Viewed more broadly, cognitive dissonance theory is essentially a theory about sense making: how people try to make sense out of their environment and their behavior and, thus, try to lead lives that are (at least in their own mind) sensible and meaningful.

As I implied above, one of the theory's most important aspects was in the challenge it presented to the long-standing dominance of reinforcement theory as an all-purpose explanation for social psychological phenomena. To illustrate this challenge (as well as its importance), I put forth the following scenario: A young man performs a monotonous, tedious task as part of an industrial relations experiment. After completing it, he is informed that his participation as a participant is over. The experimenter then appeals to him for help. He states that his research assistant was unable to be there and asks the participant if he would help run the experiment. The experimenter explains that he is investigating the effect of people's preconceptions about their performance of a task; specifically, he wants to see if a person's performance is influenced by whether he or she is told either positive things about the task (in advance), negative things about the task (in advance), or nothing at all about the task. The next participant, who is about to arrive, is assigned to be in the favorable-information condition. The experimenter asks the participant if he would tell the incoming participant that he had just completed the task (which is true) and that he found it to be an exceedingly enjoyable one (which is not true, according to the participant's own experience). The participant is offered either $1 or $20 for telling this lie and for remaining on call in case the regular assistant cannot show up in the future.

The astute reader will recognize this as the scenario of the classic experiment by Festinger and Carlsmith (1959). I regard this experiment, because of the enormous impact it had on the field, as the single most important study ever done in social psychology. The results were striking. The participants who said that they found the task enjoyable to earn the paltry payment of $1 came to believe that it actually was enjoyable to a far greater extent than those who said it to earn the princely payment of $20. The experiment was a direct derivation from the theory of cognitive dissonance. Needless to say, reinforcement theory would suggest that if you reward individuals for saying something, they might become infatuated with that statement (through secondary reinforcement). But dissonance theory makes precisely the opposite prediction. If I were a participant in the Festinger–Carlsmith experiment, my cognition that the task I performed was boring would be dissonant with the fact that I informed another person that it was enjoyable. If I were paid $20 for making that statement, this cognition would provide ample external justification for my action, thus reducing the dissonance. However, if I were paid only $1, I would lack sufficient external justification for having made the statement (I would be experiencing the discomfort of dissonance) and would be motivated to reduce it. In this situation, the most convenient way to reduce dissonance would be for me to try to convince myself that the task was somewhat more inter-esting than it seemed at first. In effect, in the process of persuading myself that the task was actually interesting, I would convince myself that my statement to the other student was not a great lie.

Similarly, in another early experiment aimed at testing dissonance theory, Aronson and Mills (1959) demonstrated that people who go through a severe initiation, to gain admission to a group, come to like that group better than people who go through a mild initiation to get into the same group. Reinforcement theory would suggest that we like people and groups that are associated with reward; dissonance theory led Aronson and Mills to the prediction that we come to like things for which we suffer. All cognitions having to do with the negative aspects of the group are dissonant with the cognition that we suffered to be admitted to the group; therefore, they get distorted in a positive direc-tion, effectively reducing the dissonance.

Even in the early years, it was crystal clear that dissonance-generated attitude change was not limited to such trivial judgments as the dullness of a boring task or the attractiveness of a discussion group. The early researchers extended the theory to much more important opinions and attitudes, such as a striking reassessment of the dangers of smoking marijuana among students at the University of Texas (Nel, Helmreich, & Aronson, 1969), and the softening of Yale students' negative attitudes toward the alleged antistudent brutality of the New Haven police (Cohen, 1962).

IMPACT ON THE FIELD

It is hard to convey the impact these early experiments had on the social psychological community at the time of their publication. The findings startled a great many social psychologists largely because they challenged the general orientation accepted either tacitly or explicitly by the field. These results also generated enthusiasm among most social psychologists because, at the time, they represented a striking and con-vincing act of liberation from the dominance of a general reward–reinforcement theory. The findings of these early experiments demonstrated dramatically that at least under certain conditions, reward the-ory was inadequate. In doing so, dissonance research sounded a clarion call to cognitively oriented social psychologists, proclaiming in the most striking manner that human beings think, they do not always behave in a mechanistic manner. It demonstrated that human beings engage in all kinds of cognitive gymnastics aimed at justifying their own be-havior.

Perhaps most important, dissonance theory inspired an enormous number and variety of hypotheses that were specific to the theory and could be tested in the laboratory. The wide array of research that dis-sonance theory has produced is truly astonishing. Dissonance research runs the gamut from decision making to color preferences, from the socialization of children to curing people's snake phobias, from inter-personal attraction to antecedents of hunger and thirst, from the pros-elytizing behavior of religious zealots to the behavior of gamblers at racetracks, from inducing people to conserve water by taking showers to selective informational exposure, from helping people curb their temptation to cheat at a game of cards to inducing people to practice safer sex.

The impact of dissonance theory went even beyond the generation of new and exciting knowledge. Given the nature of the hypotheses we were testing, dissonance researchers were forced to develop a new ex-perimental methodology—a powerful, high-impact set of procedures that allowed us to ask truly important questions in a very precise man-ner. As we all know, the laboratory tends to be an artificial environment. But dissonance research made it necessary to overcome that artificiality by developing a methodology that would enmesh participants in a set of events—a drama, if you will—which made it impossible for them to avoid taking these events seriously.

In my writing on research methods (Aronson & Carlsmith, 1968; Aronson, Ellsworth, Carlsmith, & Gonzales, 1990) I have referred to this strategy as establishing *experimental reality* where, within the ad-mittedly phony confines of the lab, the experimenter makes certain that real things are happening to real people. Because of the nature of our hypotheses, we could not afford the luxury, so common in contemporary research, of having participants passively look at a videotape of events happening to someone else and then make judgments about them. Rather, our research questions required the construction of an elaborate scenario in which participants became immersed. Thus, what dissonance research brought into focus more clearly than any other body of work is the fact that the social psychological laboratory, with all of its contrivances and complex scenarios, can produce clear, powerful effects that are conceptually replicable in both the laboratory and the real world.

DISSONANCE AND THE SELF: THE POWER OF SELF-PERSUASION

Research has shown that the persuasive effects in the experiments discussed previously are more powerful and more persistent than those resulting from persuasion techniques based on rewards, punishments, or source credibility (see, e.g., Freedman, 1965). The major reason is that the arousal of dissonance always entails relatively high levels of personal involvement and, therefore, the reduction of dissonance requires some form of self-justification. From the very outset, some of us who were working closely with the theory felt that at its core it led to clear and unambiguous predictions, but around the edges it was a little too vague. Several situations arose in which it was not entirely clear what dissonance theory would predict or, indeed, whether dissonance theory even made a prediction. Around 1958, the standing joke among Festinger's research assistants was, "If you really want to be sure whether *A* is dissonant with *B*, ask Leon!" Although this was said with our tongues firmly planted in our cheeks, it reflected the fact that we argued a lot about whether dissonance theory applied in a wide variety of situations.

What comes to mind most specifically are two strenuous running arguments that Festinger and I had about two of his classic examples. The first involved a person stepping outside in a rainstorm and not getting wet. Festinger was convinced that this would arouse a great deal of dissonance, whereas I had considerable difficulty seeing it. My disagreement went something like this: "What's that got to do with *him*? It's a strange phenomenon, all right, but unless he feared he was losing his mind, I don't see the dissonance."

The second was Festinger's classic example of a situation in which dissonance theory did not apply. This was the case of a man driving, late at night, on a lonely country road and getting a flat tire (Festinger, 1957, pp. 277–278). Lo and behold, when he opened the trunk of his car, he discovered he did not have a jack. Leon maintained that although the person would experience frustration, disappointment, and perhaps even fear, there were no dissonant cognitions in that situation. My argument was succinct: "Of course there is dissonance! What kind of idiot would go driving late at night on a lonely country road without a jack in his car?" "But," Leon countered, "where are the dissonant cognitions?"

It took me a couple of years, but it gradually dawned on me that what was at the heart of my argument in both of those situations was the self-concept. That is, when I said above that dissonance theory made clear predictions at its core, what I implicitly meant by *at its core* were situations in which the person's self-concept was at issue. Thus, in the raindrop situation, as far as I could judge, the self was not involved. In the flat tire situation, the self-concept was involved; what was dissonant was (a) the driver's cognition about his idiotic behavior with (b) his self-concept of being a reasonably smart guy. Accordingly, I wrote a monograph (Aronson, 1960), in which I argued that dissonance theory makes its strongest predictions when an important element of the self-concept is threatened, typically when a person performs a behavior that is inconsistent with his or her sense of self. Initially, I intended this not to be a major modification of the theory, but only an attempt to tighten the predictions a bit. That is, in my opinion, this tightening retained the core notion of inconsistency but shifted the emphasis to the self-concept—thus, clarifying more precisely when the theory did or did not apply. I believe that this apparently minor modification of dissonance theory turned out to have important ramifications inasmuch as it increased the predictive power of the theory without seriously limiting its scope.

In addition, this modification uncovered a hidden assumption contained in the original theory. Festinger's original statement and all of the early experiments rested on the implicit assumption that people have a reasonably positive self-concept. But if a person considered himself or herself to be a "schnook," he or she might expect to do schnooky things—like go through a severe initiation to get into a group or say things that he or she didn't quite believe. For such people, dissonance would not be aroused under the same conditions as for people with a favorable view of themselves. Rather, dissonance would occur when negative self-expectancies were violated, that is, when the person with a poor self-concept engaged in a behavior that reflected positively on the self.

To test this assumption, Merrill Carlsmith and I conducted a simple little experiment that demonstrated that under certain conditions, college students would be made uncomfortable with success; that they would prefer to be accurate in predicting their own behavior, even if it meant setting themselves up for failure. Specifically, we found that students who had developed negative self-expectancies regarding their performance on a task showed evidence of dissonance arousal when faced with success on that task. That is, after repeated failure at the task, participants who later achieved a successful performance actually changed their responses from accurate to inaccurate ones, to preserve a consistent, though negative, self-concept (Aronson & Carlsmith, 1962). (In recent years, Swann and his students have confirmed this basic finding in a number of experiments and quasi-experiments; Swann, 1984, 1991, 1996; Swann & Pelham, 1988; Swann & Read, 1981).

A few years later, I carried this reasoning a step further (Aronson, 1968; Aronson, Chase, Helmreich, & Ruhnke, 1974), elaborating on the centrality of the self-concept in dissonance processes and suggesting that in this regard, people generally strive to maintain a sense of self that is both consistent and positive. That is, because most people have relatively favorable views of themselves, they want to see themselves as (a) competent, (b) moral, and (c) able to predict their own behavior.

In summary, efforts to reduce dissonance involve a process of self-justification because, in most instances, people experience dissonance after engaging in an action that leaves them feeling stupid, immoral, or confused (see Aronson et al., 1974). Moreover, the greater the personal commitment or self-involvement implied by the action and the smaller the external justification for that action, the greater the dissonance and, therefore, the more powerful the need for self-justification. Thus, in the Festinger–Carlsmith experiment, the act of deceiving another person would make one feel immoral or guilty. To reduce that dissonance, one must convince oneself that little or no deception was involved, in other words, that the task was, in fact, a rather interesting activity. By justifying one's actions in this fashion, one is able to restore a sense of self as morally good. In the Aronson and Mills experiment, going through hell and high water to gain admission to a boring discussion group was dissonant with one's self-concept as a smart and reasonable person, who makes smart and reasonable decisions.

SCOPE VERSUS TIGHTNESS IN THEORY BUILDING

All theories are lies. That is, all theories are only approximations of the empirical domain they are trying to describe. Accordingly, it is inevitable that theories will evolve and change to accommodate new data that are being generated. Indeed, it is the duty of theorists to modify their theory in the face of new data and new ideas. Festinger understood this better than most theorists. At the same time, understandably, he was deeply enamored of both the elegant simplicity and the breadth of his original theoretical statement. When I first came out with the self-concept notion of dissonance, Festinger was not pleased. He felt that although my revision had led to some interesting research, conceptually, I was limiting the scope of the theory far too much. I agreed that the scope was a bit smaller, but I believed that the increased accuracy of prediction (the added tightness) was worth the slightly more limited scope. In 1987, while serving as a discussant at the American Psychological Association symposium on cognitive dissonance, Festinger acknowledged the dilemma of the theorist who has a hard time seeing his theory change yet knows that change it must. (One might say that this is a situation bound to produce considerable dissonance in the theorist!). In typical fashion, Leon poked fun at himself for trying to cling to the original conceptualization even though he knew better (see Appendix B, this volume, for the complete transcript of this talk):

> No theory is going to be inviolate. Let me put it clearly. The only kind of theory that can be proposed and ever will be proposed that absolutely will remain inviolate for decades, certainly centuries, is a theory that is not testable. If a theory is at all testable, it will not remain unchanged. It has to change. All theories are wrong. One doesn't ask about theories, can I show that they are wrong or can I show that they are right, but rather one asks, how much of the empirical realm can it handle and how must it be modified and changed as it matures?
>
> As a lot of people know, I ended up leaving social psychology, meaning dissonance theory, and I want to clarify that. Lack of activity is not the same as lack of interest. Lack of activity is not desertion. I left and stopped doing research on the theory of dissonance because I was in a total rut. The only thing I could think about was how correct the original statement had been ... how every word in that book was perfect. So to me, I did a good thing for cognitive dissonance by leaving it. I think if I had stayed in it, I might have retarded progress for cognitive dissonance for at least a decade. (pp. 382–383)

In theory building, there is always a tension between scope and precision; generally speaking, one usually gains precision at the price of scope. The self-concept notion strikes a pretty good balance between scope and precision. My guess is that sooner or later, someone will come along with a richer conceptualization that will strike a better balance. When that happens, I hope I will have the good grace to applaud.

THE SELF-CONCEPT AND THE INDUCTION OF HYPOCRISY

In recent years, the self-concept notion of dissonance has led us into areas of investigation that would not have been feasible under the rubric of Festinger's initial formulation. One of these involves the induction of feelings of hypocrisy. This discovery came about quite by accident. At the time, I was not even thinking about theory development but was struggling to find an effective way to convince sexually active college students to use condoms in this, the era of AIDS. The problem is not an easy one to solve, because it transcends the simple conveying of information to rational people. College students already have the requisite information, that is, virtually all sexually active college students know that condoms are an effective way to prevent AIDS. The problem is that the vast majority are not using condoms, because they consider them to be a nuisance, unromantic, and unspontaneous. In my research, I had run into a stone wall; I had tried several of the traditional, direct persuasive techniques (powerful videos, aimed at arousing fear or at eroticizing the condom) with very limited success. Whatever impact my videos did have was of very short duration; our participants would try condoms once or twice and then stop using them.

Eventually, I thought about using the counterattitudinal attitude paradigm. That is, why not try to get people to argue against their own attitudes, as in the Festinger–Carlsmith (1959) experiment? On the surface, it seemed like a great idea. After all, we had found that this strategy was powerful and, when judiciously applied, had long-term effects on attitudes and behavior—precisely what was needed in this societal situation. But wait a minute: In the condom use situation, there were no counterattitudinal attitudes to address. That is, our surveys and interviews had demonstrated that sexually active young adults already were in favor of people using condoms to prevent AIDS. They simply weren't using them. They seemed to be in a state of denial: denying that the dangers of unprotected sex applied to them in the same way they applied to everyone else. How could we invoke the counterattitudinal attitude paradigm if there was no counterattitude to invoke?

It occurred to me that the solution had to come from the self-concept, because being in denial is not an attractive thing to be doing. The challenge was to find a way to place the person in a situation where the act of denial would be unfeasible because it would conflict, in some way, with his or her positive image of theirselves. And then it struck me. Suppose you are a sexually active college student and, like most, (a) you do not use condoms regularly and (b) being in denial, you have managed to ignore the dangers inherent in having unprotected sex. Suppose, on going home for Christmas vacation, you find that Charlie, your 16-year-old brother has just discovered sex and is in the process of boasting to you about his many and varied sexual encounters. What do you say to him? Chances are, as a caring, responsible older sibling, you will dampen his enthusiasm a bit by warning him about the dangers of AIDS and other sexually transmitted diseases and urge him to, at least, take proper precautions by using condoms.

Suppose that I am a friend of the family who was invited to dinner and who happened to overhear this exchange between you and your brother. What if I were to pull you aside and say, "That was very good advice you gave Charlie. I am very proud of you for being so responsible. By the way, how frequently do you use condoms?" In other words, by getting you to think about that, I am confronting you with your own hypocrisy. According to the self-concept version of the theory, this would produce dissonance because you are not practicing what you are preaching. That is, for most people, their self-concept does not include behaving like a hypocrite.

My students and I then proceeded to design and conduct a simple little experiment following the scenario outlined above (Aronson, Fried, & Stone, 1991). In a 2 × 2 factorial design, in one condition, college students were induced to make a videotape in which they urged their audience to use condoms; they were told that the video would be shown to high school students. In the other major condition, the college students simply rehearsed the arguments without making the video. Cutting across these conditions was the "mindfulness" manipulation: In one set of conditions, our participants were made mindful of the fact that they themselves were not practicing what they were preaching. To accomplish this, we asked them to think about all those situations where they found it particularly difficult or impossible to use condoms in the recent past. In the other set of conditions, we did nothing to make the students mindful of their past failures to use condoms.

The one cell we expected to produce dissonance was the one high in hypocrisy, that is, where participants made the video and were given the opportunity to dredge up memories of situations where they failed to use condoms. Again, how did we expect them to reduce dissonance? By increasing the strength of their intention to use condoms in the future. And that is precisely what we got. Those participants who were in the high-dissonance (hypocrisy) condition showed the greatest intention to increase their use of condoms. Moreover, 2 months later, there was a tendency for the participants in the high-dissonance cell to report using condoms a higher percentage of the time than in any of the other three cells.

In a follow-up experiment (Stone, Aronson, Crain, Winslow, & Fried, 1994), we strengthened the manipulations of the initial experiment and used a "behavioroid" measure of the dependent variable. Specifically, in each of the conditions described above, participants were subsequently provided with an opportunity to purchase condoms at a very substantial discount (10¢ each). The results were unequivocally as predicted. Fully 83% of the participants in the hypocrisy condition purchased condoms; this was a significantly greater percentage than in each of the other three conditions, none of which were reliably different from each other. The effect was a powerful and long-lasting one: Three months after the induction of hypocrisy, a telephone survey indicated that 92% of the participants in the hypocrisy condition were still using condoms regularly, a figure that was significantly different from the control conditions.

Subsequently, we increased our confidence in the efficacy of the induction-of-hypocrisy paradigm by testing the paradigm in a different situation, one in which we could get a direct behavioral measure of the dependent variable. We found one in the shower room of our campus field house. As you may know, central California has a chronic water shortage. On our campus, the administration is constantly trying to find ways to induce students to conserve water. So we decided to test our hypothesis by using dissonance theory and the induction of hypocrisy to convince students to take shorter showers. What we discovered was that although it is impossible, within the bounds of propriety, to follow people into their bedrooms and observe their condom-using behavior, it was easily possible to follow people into the shower rooms and observe their shower-taking behavior.

In this experiment (Dickerson, Thibodeau, Aronson, & Miller, 1992), we went to the university field house and intercepted college women who had just finished swimming in a highly chlorinated pool and were on their way to take a shower. Just like in the condom experiment, it was a 2 × 2 design, in which we varied commitment and mindfulness. In the commitment conditions, each student was asked if she would be willing to sign a flyer encouraging people to conserve water at the field house. The students were told that the flyers would be displayed on posters, and each was shown a sample poster: a large, colorful, very public display. The flyer read: "Take shorter showers. Turn off water while soaping up. If I can do it, so can you!" After the student signed the flyer, we thanked her for her time, and she proceeded to the shower room, where our undergraduate research assistant (unaware of condition) was unobtrusively waiting (with hidden waterproof stopwatch) to time the student's shower. In the mindful conditions, we also asked the students to respond to a water conservation survey, which consisted of items designed to make them aware of their proconservation attitudes and the fact that their typical showering behavior was sometimes wasteful.

The results are consistent with those in the condom experiment: We found dissonance effects only in the cell where the participants were preaching what they were not always practicing. That is, in the condition where the students were induced to advocate short showers and were made mindful of their own past behavior, they took very short showers. To be specific, in the high-dissonance cell, the length of the average shower (which, because of the chlorine in the swimming pool, included a shampoo and cream rinse) averaged just over $3\frac{1}{2}$ min (that's short!) and was significantly shorter than in the control condition.

How can we be certain that dissonance is involved in these experiments? Although the data are consistent with the self-concept formulation of dissonance theory, there is another plausible interpretation. It is conceivable that the effects of the hypocrisy manipulation may have been due to the effects of priming. The combination of proattitudinal advocacy and the salience of past behavior may have served, in an additive fashion, to make participants' positive attitudes toward condom use or water conservation highly accessible, thus fostering a stronger correspondence between their attitudes and behavior (e.g., Fazio, 1989). What is needed to pin it down is evidence that the hypocrisy effect involves physiological arousal, thereby indicating the presence of dissonance rather than the mere influence of attitude salience.

An experiment by Fried and Aronson (1995) provides exactly this sort of evidence. Within the context of the hypocrisy paradigm, this experiment used a misattribution-of-arousal manipulation, a strategy brilliantly developed in earlier research to document the existence of dissonance as an uncomfortable state of arousal by Zanna and Cooper (1974). Zanna and Cooper found that when participants were given an opportunity to misattribute their arousal to a source other than their dissonance-arousing behavior—for example, to an overheated room, a placebo, or glaring florescent lights—the attitude change typically associated with dissonance reduction no longer occurs.

Using a modified version of the earlier condom experiments, Fried and Aronson's (1995) study required participants to compose and deliver proattitudinal, videotaped speeches advocating the importance of recycling. These speeches were ostensibly to be shown to various groups as part of a campaign to increase participation in recycling programs on campus and in the larger community. Hypocrisy was induced in half the participants by asking them to list recent examples of times when they had failed to recycle; the other half simply wrote and delivered the speech, without being reminded of their wasteful behavior. In addition, half the participants in each condition were given an opportunity to misattribute arousal to various environmental factors within the laboratory setting. Specifically, participants were asked to answer questions regarding the room's lighting, temperature, and noise level, including how these ambient factors might have affected them. (This was accomplished under the guise of asking participants to rate the room's suitability for use as laboratory space—a request that was made to appear unrelated to the activities in which participants were participating.) To summarize, proattitudinal advocacy was held constant, and the salience of past behavior and the opportunity for misattribution were manipulated, yielding a 2 × 2 factorial design with the following conditions: (a) hypocrisy (high salience), (b) hypocrisy with misattribution, (c) no hypocrisy (low salience), (d) no hypocrisy with misattribution. Dissonance reduction was measured by asking participants to volunteer to help a local recycling organization by making phone calls soliciting support for recycling.

The results of this experiment revealed that arousal was indeed present within the hypocrisy conditions. Hypocrisy participants who were not afforded the opportunity to misattribute the source of their arousal volunteered significantly more often, and for longer blocks of time, than participants in the other experimental conditions. Moreover, volunteer behavior for hypocrisy participants who were allowed to misattribute their arousal was no greater than for participants who were not exposed to the hypocrisy manipulation.

HYPOCRISY: DISSONANCE IN THE ABSENCE OF AVERSIVE CONSEQUENCES

As I stated above, the initial reason for the development of the hypocrisy paradigm was couched in my attempt to apply dissonance theory to the solution of a societal problem. The hidden bonus was that it also shed some light on an interesting theoretical controversy among dissonance theorists. I should say at the outset that dissonance research tends to be a family business; thus, the controversies are invariably friendly arguments, around the dinner table as it were. One such controversy involves the new look theory, developed several years ago by Cooper and Fazio (1984). In examining the early forced-compliance experiments, such as the Festinger–Carlsmith (1959) experiment and the Nel et al. (1969) experiment, Cooper and Fazio made an interesting discovery: In these experiments, participants not only experienced cognitive dissonance but also inflicted aversive consequences on the recipient of their communication; that is, lying to another person is presumed to have aversive consequences to that person. Their next step was a bold one: Cooper and Fazio asserted that dissonance was not due to inconsistent cognitions at all, but, rather, was aroused only when a person felt personally responsible for bringing about an aversive or unwanted event. Or, to put it in my terms, dissonance was caused solely by the person's doing harm to another person, which was a threat to the person's self-concept as a morally good human being.

Although I always appreciated the boldness implicit in Cooper and Fazio's (1984) theorizing, I could never bring myself to buy into the notion that aversive consequences are essential for the existence of dissonance. Moreover, in terms of my earlier discussion of scope versus tightness, it seems to me that Cooper and Fazio's conception is limiting the scope of the theory enormously while gaining nothing in tightness that wasn't already present in the self-concept notion.

How would one test this difference empirically? Several years ago, I was at a loss as to how to produce inconsistency in the Festinger and Carlsmith (1959) type of experiment without also producing aversive consequences for the recipient of one's message. That is, if you are misleading another person, by telling her or him something you believe is false, then you are always bringing about aversive consequences. But without quite realizing it, my students and I seem to have stumbled onto the solution with the hypocrisy experiments. In this procedure, the participants are preaching what they are not practicing (and are therefore experiencing dissonance), but where are the aversive consequences for the audience in the condom experiment? There are none. Indeed, to the extent that the "hypocrites" succeed in being persuasive, far from producing aversive consequences for the recipients, they may well be saving their lives. And still, it is clear from the data that our participants were experiencing dissonance. For a fuller discussion of this theoretical controversy, see Thibodeau and Aronson (1992).

SELF-JUSTIFICATION AND SELF-ESTEEM—SOME UNSUBSTANTIATED SPECULATIONS

From the very beginning, I found dissonance theory to be a powerful explanation for a wide swath of human behavior. The scientist in me was always delighted by the exciting, nonobvious predictions generated by the theory, as well as the creative experimentation used to test these predictions. But at the same time, the humanist in me was always a bit troubled by the rather bleak, rather unappetizing picture the theory painted of the human condition—forever striving to justify our actions after the fact. Over the past few years, my reasoning about dissonance and the self-concept has led me to speculate about how a person's self-esteem might interact with the experiencing and reduction of dissonance. These speculations might suggest a more complete picture of human nature. Note two intriguing experiments in the dissonance literature. First, consider an experiment I did a great many years ago with David Mettee (Aronson & Mettee, 1968), in which we demonstrated that if we temporarily raised a person's self-esteem, it would serve to insulate him or her from performing an immoral act such as cheating. We found that the higher self-esteem served to make the anticipation of doing something immoral more dissonant than it would have been otherwise. Thus, when our participants were put in a situation in which they had an opportunity to win money by unobtrusively cheating at a game of cards, they were able to say to themselves, in effect, "Wonderful people like me don't cheat!" And they succeeded in resisting the temptation to cheat to a greater extent than those in the control condition.

Now consider an experiment performed by Glass (1964). In this study, people were put in a situation where they were induced to deliver a series of electric shocks to other people. They then had an opportunity to evaluate their victims. Dissonance theory predicts that if individuals are feeling awful about having hurt someone, one way to reduce the dissonance is to convince themselves that their victim is a dreadful person who deserved to suffer the pain of electric shock. What Glass found was that it was precisely those individuals who had the highest self-esteem who derogated their victims the most. Consider the irony: It is precisely because I think I am such a nice person that if I do something that causes you pain, I must convince myself that you are a rat. In other words, because nice guys like me don't go around hurting innocent people, you must have deserved every nasty thing I did to you. On the other hand, if I already consider myself to be something of a scoundrel, then causing others to suffer does not introduce as much dissonance; therefore, I have less of a need to convince myself that you deserved your fate. The ultimate tragedy, of course, is that once I succeed in convincing myself that you are a dreadful person, it lowers my inhibitions against doing you further damage.

Aronson and Mettee (1968) showed that high self-esteem can serve as a buffer against immoral behavior, whereas Glass (1964) showed that once a person commits an immoral action, high self-esteem leads him or her into a situation where he or she might commit further mischief. In pondering these two experiments, I have come to the conclusion that it is far too simplistic to think of self-esteem as a one-dimensional phenomenon—either high or low. My reasoning here is similar to that of Baumeister (1998), Rohan (1996), Kernis, Cornell, Sun, Berry, and Harlow (1993), and Waschull and Kernis (1996). My notion is that self-esteem can be high or low and either fragile or well grounded. *Well grounded* in this context means that a positive self-image has been developed and held during a great deal of past behavior, whereas *fragile* suggests that a positive self-image has never been securely developed. People with high and well-grounded self-esteem need not be concerned with developing or verifying their self-image, and can enter situations with the confident knowledge that they are competent, moral people. On the other hand, people with high and fragile self-esteem, because of their lack of a secure self-image, are overly concerned with trying to preserve images of themselves as being competent and moral at all costs.

Typically, people with high and fragile self-esteem, in their zeal to maintain a belief in their own competence and virtue, often boast about their achievements—trying desperately to convince themselves and others that they are terrific. But their boasting behavior, their misjudgments, their errors, and the wrong turns they make because they are thinking more about themselves than the situation they are in all tend to shatter the fragile image they are trying to defend. As a result, they frequently feel like impostors and are forever trying to prove that they are not. Thus, they are trying to win every possible argument, pushing themselves to believe they are always right, justifying their behavior to themselves at every turn, and explaining away failures and mistakes instead of attending to them long enough to learn from them.

In contrast, people with high and well-grounded self-esteem are not invested in winning arguments for winning's sake, do not need to believe they are always right, do not need to explain away failures and mistakes, and do not need to engage in the almost frantic self-justification in which high and fragile self-esteem people constantly engage. Instead, when they fail or make mistakes, people with high and well-grounded self-esteem can look at their failures and mistakes and learn from them. For example, a person with high, well-grounded self-esteem can look at his or her errors and say, in effect, "I screwed up. I did a stupid (or hurtful or immoral) thing. But just because I did a stupid (or hurtful or im-moral) thing this time, this doesn't make me a stupid (or hurtful or immoral) person. Let me look at it. How did it come about? How can I make it better? What can I learn from this situation, so that I might decrease the possibility that I'll screw up in a similar way again?"

At this point, I have no idea whether the fragile and well-grounded dimension of self-esteem is normally distributed. If I were to hazard a guess, I would speculate that high, well-grounded self-esteem is not a common thing; accordingly, my guess is that the majority of people who score high on general measures of self-esteem would cluster near the fragile end of the continuum. If this were true, it would certainly account for the behavior of Glass's (1964) high-self-esteem participants who did not hesitate to derogate their victim. In contrast, people with high, well-grounded self-esteem would not use derogation of the victim as a way to reduce their dissonance; rather, they would be more likely to take responsibility for their actions and try, in some way, to make amends for their cruel behavior.

This strikes me as an important area of inquiry. Again, these are mere speculations; I have no data to confirm them. Somehow, it seems reasonable to end this chapter with unsubstantiated speculation be-cause, for me, it has always been the interesting loose ends that make science such an exciting enterprise.

REFERENCES

Aronson, E. (1960). *The cognitive and behavioral consequences of the confirmation and disconfirmation of expectancies.* Grant proposal, Harvard University.

Aronson, E. (1968). Dissonance theory: Progress and problems. In R. P. Abelson, E. Aronson, W. J. Mcguire, T. M. Newcomb, M. J. Rosenberg, & P. H. Tannenbaum (Eds.), *Theories of cognitive consistency: A sourcebook.* Chicago: Rand McNally.

Aronson, E., & Carlsmith, J. M. (1962). Performance expectancy as a determinant of actual performance. *Journal of Abnormal and Social Psychology, 65,* 178–182.

Aronson, E., & Carlsmith, J. M. (1968). Experimentation in social psychology. In G. Lindzey & E. Aronson (Eds.), *The handbook of social psychology* (2nd ed., Vol. 2, pp. 1–79). Reading, MA: Addison-Wesley.

Aronson, E., Chase, T., Helmreich, R., & Ruhnke, R. (1974). A two-factor theory of dissonance reduction: The effect of feeling stupid or feeling awful on opinion change. *International Journal for Research and Communication, 3,* 59–74.

Aronson, E., Ellsworth, P., Carlsmith, J. M., & Gonzales, M. H. (1990). *Methods of research in social psychology.* New York: McGraw Hill.

Aronson, E., Fried, C., & Stone, J. (1991). Overcoming denial and increasing the intention to use condoms through the induction of hypocrisy. *American Journal of Public Health, 81,* 1636–1638.

Aronson, E., & Mettee, D. (1968). Dishonest behavior as a function of differential levels of induced self-esteem. *Journal of Personality and Social Psychology, 9,* 121–127.

Aronson, E., & Mills, J. (1959). The effect of severity of initiation on liking for a group. *Journal of Abnormal and Social Psychology, 59,* 177–181.

Asch, S. E. (1951). Effects of group pressure upon the modification and distortion of judgments. In H. Guetzkow (Ed.), *Groups, leadership and men* (pp. 177–190). Pittsburgh, PA: Carnegie Press.

Baumeister, R. F. (1998). The self. In D. Gilbert, S. Fiske, & G. Lindzey, (Eds.), *The handbook of social psychology* (4th ed., pp. 680–740). Boston: McGraw-Hill.

Cohen, A. R. (1962). An experiment on small rewards for discrepant compliance and attitude change. In J. W. Brehm & A. R. Cohen (Eds.), *Explorations in cognitive dissonance*, (pp. 73–78). New York: Wiley.

Cooper, J., & Fazio, R. H. (1984). A new look at dissonance theory. In L. Berkowitz (Ed.), *Advances in experimental social psychology* (Vol. 17, pp. 229–266). Orlando, FL: Academic Press.

Dickerson, C., Thibodeau, R., Aronson, E., & Miller, D. (1992). Using cognitive dissonance to encourage water conservation. *Journal of Applied Social Psychology, 22*, 841–854.

Fazio, R. H. (1989). On the power and functionality of attitudes: The role of attitude accessibility. In A. R. Pratkanis, S. J. Breckler, & A. G. Greenwald (Eds.), *Attitude structure and function* (pp. 153–179). Hillsdale, NJ: Erlbaum.

Festinger, L. (1957). *A theory of cognitive dissonance*. Evanston, IL: Row, Peterson.

Festinger, L., & Carlsmith, J. M. (1959). Cognitive consequences of forced compliance. *Journal of Abnormal and Social Psychology, 58*, 203–211.

Freedman, J. (1965). Long-term behavioral effects of cognitive dissonance. *Journal of Experimental Social Psychology, 1*, 145–155.

Fried, C., & Aronson, E. (1995). Hypocrisy, misattribution, and dissonance reduction: A demonstration of dissonance in the absence of aversive consequences. *Personality and Social Psychology Bulletin, 21*, 925–933.

Glass, D. (1964). Changes in liking as a means of reducing cognitive discrepancies between self-esteem and aggression. *Journal of Personality, 32*, 531–549.

Hovland, C. I., & Weiss, W. (1951). The influence of source credibility on communication effectiveness. *Public Opinion Quarterly, 15*, 635–650.

Kernis, M., Cornell, D., Sun, C.-R., Berry, A., & Harlow, T. (1993). There's more to self-esteem than whether it is high or low: The importance of stability of self-esteem. *Journal of Personality and Social Psychology, 65*, 1190–1204.

Nel, E., Helmreich, R., & Aronson, E. (1969). Opinion change in the advocate as a function of the persuasibility of the audience: A clarification of the meaning of dissonance. *Journal of Personality and Social Psychology, 12*, 117–124.

Rohan, M. J. (1996). *The performance-integrity framework: A new solution to an old problem*. Unpublished doctoral dissertation, University of Waterloo, Waterloo, Ontario, Canada.

Stone, J., Aronson, E., Crain, A. L., Winslow, M. P., & Fried, C. B. (1994). Inducing hypocrisy as a means of encouraging young adults to use condoms. *Personality and Social Psychology Bulletin, 20,* 116–128.

Swann, W. B., Jr. (1984). Quest for accuracy in person perception: A matter of pragmatics. *Psychological Review, 91,* 457–477.

Swann, W. B., Jr. (1991). To be adored or to be known? The interplay of self-enhancement and self-verification. In R. M. Sorrentino & E. T. Higgins (Eds.), *Handbook of motivation and cognition.* New York: Guilford Press.

Swann, W. B., Jr. (1996). *Self-traps: The elusive quest for higher self-esteem.* New York: Freeman.

Swann, W. B., Jr., & Pelham, B. W. (1988). *The social construction of identity: Self-verification through friend and intimate selection.* Unpublished manuscript, University of Texas at Austin.

Swann, W. B., Jr., & Read, S. J. (1981). Acquiring self-knowledge: The search for feedback that fits. *Journal of Personality and Social Psychology 41,* 1119–1128.

Thibodeau, R., & Aronson, E. (1992). Taking a closer look: Reasserting the role of the self-concept in dissonance theory. *Personality and Social Psychology Bulletin, 18,* 591–602.

Waschull, S., & Kernis, M. (1996). Level and stability of self-esteem as predictors of children's intrinsic motivation and reasons for anger. *Personality and Social Psychology Bulletin, 22,* 4–13.

Self-Affirmation Theory:
An Update and Appraisal

Joshua Aronson, Geoffrey Cohen, and Paul R. Nail

Because the main propositions of dissonance theory have been
confirmed with sufficient regularity, there is not a great deal
to be gained from further research in this area.

E. E. Jones (1985, p. 57)

U ncharacteristically, time has proven Ned Jones (1985) wrong. Dissonance theory is now 40 years old, and as the content of this volume demonstrates, there is much to be gained from researching dissonance phenomena. Moreover, it is clear that the reports by Jones and others of waning interest in the theory were premature. This volume attests to the considerable research activity that has repopulated the journals with dissonance studies. In a computer search on *PsycINFO*, we found 68 journal articles published between 1991 and 1996 explicitly focusing on dissonance theory, a healthy increase from the 38 articles published between 1985 and 1990.

In this chapter, we discuss *self-affirmation theory* (Steele, 1988), a

---

The writing of this chapter benefited greatly from many delightful conversations with Claude Steele.

theoretical development that we see as a major force in sparking the resurgent interest and progress in the study of dissonance processes. Although it is a broad theory, addressing self-esteem maintenance processes underlying an array of phenomena, a good deal of the published research on self-affirmation theory has sought to provide alternative explanations for dissonance effects. We do not argue that self-affirmation theory is a more correct statement about human thought and action than Festinger's original theory (see Steele, 1988, Steele & Spencer, 1992; Steele, Spencer, & Lynch, 1993) or than other revisions of the theory (e.g., Cooper & Fazio, 1984; Thibodeau & Aronson, 1992). Instead, we hope to show that the self-affirmation perspective is particularly valuable in the way that Festinger's original formulation was valuable—in its simplicity, scope, and richness as a source of new, interesting, and testable hypotheses. In addition to celebrating its progress, we discuss a few of the challenges posed to the theory by recent data on the role of the self-concept in dissonance phenomena.

THE THEORY IN A NUTSHELL

According to self-affirmation theory, thought and action are guided by a strong motivation to maintain an overall self-image of moral and adaptive adequacy. We want to see ourselves as good, capable, and able to predict and control outcomes in areas that matter. Awareness of information that threatens this image motivates us to restore it to a state of integrity. Like dissonance motivation, the self-affirmation drive can be strong or weak, depending on the size of the threat to the self-image. But because the objective is global self-worth and not cognitive consistency, we have tremendous flexibility in satisfying the need to restore a sense of general goodness. Self-worth derives from many resources, the myriad self-conceptions that are hypothesized to constitute a larger self-system. Thus, the larger self can be reaffirmed by thought or action addressed to one or more of these self-resources. So long as the affirming self-conception is important enough, this manner of restoring feelings of self-integrity can obviate the need to resolve the provoking inconsistency or threat, because "it is the war, not the battle, that orients this [self] system" (Steele, 1988, p. 289). For instance, a person does not have to rationalize a regrettable decision at work if his or her global sense of self-worth is secured by being a good parent or community member. Nor do cigarette smokers need to deny the risks of their self-incriminating habit if they can find other ways to bolster the global self, say, by affirming their capacities and worth in the workplace.

On the basis of this logic, Steele and Liu (1983) predicted that people would have no problem tolerating cognitive inconsistency in a forced-compliance paradigm, provided that the experimental procedure gave them the opportunity to affirm some important feature of the self—in this case, a cherished value. Students wrote essays in favor of a large tuition increase at their university. Immediately after writing the essay but before a measure of their attitudes, some participants were reminded of an important aspect of their self-concept by completing an aesthetic-values scale (value-oriented participants). Other participants went through the same procedure, but they were chosen for the study because aesthetic values were unimportant to them (non-value-oriented participants). As predicted, filling out the values scale eliminated dissonance—there was no attitude change in the direction of the essay—but only among value-oriented participants. According to Steele and Liu, these findings support self-affirmation theory over Festinger's (1957) consistency-based explanation because completing the values scale did nothing to reduce attitude–behavior inconsistency, yet the values-oriented participants showed no need to rationalize their behavior. In subsequent studies, "value affirmation" also has been shown to reduce rationalizing in the free-choice paradigm (Steele, Hopp, & Gonzales, [cited in Steele, 1988]).

In more recent work, Steele and his colleagues (Steele, Spencer, & Lynch, 1993) carried the self-affirmation logic a step further, to make an additional prediction about the role of dispositional self-esteem in dissonance processes. People with high self-esteem, they argued, should be less inclined to rationalize in dissonance-inducing situations than people with low self-esteem. Why? Because people with high self-esteem presumably have more internal resources, that is, more favorable self-concepts, with which to affirm away the self-esteem threat inherent in the dissonance-arousing episode. The simple version of this hypothesis was not supported in Steele et al.'s research. That is, people with high self-esteem were no less likely to rationalize in a standard dissonance procedure than people with low self-esteem. But the hypothesis was confirmed if just before the dissonance manipulation, participants' self-concepts were made salient by having them complete a self-esteem measure. In this scenario, only low-self-esteem individuals rationalized, whereas their high-self-esteem counterparts showed no evidence of rationalization. This last finding provides strong support for the resource model of dissonance reduction.

The student of dissonance theory may note that the results of the Steele et al. (1993) study fly in the face of the *self-consistency* reformulation of dissonance (E. Aronson, 1968; chap. 5, this volume). Like self-affirmation theory, the self-consistency model sees dissonance as mediated by the ego and not in a freestanding need for cognitive consistency (see Greenwald & Ronis, 1978, p. 55). However, unlike the self-affirmation model, the self-consistency model still puts the need for consistency at the heart of dissonance. In this view, a given cognition arouses dissonance because it is inconsistent with a self-concept—that is, people experience dissonance because they perceive an inconsistency between a behavior (e.g., writing a counterattitudinal essay) and a valued self-concept (being an honest person; see E. Aronson, chap. 5, this volume, for a complete discussion). Thus, self-affirmation and self-consistency theories make opposite predictions with regard to whether low- or high-self-esteem individuals will be more likely to rationalize a dissonant action. Self-affirmation theory predicts that low-self-esteem individuals will rationalize more, because they have fewer esteem-saving resources with which to counter a threatening inconsistency. By contrast, self-consistency theory predicts that high self-esteem individuals will rationalize more, because their positive self-concept will be more inconsistent with the dissonant act. Thus, the Steele et al. (1993) finding that people with low self-esteem rationalize more than those with high self-esteem is an important theoretical advance—both for dissonance theory and for the study of the role of the self-concept in social cognition.

ANALYSIS: SOME EMERGENT THEORETICAL ISSUES

Do We Need a New Theory?

Notwithstanding the impressive support for self-affirmation theory provided by Steele and his colleagues (e.g., Steele & Liu, 1983; Steele et al. 1993) and others (e.g., Tesser & Cornell, 1991), some dissonance theorists have questioned the need for a new and separate theory to explain the results of self-affirmation studies (e.g., E. Aronson, chap. 5 this volume; Beauvois & Joule, 1996; Simon, Greenberg, & Brehm, 1995; Thibodeau & Aronson, 1992). For example, Thibodeau and Aronson (1992) remind us that one of Festinger's (1957) hypothesized modes of dissonance reduction is adding new, consonant cognitions to the dissonant elements. Presumably these cognitions are postulated to reduce dissonance because the magnitude of dissonance is defined by the ratio of dissonant elements to dissonant plus consonant elements $[D/(D + C)]$. Thibodeau and Aronson asserted that once participants' central values have been affirmed, they have little need for attitude change because affirmation reminds them of valued, self-relevant cognitive elements that are consonant with a positive self-concept. Once these consonant elements are added to the dissonance equation, the magnitude of dissonance is reduced. Thus, the self-affirmation findings, one could argue, can be readily accommodated by the original dissonance formulation.

However, the strong version of this argument is challenged by the results of Steele et al. (1993), which suggest that reminding people of their self-concepts not only alleviates rationalization among high-self-esteem individuals but also tends to exacerbate it among low-self-esteem individuals. Thibodeau and Aronson (1992) have predicted the opposite with regard to low-self-esteem participants. Among these participants, completing the self-esteem scale decreased the magnitude of dissonance by reducing the number of cognitions consonant with a positive self-image. In any event, one strategy to illuminate this theoretical tension is to examine whether an irrelevant esteem threat increases or decreases rationalization in a dissonance paradigm. An increase would support the resources model; a decrease would support the original consistency formulation. To our knowledge, no direct test of this question exists.

In a slightly different vein, Simon et al. (1995) have proposed that self-affirmation interventions may eliminate the need for dissonance reduction not because they restore one's self-image, but because they establish a trivializing frame of reference whereby the relative importance of dissonant elements is reduced. One of Festinger's (1957) proposed methods of dissonance reduction was to decrease the importance of dissonant cognitions. Simon et al. found that reminding participants of a generally important issue (e.g., world hunger) after counterattitudinal behavior eliminated the need for dissonance reduction. This occurred regardless of the issue's personal importance to the participants. This finding contradicts self-affirmation theory because, by definition, an issue cannot be self-affirming unless it is of high personal importance.

Effects of Dispositional Self-Esteem

Another theoretical problem concerns the data discussed regarding the *resources* model and the role of self-esteem. As noted, the self-esteem differences predicted by self-affirmation theory emerge only when steps are taken to remind participants of their resources. When people are made mindful of their resources, the model works. But some recent evidence by Stone and his colleagues (see Stone, chap. 8, this volume) suggests a new twist. This research showed that people with high self-esteem actually rationalize more than people with low self-esteem if the self is brought on-line *after* dissonance has been aroused—in direct opposition to the resources model. When self-focus precedes the dissonance-arousing act, the self-affirmation resources model is supported; when self-focus follows the dissonance manipulation, the self-consistency model holds.

Moreover, some studies have shown that self-affirmation, under certain circumstances, can backfire—that positive feedback can increase rationalization if it focuses attention onto the domain threatened by dissonant behavior (J. Aronson, Blanton, & Cooper, 1995; Blanton, Cooper, Skurnik, & Aronson, 1997). For example, Blanton et al. had college students write dissonant essays arguing against increased university funding to help students with disabilities, a topic designed to impugn the essay writer's self-image as compassionate. After writing the essay, participants received feedback from a bogus personality test they had taken earlier. In one condition of the experiment, the feedback extolled the essay writer's compassion (thus, it was relevant to the uncompassionate essay the participant had written); in the other condition, the feedback praised the participant's creativity (irrelevant feedback). After reading the feedback, participants' attitudes toward the funding issue were assessed. The results showed that relevant affirmations—that is, affirming the writers' compassion after the noncompassionate act— exacerbated dissonance, causing them to change their attitude in the direction of the essay more than participants who received no affirmation. In the irrelevant-feedback condition, there was no such rationalizing attitude change. Clearly, then, there are some constraints on the self-affirmation process; it appears that to reduce dissonance, the affirmation may need to be irrelevant rather than relevant to the dissonance-arousing act.

It is unclear what this research implies for dissonance reduction in the real world, where no one else may be around to focus a person on his or her resources—relevant or irrelevant, before or after the fact. Outside of the laboratory, does high self-esteem lead to less rationalizing? A recent study by Gibbons, Eggleston, and Benthin (1997) suggests not. Gibbons et al. looked at the rationalizations of nonsmokers who fell off the wagon and started smoking again. Contrary to self-affirmation predictions, it was the high-self-esteem relapsers who were most likely to rationalize their renewed habit by denying the risks of smoking. The relapsers with low self-esteem behaved as self-consistency theory would predict: They seemed to accept their failure as befitting their low self-image.

What can be made of the difficulty in making clear predictions about the role of dispositional self-esteem and dissonance or, more specifically, of results suggesting that affirmations sometimes reduce but at other times exacerbate dissonance? What can dissonance theorists conclude about the relative merits of self-affirmation theory and more conventional self-consistency theories? The self-image may at times serve as a standard of conduct, evoking dissonance when behavior fails to meet this standard. And at other times, the self-concept may serve as a resource, replenishing self-worth in the wake of a threat. Various factors (such as the relevance and timing of the affirmation) will influence whether the self functions as a standard or resource.

In support of this argument, one study examined whether people avoid affirmations that are relevant to a dissonance-arousing act (J. Aronson et al., 1995). J Aronson et al. reasoned that relevant affirmations provide a threatening reminder of one's failure to live up to a valued standard of conduct. Accordingly, after behaving in an uncompassionate manner, people were found to eschew personality-test feedback that extolled their compassion. Although such feedback was flattering, it nonetheless was threatening, because it reminded participants that they had violated their usual standards of compassionate behavior and it thus intensified the dissonance induced by their earlier unsympathetic actions.

Thus, positive self-conceptions can function both as resources (as in Steele et al., 1993) and as standards of conduct (as in J. Aronson et al., 1995), depending on the particulars of the situation. As the Stone, Cooper, Galinsky, and Kelly (1997) research demonstrates, the timing of an affirmation, like its relevance, may also be an important determinant of when a self-concept will function as an affirmational resource. There are undoubtedly other factors—such as the severity of the threat presented in the experiment—that must matter a great deal. The effect of self-image motivations on thought and behavior depends on several factors, and neither self-affirmation nor self-consistency offers a complete picture of the complex and manifold ways in which people regulate to their self-concepts. A straightforward calculus of the amount of dissonance from the number of positive self-conceptions may be impossible given the importance of the situation in determining whether a particular self-conception will be a source of pride or shame.

This last point raises a broader critique of dissonance research. Many investigators presume, either explicitly or implicitly, a general, universal, invariant process underlying all cognitive dissonance phenomena. This is a delusion; the form of the process, we believe, will depend on the specifics of the situation. Accordingly, the preconditions for dissonance will vary across contexts; sometimes freely chosen decisions whose outcomes are aversive will be necessary (Cooper & Fazio, 1984), and sometimes they will not be necessary (Thibodeau & E. Aronson, 1992; Harmon-Jones, chap. 4, this volume). There may be situational regularities common to dissonance phenomena, such as the perception of self-threat. But the process that creates this threat, and the strategies people deploy for reducing it, will vary a great deal depending on the nature of the situation. The delusion of a single pristine and precise mental process fuels much research both in the dissonance tradition and in other areas of psychological inquiry. It derives from an implicit assumption in general psychology that there is an abstract central processing unit (CPU) called *mind* and that it is the task of researchers to discern its properties and algorithms with more and more precise laboratory methods (Shweder, 1991). Because the goal is understanding the nature of this disembedded, context-free CPU, researchers assume that they can stick to one paradigm and through systematic variations on this paradigm, they will eventually divine the exact nature of the universal psychological processes—the fundamental laws—underlying psychological phenomena, in this case, cognitive dissonance phenomena. It is assumed that these processes will apply to all situations everywhere. But a great deal of evidence has accumulated suggesting that the nature of the psychological process depends on the content of the situation—a critique made time and again by researchers in cultural psychology (e.g., Shweder, 1991).

SYNTHESIS AND SOME NEW DIRECTIONS

Cognitive dissonance theory was inspiring in part because it encompassed so many different phenomena. It gave a way of understanding and talking about a vast array of human behavior with a relatively simple construct. For example, it could explain patterns of rumor transmission after catastrophes (Festinger, 1957) or the behavior of cultists (Festinger, Reicken, & Schachter, 1956). It helped us understand why people come to love the things they suffer for (E. Aronson & Mills, 1959) and hate the people they inflict suffering on (Glass, 1964). It offered useful techniques for parenting, for example, how to get children to learn to like their vegetables (Brehm, 1959), or how to get them to dislike a forbidden toy (E. Aronson & Carlsmith, 1962). Other topics within dissonance's explanatory purview included defensive projection (Bramel, 1962), consumer behavior (Doob, Carlsmith, Freedman, Landauer, & Tom, 1969), and the treatment of phobias (Cooper, 1980) and obesity (Axsom & Cooper, 1985). In short, it was synthetic rather than analytic. That is, it opened doors to new and unthought-of manifestations of a process rather than cautiously describing the boundary conditions of a theoretical process. Perhaps spurred by theoretical critiques (e.g., Bem, 1967) and the rise of the cognitive approach, dissonance research became more and more analytic and less and less synthetic (Berkowitz & Devine, 1989).

One downside of the analytic approach has been that theory testing tends to limit itself to one or two paradigms, leading to the mistaken idea that a theory largely applies to processes occurring in those paradigms. In the case of dissonance theory, most of the studies conducted after the early 1970s used the *induced-compliance* paradigm, a state of affairs that created the false impression that dissonance theory was mostly about what happened to people's attitudes after being induced to contradict those attitudes by writing an essay that argued against one's true beliefs. For example, Cooper and Fazio's (1984) reformulation of dissonance theory refers exclusively to the studies using the induced-compliance paradigm, focusing on the necessary preconditions for creating sufficient dissonance to induce attitude change (e.g., foreseeable, aversive consequences). Gone was dissonance theory's enormous scope.

Self-affirmation theory has had tremendous value in moving the study of dissonance—or at least dissonance-like—phenomena in the direction of synthesis and in uncovering new areas in which self-image maintenance affects beliefs and behavior. Self-affirmation theory provides a theoretical framework that like Festinger's original theory, captures many disparate phenomena with a single, compelling formulation. Unfettered by the excess baggage that the definition of *dissonance* has picked up in the last four decades and equipped with new methodological techniques derived from the dissonance-as-self-threat perspective, self-affirmation theory is reexamining some old terrain with a fresh perspective. Below, we offer a few examples of recent research derived from the logic of self-affirmation theory. Note that very little if any of the hypotheses could have been derived from the version of dissonance that was predominant when Jones (1985) declared that dissonance had ceased to bear fruit. Note also the return of motivation to phenomena, like prejudice and inferential biases, that for the past few decades have been understood from a primarily cognitive perspective. Self-affirmation theory offers both a conceptual framework and a methodological technique for demonstrating the influence of motivation on cognition and behavior.

Self-Affirmation and Prejudice

Reasoning that people make themselves feel better about themselves by putting down members of socially devalued groups, Fein and Spencer (1997) asked whether affirming people's self-concepts might reduce their tendency to evaluate members of stereotyped groups negatively. Participants in their study evaluated a job candidate who, by manipulating her last name and showing her with or without a Star of David or a Crucifix, was either presented as a member of a negatively stereotyped group (a "Jewish American princess") or was not (an Italian American woman). Despite having identical credentials, the Jewish woman received significantly lower ratings than the Italian American woman when evaluated by participants asked to rate her personality. However, half of Fein and Spencer's particpants were given the opportunity to affirm their self-concepts by writing about an important value (e.g., art, music, or theater). These affirmed participants were not influenced by the stereotype, that is, they did not give negative ratings to the Jewish woman; they saw her as just as nice, honest, and intelligent as when she was portrayed as Italian American. In a subsequent study,

Fein and Spencer (1997) showed that threatening people's self-esteem by giving them negative feedback on a bogus test of intelligence increased their prejudiced reactions to a stereotype target, in this case, a presumably gay man. The negative feedback had no effect on their evaluations of the same person when he was not presented as gay. This work is the first empirical demonstration of the motivational forces underlying prejudice: It suggests that negative stereotypes provide a "cognitively justifiable" means to bolster self-regard.

Self-Affirmation and Health

Drawing from the increased awareness of the link between stress and physical illness, Keough, Garcia, and Steele (1997) reasoned that the net effect of one's daily self-esteem threats could be reduced health. Drawing from the work on self-affirmation theory, they tested this notion by affirming a group of undergraduate students over a period of time and then comparing their health (as measured by a number of self-report instruments) to a control group of unaffirmed students. Specifically, during an academic vacation, affirmed students wrote about their daily experiences and about their feelings about those experiences with regard to a centrally important personal value. The results showed that compared with two other writing control conditions, those who completed the affirmation assignments were physically healthier at the end of the vacation than those who wrote about things that made them feel good or about their friends' activities. This research ruled out other, more conventional explanations (such as mood effects or the importance of positive thoughts) and suggested that it was the unique exercise of integrating daily experiences into a personally important value, rather than simply reflecting on happy events, that improved health.

Biases in Persuasion and Negotiation

People with strong beliefs on a topic tend to cling to their attitudes in the face of ambiguous and even well-reasoned disconfirming information. They tend also to see people who espouse opposing views as misguided. This tendency has typically compelled nonmotivational explanations (e.g., Lord, Ross, & Lepper, 1979). Cohen, Aronson, and

Steele (1997) wondered if part of the reason that people dig in their heels and refuse to change their minds is because it is self-threatening —or dissonant—to do so, because these opinions are self-defining. The hypothesis was straightforward. Partisans of a particular belief (e.g., advocates of the abortion issue or opponents and proponents of capital punishment) would be more open to arguments against their position if they were given an affirmation of an alternative source of identity or self-worth. In a series of studies, this hypothesis was supported. In one study, opponents and proponents of capital punishment were more persuaded by an article impugning their views when, before reading the article, they were given a self-affirmation in the form of positive feedback on their social perceptiveness skills. Self-affirmed partisans also were less likely to dismiss advocates of opposing views as political extremists, and they even became more critical in their evaluation of evidence that confirmed their own preexisting beliefs. In another study, a self-affirmation procedure reduced people's tendency to engage in "reactive devaluation"—the problematic impulse of negotiators to derogate a concession that has been offered relative to one that has been withheld (Atkins, Ward, & Lepper, 1997). Although an extension of self-affirmation theory, this research also begins to resolve classic issues in social psychology regarding the effect of motivational forces on cognitive biases (see also Dunning, Leuenberger, & Sherman, 1995; Kunda, 1987).

Self-Affirmation and the Academic Underperformance of Black Students

The underperformance of Blacks on standardized tests and in school has been explained in terms ranging from the *sociological disadvantage* (Bereiter & Engleman, 1966) to *genetic differences* in intelligence (e.g., Benbow & Stanley, 1980; Herrnstein & Murray, 1994; Jensen, 1969). Noting the insufficiency of these explanations, Steele and his colleagues, (J. Aronson, Quinn, & Spencer, 1997; Spencer, Steele, & Quinn, 1997; Steele, 1997; Steele & Aronson, 1995) drew on self-affirmation logic to offer a new explanation. They hypothesized that being the target of a negative stereotype (e.g., "Black people are unintelligent") in a situation where that stereotype is relevant (e.g., taking a test of intelligence) functioned as a self-threat, with some of the same arousal properties. They further reasoned that the underperformance of Blacks (and of women in mathematics) might be due in part to the extra test anxiety brought on by this sense of "stereotype threat." In one series of studies testing this reasoning (Steele & Aronson, 1995), Black and White college students were given a difficult standardized test (the Verbal Ability subscale of the Graduate Record Examinations) under conditions designed to either eliminate or exacerbate this stereotype threat. When stereotype threat was increased by underscoring the evaluative nature of the test, the Black students performed much worse than the White students. But when stereotype threat was minimized by introducing the same test as nonevaluative, the Black students performed just as well as the White students.

Despite the fact that the stereotype-threat situation bears no resemblance to a traditional dissonance—self-affirmation paradigm, thinking about the test-taking situation in those terms has been extremely useful. In a recent study (J. Aronson & Damiani, 1997), we tested whether self-affirmations could mitigate the underperformance engendered by the stereotype threat. In essence, we asked if being reminded of one's general sense of goodness could protect one from the threatening and performance-disruptive implications of a negative stereotype about one's intellectual abilities. Could we help a Black test taker to perform better by affirming him or her in some valued domain of the self-concept? To find out, we replicated the Steele and Aronson procedure described above. But in this experiment, half of the test takers received a self-affirmation just before starting the test. For one group, the affirmation was relevant: We affirmed their verbal skills. The other two groups received an irrelevant affirmation (of either their social skills or their ethnic identity). The results were very clear. The only affirmation that benefited the test takers was the affirmation of their verbal skills. Relevance, in this instance, buffered participants against a self-threat.

Self-Affirmation and the Effect of Positive Role Models

Reading through the literature on academic underperformance, one frequently confronts the role model argument: Why do Black and Latino students fail to do as well as White students in school? One explanation is that they lack adequate Black and Latino role models, who demonstrate, by example, that people of their race can succeed in academics. This argument also surfaces frequently during discussions of affirmative action. But despite the intuitive appeal of this argument, evidence that the presence of minority role models improves the outcomes of minority students is hard to come by. It is not at all clear, for example, that on integrated college campuses, there is a correlation between the number of Black professors and the academic performance of the Black student body (J. Aronson & Disko, 1997).

In a recent study, we (J. Aronson & Disko, 1997) examined the hypothesis, derived from self-affirmation theory, that role models can actually be threatening if they excel in domains where a person feels threatened. As a result, we may denigrate rather than identify with such role models. To test this reasoning, we gave students a test of either their verbal skills or their hand−eye coordination skills. Regardless of experimental condition, the students were made to feel that they had performed poorly on the test. Later, in the context of a supposedly unrelated survey, we told students that we needed their help in putting together some interventions aimed at motivating high school students to excel in academics. Specifically, we asked them to rate the suitability of various role models who could be used as spokespeople for this cause. The list of role models they rated came from various walks of life: famous scientists, athletes, politicians, writers, and so on. Our key hypothesis centered on the ratings of the writers on our list (e.g., Stephen King and Anne Rice) because they represented the category of people with excellent verbal skills, the same skills that half of our participants were presumably doubting because of their failure in the first part of the study. As predicted, the participants in the verbal-skills-failure condition gave much more negative ratings to the writers than they did to the other role model candidates. This pattern of role model bashing did not occur for participants in the hand−eye-coordination condition. This study, we believe, helps to explain why the mere presence of positive role models may not be enough. Students may feel threatened, rather than inspired, by excellent role models, especially in domains where they feel under suspicion.

Self-Concept Change Through Disidentification

One additional advantage of the self-affirmation approach is that it considers the self as an element in the dissonance process. Because the self is an element, changing one's self-concept may be an effective means to reduce dissonance. According to this reasoning, when one's behavior or performance in a domain casts a negative light on oneself, one can maintain global self-esteem by disidentifying with the domain in question. For example, we (J. Aronson & Fried, 1997) have found that Blacks with relatively low academic performance in school cope by making academics less important to their self-concepts, that is, they rationalize their lower achievement by reorganizing their priorities (see also Steele, 1997). We have studied the *disidentification* hypothesis in the domain of moral goodness as well. For example, J. Aronson et al. (1995) found that after behaving uncompassionately, participants attempted to affirm themselves by denying the importance of compassion to their self-concepts. Although such effects were certainly conceivable under the older formulations of dissonance theory, the effect of dissonance on the self was never a focal point. In a conceptually related study, it was found that in the face of a self-threat, people recruited lost self-esteem by heightening their identification with a valued reference group, a defensive reaction that was attenuated when people were able to affirm another unrelated aspect of their self-concept. This research demonstrates how identification and disidentification processes may produce changes in self-concept—a finding that poses serious challenges for conventional theories that view social identity as fixed rather than malleable (Garcia & Steele, 1997).

CONCLUSION

Self-affirmation theory contributed a great deal to bringing dissonance and motivational processes back to the analysis of significant social psychological phenomena. Like the early version of dissonance theory, self-affirmation theory lacks precision with regard to some of its postulates and with regard to the mediating process. But, like dissonance theory, this imprecision comes with the benefit of an expansive range of application. It is a useful tool for examining a broad range of phenomena where self-protective motivations play a role, and it pushes dissonance theory beyond the consideration of simple consistency drives to a broader and richer territory. That is, self-affirmation theory directs our attention to the many manifestations and implications of the motivation to manage and protect self or identity. How this motivation plays out depends on the opportunities and threats presented by a particular situation, whether it be a dissonance paradigm (Steele & Liu, 1983), the more common daily stressors people face in their lives (Keough et al., 1997), the context of debate or negotiation (Atkins et al., 1997; Cohen et al., 1997), or the schooling environment (Steele & Aronson, 1995).

This synthetic approach of applying self-affirmation theory to new phenomena is likely to shed light on the processes underlying these phenomena (including stress and illness, stereotyping and inferential biases, and academic identification). But it is also likely to provide insights into the nature of dissonance processes, especially when such synthesis is tempered by a consideration of the constraints and limiting conditions uncovered by more analytically inclined experimenters. For example, one message of self-affirmation research is that self-image motivations permeate a wide range of phenomena, even very basic and everyday tasks like causal attribution (e.g., Liu & Steele, 1986). Thus, it may be premature to assert that the precondition for all dissonance phenomena is the commission of a freely chosen act with aversive, foreseeable consequences (Cooper & Fazio, 1984). Although in some situations, this may hold, in other situations, different factors may create self-threat and arouse dissonance.

At present, using self-affirmation theory as opposed to a more analytic theory is a bit like trading in a fine-tuned sports sedan for an all-terrain vehicle with huge tires and a bulky suspension system. One sacrifices the ability to sense slight variations in the texture of the road for the ability to venture into uncharted, unpaved territory. As research continues and the theory becomes more precise, the trade-off will become less and less significant.

REFERENCES

Aronson, E. (1968). Dissonance theory: Progress and problems. In R. Abelson, E. Aronson, W. McGuire, T. Newcomb, M. Rosenberg, & P. Tannenbaum (Eds.), *Theories of cognitive consistency: A sourcebook* (pp. 5–27). Chicago: Rand McNally.

Aronson, E. (1992). The return of the repressed: Dissonance theory makes a comeback. *Psychological Inquiry, 3,* 303–311.

Aronson, E., & Carlsmith, J. M. (1962). Performance expectancy as a determinant of actual performance. *Journal of Abnormal and Social Psychology, 65,* 178–182.

Aronson, E., & Mills, J. (1959). The effects of severity of initiation on liking for a group. *Journal of Abnormal and Social Psychology, 59,* 177–181.

Aronson, J., Blanton, H., & Cooper, J. (1995). From dissonance to disidentification: Selectivity in the self-affirmation process. *Journal of Personality and Social Psychology, 68,* 986–996.

Aronson, J., & Damiani, M. (1997). *Stereotype threat, attributional ambiguity and fragile self-competence.* Unpublished manuscript, University of Texas at Austin.

Aronson, J., & Disko, D. (1997). *Why role models aren't enough: The influence of self-affirmation processes on positive social influence.* Paper presented at the 77th annual meeting of the Western Psychological Association, Seattle.

Aronson, J., & Fried, C. (1997). *Reducing disidentification and boosting the academic achievement of stereotype vulnerable students: The role of theories of intelligence.* Unpublished manuscript, University of Texas at Austin.

Aronson, J., Quinn, D., & Spencer, S. (1997). Stereotype threat and the academic performance of minorities and women. In J. Swim & C. Stangor (Eds.), *Prejudice: The target's perspective* (83–103). San Diego, CA: Academic Press.

Atkins, D., Ward, A., & Lepper, M. (1997). *Reducing reactive devaluation with a self-affirmation.* Unpublished manuscript, Stanford University, Palo Alto, CA.

Axsom, D., & Cooper, J. (1985). Cognitive dissonance and psychotherapy: The role of effort justification in inducing weight loss. *Journal of Experimental Social Psychology, 21*, 149–160.

Bem, D. J. (1967). Self-perception: An alternate interpretation of cognitive dissonance phenomena. *Psychological Review, 74*, 183–200.

Benbow, C. P., & Stanley, J. C. (1980). Sex differences in mathematical ability: Fact or artifact? *Science, 210*, 1262–1264.

Bereiter, C., & Engleman, S. (1966). *Teaching disadvantaged children in the preschool*. Englewood Cliffs, NJ: Prentice-Hall.

Berkowitz, L., & Devine, P. G. (1989). Research traditions, analysis, and synthesis in social psychological theories: The case of dissonance theory. *Personality and Social Psychology Bulletin, 15*, 493–507.

Blanton, H., Cooper, J., Skurnik, I., & Aronson, J. (1997). When bad things happen to good feedback: Exacerbating the need for self-justification with self-affirmations. *Personality and Social Psychology Bulletin, 23*, 684–692.

Bramel, D. (1962). A dissonance theory perspective on defensive projection. *Journal of Abnormal and Social Psychology, 64*, 121–129.

Brehm, J. (1959). Increasing cognitive dissonance by a fait accompli. *Journal of Abnormal and Social Psychology, 58*, 379–382.

Cohen, G. L., Aronson, J., & Steele, C. M. (1997). *When beliefs yield to evidence: Reducing biased evaluation by affirming the self.* Manuscript submitted for publication.

Cooper, J. (1980). Reducing fears and increasing assertiveness: The role of dissonance reduction. *Journal of Experimental Social Psychology, 16*, 199–213.

Cooper, J., & Fazio, R. H. (1984). A new look at dissonance theory. In L. Berkowitz (Ed.), *Advances in experimental social psychology* (Vol. 17, pp. 229–262). Hillsdale, NJ: Erlbaum.

Doob, A., Carlsmith, J., Freedman, J., Landauer, T., & Tom, S. (1969). Effect of initial selling price on subsequent sales. *Journal of Personality and Social Psychology, 11*, 345–350.

Dunning, D., Leuenberger, A., & Sherman, D. A. (1995). A new look at motivated inference: Are self-serving theories of success a product of motivational forces? *Journal of Personality and Social Psychology, 69*, 58–68.

Festinger, L. (1957). *A theory of cognitive dissonance*. Stanford, CA: Stanford University Press.

Festinger, L., Reicken, H. W., & Schachter, S. (1956). *When prophecy fails.* New York: Harper & Row.

Garcia, J., & Steele, C. M. (1997). *Social identity and self-affirmation.* Manuscript submitted for publication.

Gibbons, F. X., Eggleston, T. J., & Benthin, A. C. (1997). Cognitive reactions to smoking relapse: The reciprocal relation between dissonance and self-esteem. *Journal of Personality and Social Psychology, 72,* 184–195.

Glass, D. (1964). Changes in liking as a means of reducing cognitive discrepancies between self-esteem and aggression. *Journal of Personality, 32,* 531–549.

Greenwald, A. G., & Ronis, D. L. (1978). Twenty years of cognitive dissonance: Case study of the evolution of a theory. *Psychological Review, 85,* 53–57.

Herrnstein, R. J., & Murray, C. (1994). *The bell curve: Intelligence and class structure in American life.* New York: Free Press.

Jensen, A. R. (1969). How much can we boost I.Q. and scholastic achievement? *Harvard Educational Review, 39,* 1–123.

Jones, E. E. (1985). Major developments in social psychology during the past five decades. In G. Lindzey & E. Aronson (Eds.), *The handbook of social psychology* (3rd ed., Vol. 1, pp. 47–108). New York: Random House.

Keough, K. A. (1997). *When the self is at stake: Integrating the self into stress and physical health research.* Unpublished manuscript, University of Texas at Austin.

Keough, K. A., Garcia, J., & Steele, C. M. (1997). *Reducing stress and illness by affirming the self.* Unpublished manuscript, University of Texas at Austin.

Kunda, Z. (1987). Motivated inference: Self-serving generation and evaluation of causal theories. *Journal of Personality and Social Psychology, 53,* 37–54.

Liu, T. J., & Steele, C. M. (1986). Attributional analysis as self-affirmation. *Journal of Personality and Social Psychology, 51,* 531–540.

Lord, C. G., Ross, L., & Lepper, M. R. (1979). Biased assimilation and attitude polarization: The effects of prior theories on subsequently considered evidence. *Journal of Personality and Social Psychology, 37,* 2098–2109.

Shweder, R. A. (1991). *Thinking through cultures: Expeditions in cultural psychology.* Cambridge, MA: Harvard University Press.

Simon, L., Greenberg, J., & Brehm, J. (1995). Trivialization: The forgotten mode

146

of dissonance reduction. *Journal of Personality and Social Psychology, 68,* 247–260.

Spencer, S. J., Steele, C. M., & Quinn, D. M. (1997). *Stereotype threat and women's math performance.* Unpublished manuscript, University of Waterloo, Waterloo, Ontario, Canada.

Steele, C. M. (1988). The psychology of self-affirmation: Sustaining the integrity of the self. In L. Berkowitz (Ed.), *Advances in experimental social psychology* (Vol. 21, pp. 261–302). Hillsdale, NJ: Erlbaum.

Steele, C. M. (1997). A threat in the air: How stereotypes shape intellectual identity and performance. *American Psychologist, 52,* 613–629.

Steele, C. M., & Aronson, J. (1995). Stereotype threat and the intellectual test performance of African Americans. *Journal of Personality and Social Psychology, 69,* 797–811.

Steele, C. M., & Liu, T. J. (1983). Dissonance processes as self-affirmation. *Journal of Personality and Social Psychology, 45,* 5–19.

Steele, C. M., & Spencer, S. J. (1992). The primacy of self-integrity. *Psychological Inquiry, 3,* 345–346.

Steele, C. M., Spencer, S. J., & Lynch, M. (1993). Dissonance and affirmational resources: Resilience against self-image threats. *Journal of Personality and Social Psychology, 64,* 885–896.

Stone, J., Cooper, J., Galinsky, A., & Kelly, K. (1997). *Self-attribute accessibility in dissonance: The mirror has many faces.* Manuscript submitted for publication.

Tesser, A., & Cornell, D. P. (1991). On the confluence of self processes. *Journal of Experimental Social Psychology, 27,* 501–526.

Thibodeau, R., & Aronson, E. (1992). Taking a closer look: Reasserting the role of the self-concept in dissonance theory. *Personality and Social Psychology Bulletin, 18,* 591–602.

7

Unwanted Consequences and the Self: In Search of the Motivation for Dissonance Reduction

Joel Cooper

M ore than 40 years ago, Leon Festinger (1957) made the marvelously elegant suggestion that inconsistency between pairs of cognitive elements causes the psychological discomfort known as *cognitive dissonance*. That statement, and a modest number of supporting postulates, spawned more than 2,000 empirical investigations examining the nonobvious predictions of the theory and expanding its reach into new areas of applicability.

The longevity of dissonance at or near the center stage of social psychology is impressive. The early days of dissonance research were characterized by novel, high-impact experimentation conducted by clever and intuitive experimenters. But this alone could not have been sufficient to carry the dissonance tradition through 4 decades. More impressive than the impact of the original experiments was Festinger's foresight to recognize the careful interplay between motivation and cognition. Festinger recognized, before it was fashionable, that knowledge of the environment and knowledge of one's own behaviors, attitudes, and emotions were represented cognitively and that it was the relation-

---

I gratefully acknowledge the help of Adam Galinsky in the preparation of this chapter.

ship among the cognitive representations that prompted motivation. Thus, when social psychology strayed toward the purely motivational, dissonance theory was present to remind the field of the importance of cognitive representations of the person and the environment. Similarly, and perhaps more important, when social psychology strayed toward the purely cognitive, dissonance theory reminded us that cognitive representations lead to motivation and that motivation affects the representations themselves (cf. Kunda, 1990). Thus, in addition to being a provocative theory in its own right, dissonance's reliance on the cognitive and the motivational provided an important middle ground to which social psychology could consistently return.

In this chapter, I examine the motivational basis of dissonance reduction. Why does inconsistency motivate people to go about the difficult task of cognitive change? What makes people experience arousal and negative affect? For Festinger, the answer lay in the mere presence of inconsistency. But more recent work has suggested alternative mechanisms for change, including the elimination of aversive consequences and the bolstering of the self-concept. In the current chapter, I consider the difference between motivational views that focus on the self and those that focus on behavioral consequences. Although there is considerable wisdom drawn from the representation of the self, I argue that the motivation for dissonance reduction arises from the perception of aversive consequences and that changes of attitudes that generally follow from dissonance arousal are at the service of rendering those consequences nonaversive.

CURING THE "BUT ONLYS": FROM INCONSISTENCY TO AVERSIVE OUTCOMES

When dissonance theory was merely 25 years old, Russell Fazio and I set out to put together much of the research that had accumulated over dissonance's first quarter-century. We wanted to see if comprehensive sense could be made of a theory that had an impressive history but that was saddled with a bad case of the "but onlys." Dissonance arose from inconsistent cognitions, *but only* if there was free choice to act counterattitudinally; *but only* if there was commitment to the counterattitudinal act; *but only* if an unwanted consequence had occurred; *but only* if the consequence was foreseeable, and so forth.

Fazio and I wanted to see if we could plot the best fitting theoretical curve that passed through the numerous replications of dissonance and the impressive list of "but only" exceptions. In the end, we concluded that the best fitting curve did not pass through cognitive inconsistency at all (Cooper & Fazio, 1984). Rather, we concluded that dissonance was a state of arousal caused by behaving in such a way as to feel personally responsible for bringing about an aversive event. If that arousal was not misattributed to another source or reduced in some other way, dissonance arousal became *dissonance motivation,* an instigation to engage in cognitive changes for the fundamental purpose of rendering the consequence nonaversive. That is why the consequence, the unwanted result of a person's behavior, is so critical in driving the dissonance engine. It is the essential ingredient, the primary reason for people engaging in the effort of dissonance reduction.

The new look model was intended not as a new theory, but rather as a change in emphasis of a venerable theory. We suggested that the emphasis on inconsistency in causing dissonance arousal had been misplaced. Because acting inconsistently usually has the potential to result in an aversive or unwanted consequence, inconsistency is a reasonable stand-in variable for aversive consequences in producing dissonance. However, it is not the inconsistency per se that causes the arousal, but rather the result of that inconsistency, the unwanted consequence. When viewed this way, the "but onlys" fall into place, not as exceptions to the theory, but as explicable and important components of dissonance.

Nonetheless, the difference in the two approaches is not trivial. On those occasions in which inconsistency can be separated from aversive consequences, it is the latter and not the former that holds up to empirical test. Cooper and Worchel (1970) showed that inconsistency is not a sufficient condition for dissonance arousal if aversive consequences are lacking. Scher and Cooper (1989) showed that inconsistency is neither sufficient nor necessary for dissonance arousal if the production of aversive consequences is carefully disentangled from the cognitive inconsistency.

WHAT IS AN AVERSIVE CONSEQUENCE?

Meeting the Positivistic Test

In our new look paper (1984), Fazio and I defined aversive consequences *positivistically* rather than a priori. According to the positivistic view, the ultimate authority for theoretical terms is how they are experienced by the perceiver. Similarly, in our view, *aversive* consequences are best defined by the way they are experienced by the actor rather than by an abstract definition in advance of an act that fails to consider the actor's experience. We defined an *aversive* consequence as the real or potential result of behavior that a person would rather have not brought about. The emphasis in this definition is on the actor who determines, by his or her experience of an event, whether it is wanted or unwanted. What makes a consequence aversive is the way an outcome of an act is perceived by the actor. If the actor perceives the consequence as unwanted, then it successfully meets the test of being an aversive consequence.

The experiment by Cooper and Worchel (1970) established a procedure that perhaps became the paradigmatic example of an aversive consequence. Worchel and I had student volunteers participate in a procedure substantially similar to the original well-known induced-compliance experiment of Festinger and Carlsmith (1959). In the original study, participants engaged in a truly boring task and then were induced, for either a low or high monetary inducement, to tell a waiting participant (actually, a confederate of the experimenter) that the task was truly exciting and interesting. Festinger and Carlsmith had reasoned that the inconsistency between saying the task was interesting while privately believing that the task was deadly dull was sufficient to cause dissonance. As is well known, they also established and confirmed the nonobvious prediction that acting inconsistently for a small monetary inducement would create more dissonance and thus lead to more attitude change than acting inconsistently for a large inducement. People came to believe that the task was more interesting if they had lied to the waiting participant for only a meager amount of financial inducement.

Worchel and I argued that it was not the inconsistency between saying the task was interesting and believing it was dull that led to dissonance, but rather the unwanted event of having duped a fellow student to look forward to an exciting experience. The participant knew full well that the waiting participant was in for an immense letdown. Indeed, we found that if the student who was waiting explicitly stated that he believed the participant and was looking forward to performing the task, there was dissonance-produced attitude change. But if that consequence was removed by the waiting confederate, indicating that he did not believe the participant, then, despite the participant's having behaved inconsistently, his actions produced no dissonance.

From that study, and several others that confirmed its basic tenet (e.g., Hoyt, Henley, & Collins, 1972; Cooper, Zanna, & Goethals, 1974), it appeared that an aversive consequence would be characterized as doing something bad to someone else, like duping a fellow student, or bringing about an unwanted policy which could harm hundreds of students. Undoubtedly, these are unwanted consequences for most people and serve to initiate the arousal of dissonance. However, causing negative consequences to others and bringing about unwanted political ends are but two of the myriad behavioral outcomes that a person may find aversive. Rejecting a particular consumer item in the research procedure made famous by Brehm (1956) and his colleagues causes the potentially aversive consequence to oneself of giving up the positive benefits associated with that choice and accepting all of the negative features associated with the chosen alternative. Indeed, people may differ in their opinions of the kinds of consequences they find aversive. My list may bear significant similarities to yours, although differences would almost certainly exist. I may think it is particularly aversive to dupe a fellow student, but someone else may find it pleasant to have successfully completed a task requested by the experimenter.

Normative and Ideographic Standards

The fact that people may differ in what they find aversive does not plunge us toward definitional chaos. Regularities exist. Some behavioral outcomes violate generally shared expectations of what is appropriate in a particular situation. That is, they violate normative standards of behavior. Most people in a culture know that it is unacceptable to bring harm to others or knowingly and freely create harmful policies that affect one's university, society, or social group. As Cooper (1997) and Stone (chap. 8, this volume) have argued, the discrepancy between one's behavioral outcome and the normative standard gives that behavior its psychological meaning. For most people, violating normative standards designates the consequence as aversive and unwanted and drives the arousal of dissonance.

On the other hand, behavior can also be discrepant from *ideographic*, or personal standards, and the violation of personal standards also can create dissonance. Years ago, Cooper and Scalise (1974) showed that introverts, as measured by the Myers–Briggs Type Indicator, experience dissonance from different behavioral outcomes than do extraverts. To the extent that personal, ideographic standards are made salient, behavioral outcomes that violate those standards serve as unwanted consequences. The standard that is made accessible in the situation gives meaning to a particular behavioral outcome. If normative standards are most easily accessible,—and they usually are—then behavioral outcomes that violate those standards will cause dissonance. If personal standards become accessible, then behaviors that violate such standards will be considered aversive and lead to the arousal of dissonance.

In essence, then, a behavioral consequence is aversive only when it is psychologically measured against a standard. Typically, that standard is defined by cultural and societal norms, meaning that it is consistent with what most people find aversive about a particular outcome. Occasionally, through chronic accessibility of a personal standard or through an environmental prime, a personal standard becomes highly accessible and then that standard functions as the measuring stick for determining aversiveness.

THE ROLE OF THE SELF IN DISSONANCE

What systematic role does the self play in the dissonance process? There have been several fascinating and provocative theoretical accounts that have implicated self-esteem in the dissonance process. For Aronson (1968, 1992), a person's perception of him- or herself as a competent and moral person necessarily forms one of the cognitions that lead to dissonance arousal. The inconsistent cognition arises from the representation of behavior that compromises or threatens the person's preferred assessment of being a highly moral and competent individual. For Steele and his colleagues (e.g., Steele, 1988; Steele & Liu, 1983), *dissonance reduction* is a strategy designed to protect a person's global feeling of self-worth and self-esteem. Counterattitudinal behavior threatens the self and thus needs to be dealt with, often through attitude change. Ironically, these two versions of the role of self-esteem have made dramatically different predictions. Aronson's *self-consistency* view argues that the typical dissonance situation is arousing only for people with high self-esteem, whereas *self-affirmation* theory argues that people with low self-esteem are primarily upset or threatened by attitude-inconsistent behavior (Steele, Spencer, & Lynch, 1993). These predictions stem from fundamentally different views of the self. Self-consistency views the self as an expectancy, with high self-esteem serving as a more exacting and stringent expectation for one's behavior. For self-affirmation, high self-esteem is a resource that can be brought to bear to buffer the actor against the experience of discomfort.

In my view, there is no consistent or systematic role for the self in the dissonance process. By this I mean that dissonance is not confined to people with one type of self-conception or another. That is, dissonance is not limited to people of high self-esteem, as suggested by self-consistency, nor is it limited to people with low self-esteem, as indicated by self-affirmation. It is not a process that occurs only for introverts, high achievers, or people high in nurturance needs, and so forth. To the contrary, dissonance is a process that is aroused in all people whenever they are responsible for bringing about an aversive consequence. As I suggested previously, the self may become involved in helping to determine when a behavioral consequence is considered aversive. If a personal, self-relevant standard is promoted to a position of high accessibility in a person's cognitive field, then behavioral outcomes that are at variance with the self-standard will create dissonance. But this is a very different view from the totalitarian sense of self in which one aspect of self (e.g., self-esteem) dominates and determines the existence of dissonance.

A CASE IN POINT: IS DISSONANCE SELF-AFFIRMATION?

The general proposition of self-affirmation is that people are concerned with the integrity of their self-worth and will take great pains to protect it. There is nothing in dissonance theory that contradicts this important message. The question at issue is whether dissonance reduction may be conceived solely as a strategic maneuver to accomplish self-affirmation. What Steele and his colleagues have contended is that participants' changes of the representations of their attitudes in dissonance experiments are merely strategic maneuvers to satisfy the self-affirmation motive. The theory holds that people who commit counterattitudinal acts see that they have compromised their integrity. There is nothing special about a dissonant act; it is simply one more way that people can have their self-integrity threatened.

In self-affirmation's view, people with shaky self-concepts (i.e., people with low self-esteem) are the ones most threatened. They will be most in need of finding a way to restore their self-integrity. However, in dissonance experiments, there is only one way provided for them: They can change their attitudes, so that their behavior no longer seems like a compromise to their integrity. Coming to believe what they said is a way for participants in a dissonance experiment to restore their self-integrity and to accomplish the task of self-affirmation. There are other ways that the self can be affirmed if people are given the opportunity. If, after performing some dastardly, consequential counterattitudinal act, one can think of positive features that support her or his self-integrity, then, according to the self-affirmation approach, consequential counterattitudinal behavior will not lead to attitude change.

Thus, Steele and Liu (1983) found that if people are reminded of their basic and important values by, for example, filling out an Allport–Vernon–Lindzey Study of Values (AVL), then counterattitudinal behavior does not lead to dissonance-produced attitude change.

If it were true that merely thinking about one's good attributes eliminates cognitive dissonance, it would be a major challenge to the new look model. This is not just because it was unpredicted, but because it is at variance with the presumed motivational underpinning of dissonance. Why do people change their attitudes after counterattitudinal advocacy or after making difficult decisions among choice alternatives? As mentioned previously, it is to render the consequence of the behavior nonaversive. If you convince fellow voters to elect a disliked candidate to your city council, for example, thinking about how good a tennis player you are hardly solves the dilemma in which you placed yourself—assuming the dilemma is that the wrong councilperson has been elected. Only changing your attitude to favor the newly elected councilperson will render the outcome nonaversive. Of course, that is the crux of the theoretical difference: Is dissonance reduction a way to deal with the arousal created by the behavioral outcome, or is it merely a strategy of self-affirmation?

Consider the following thought-experiment: You are a person who thinks it is important to provide services for the handicapped. Nonetheless, an experimenter convinces you to write an essay advocating a cut in handicapped services at your university. You feel upset and negatively aroused at what you have done. If the motivation posited by self-affirmation is correct, you have all the wherewithal at your disposal to reduce your discomfort and reaffirm yourself any time you wish to do it. All of the ingredients you need are currently in your head. There are values you possess, abilities you have, accomplishments you have produced—all of these and more are waiting for you in memory if you only choose to use them. Any of those mnemonic cognitions can be used for self-affirmation and should be every bit as good as, for example, the filling out of an AVL, which forms the self-affirmation manipulation in Steele and Liu's (1983) experiment. The question is, will you use these memory traces? Will you end your discomfort by conjuring up the recollection of some of your positive values or achievements?

Most probably, this would not happen. The results of so many experiments in which people advocated attitude-discrepant positions argue that people will not make use of the potentially self-affirming cognitions they already possess in memory. If they did—and surely such cognitions were available for use—then counterattitudinal advocacy would never lead to attitude change. It would seem so much more efficient and require so little effort to think quickly of your prowess at tennis or of the great meal you cooked the other night. Even these thoughts are only indirect ways of restoring the self-concept that was threatened by your heartless, noncompassionate essay. It would seem so much more effective to take a frontal attack on your seeming lack of concern for the handicapped by remembering how compassionate you typically have been toward people in need. There must have been some occasion in which your compassion and concern come to mind. However, we know that people do not conjure up such cognitions because cognitions that could provide such direct self-affirming information are always available in memory but are not used by people in any of the research in counterattitudinal advocacy.

It could be argued that, although they are potentially available, such cognitions are largely inaccessible in the context of a psychology experiment. You chose to make a speech, you wove an argument in support of your disliked position, you risked bringing about an unwanted consequence, and you were then given an attitude scale. Perhaps there was no opportunity for your compassionate memories to become accessible in memory.

Avoidance of Relevant Affirmations

Joshua Aronson, Hart Blanton, and I decided to assess this possibility (Aronson, Blanton, & Cooper, 1995). It was our plan to place people in a dissonant situation, make self-affirming cognitions readily accessible, and examine their impact on the dissonance process. It was not at all clear to us that making cognitions accessible that were directly related to the self-concept dimension threatened by the counterattitudinal advocacy would make people more comfortable. Although directly self-affirming on the threatened dimension, such cognitions might make the behavioral outcome seem worse and increase, rather than decrease, the uncomfortable arousal state of dissonance. Thus, such cognitions might be avoided rather than sought and not lower the need for dissonance-reducing attitude change.

In our study, we had volunteers participate in an experiment described as a study in personality structure. Participants were seated by a computer and were asked to respond on-line to the items generated on the screen. When they had completed the inventory, they were told that it would take approximately 15 min for the computer to analyze their responses and present a personality profile.

The study used a two-experimenter procedure, with participants being ushered into the office of a second experimenter while waiting for the computer to analyze the personality results. The second experimenter explained that he was working with the university on research about handicapped facilities on campus. He explained that the university was considering curtailing some of its services for the handicapped and that the policymakers wanted to study students' opinions. In keeping with procedures that have often been used in counterattitudinal advocacy research, the experimenter explained that one of the best ways to obtain people's thoughts on both sides of an issue was to have people write strong and forceful essays favoring one of the two sides. He explained that he had plenty of essays opposing any curtailing of services for the handicapped and that what he needed now were essays taking the strong and forceful position that services should be reduced. The first independent variable was the magnitude of the choice that participants were given to write the essay. In the high-choice conditions, participants were told that the choice to write this essay was completely their own, whereas in the low-choice conditions, they were merely told to write the anti-handicapped services essay.

When the essay was completed and before any assessment of the participant's attitudes, the participant was sent back to the office of the first experimenter to complete the personality structure research. The timing of the attitude assessment, relative to the participant's opportunity to learn how compassionate he or she was, served as the second independent variable in the study. In the attitude-first condition, the second experimenter immediately knocked on the first experimenter's door. Embarrassed and somewhat out of breath, he explained that he had forgotten to give the participant a questionnaire that the university needed. This questionnaire contained the crucial measurement of the participant's opinion about reducing handicapped funding. In the attitude-second condition, the embarrassed first experimenter knocked on the door after the participant's opportunity to receive information on how highly compassionate he or she was.

The first experimenter explained to all participants that the feedback from the personality profile was ready and there was both good news and bad news. The good news was that the computer had identified a large number of factors on which the participant scored greater than the median. The computer printed a paragraph describing the participant's personality profile on all items in which he or she scored above the median. The bad news was that so many items had been identified, there was not time to read all of them. Thus, the participant was told he or she would have to choose which of 10 personality dimensions to read. Would the participants seek or avoid the directly affirming paragraphs that identified him or her as high in compassion? The participants' choice of which paragraphs to read served as a second important dependent measure.

First, let us look at the attitude measure. Recall that in the attitude-first condition, participants had their attitudes assessed before receiving any feedback that could have served as self-affirmation. Both self-affirmation theory and dissonance theory would predict greater opinion change for high-choice than for low-choice participants (i.e., the typical induced-compliance effect found in many studies). However, in the attitude-second condition, participants had already had an opportunity to read about their good qualities, including—if they so desired—direct confirmation of their goodness in the area of compassion. This manipulation made positive self-information both available and accessible and should have provided ample opportunity for self-affirmation. Nonetheless, Figure 1 shows that reading about one's good personality

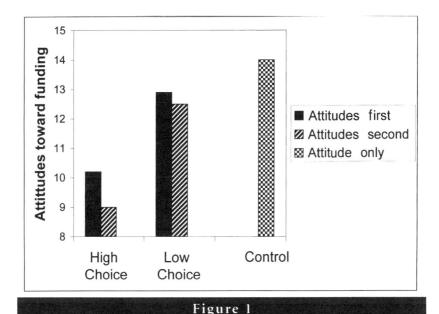

Figure 1

Attitudes toward handicapped funding after counterattitudinal behavior. Low numbers indicate greater attitude change. From "Dissonance to Disidentification: Selectivity in the Self-Affirmation Process," J. Aronson, H. Blanton, and J. Cooper, 1995. *Journal of Personality and Social Psychology, 68,* p. 989. Copyright 1995 by the American Psychological Association.

traits had absolutely no effect on attitudes. In the attitude-second condition, just like the attitude-first condition, high-choice participants expressed attitudes that were significantly more in favor of reducing handicapped funding than did participants in an attitude-only control condition in which attitudes were assessed without any experimental manipulations. Low-choice participants, however, did not differ from the control. The analysis of the data revealed a main effect for choice and significant simple effects for choice within the attitude-first and attitude-second conditions. Simply put, the opportunity to self-affirm had no impact on reducing the need to change attitudes following freely chosen, counterattitudinal advocacy.[1]

---

[1]In this study, as in many studies in the dissonance tradition, attitude change is inferred from differences in attitude scores between the experimental and control conditions.

We now address a related question: Did participants even want to see how compassionate they were? It follows from the basic assumptions of self-affirmation that people who have had their compassionate selves compromised by their counterattitudinal advocacy should jump at the opportunity to reinstate their compassion. The results, presented in Figure 2, showed that this did not happen. To the contrary, a main effect for choice showed that the more dissonance the participants had, the less they wanted to read about their compassion. And within the attitude-second condition, high-choice participants particularly wanted no part of learning about their compassion, showing the greatest avoidance of the compassion paragraphs of all the participants in the study.

From this study, conducted at Princeton University, and a nearly

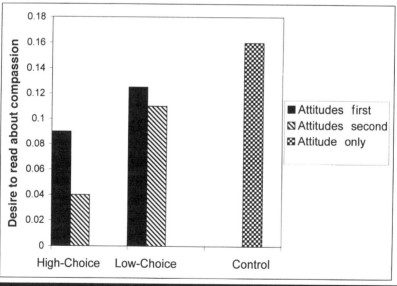

Figure 2

Interest in reading affirming information about compassion as a function of choice and affirmation opportunity. Dependent measure is the proportion of paragraphs chosen about compassion relative to the total number of paragraphs chosen. From "Dissonance to Disidentification: Selectivity in the Self-Affirmation Process," by J. Aronson, H. Blanton, and J. Cooper, 1995, *Journal of Personality and Social Psychology, 68*, p. 990. Copyright 1995 by the American Psychological Association.

identical replication run at Stanford University, we have learned a number of important facts: First, when in the throes of cognitive dissonance, people do not want to know about affirming, positive information relevant to the attribute that has been challenged by the potential consequences of their counterattitudinal behavior. Second, not only do participants not want such information, but its increased accessibility does not alter their need to reduce dissonance. Instead, participants continue to deal with the unwanted consequences of their behavior by changing their attitudes, presumably to render those consequences less aversive than they otherwise would have been.

Confronting People With Affirmation

The next question that my colleagues and I tried to answer was the effect of confronting people directly with self-affirming information (Blanton, Cooper, Skurnik, & Aronson, 1997). The previous study had shown that people who are experiencing dissonance avoid information that could directly affirm the valued personality trait that had been compromised by their counterattitudinal behavior. What would happen if people were presented with the information that showed that they were indeed compassionate, helpful people? Would making such praiseworthy information immediately salient help to reduce people's discomfort, that is, would it reduce the need for attitude change?

Our prediction was that although a directly relevant affirmation might bolster a person's self-esteem, it also could make salient a personal standard to which the behavioral outcome of an action could be compared. If people were forced to consider that they are helpful, compassionate people, that might cause the ideographic, personal standard to be brought to bear on the dissonant act.

Now, writing an essay against funding for the handicapped is aversive when considered against the normative standard and when considered against the personal standard of compassion. If compassionate people bring about effects that are antithetical to compassion, then the counterattitudinal behavior would be especially aversive. In summary, supplying a person with relevant, self-affirming information can lead to greater dissonance because the accessible personal standard makes the behavioral outcome seem even more noxious and aversive than when considered against the normative standard alone.

As in the previous study, Blanton et al. (1997) had participants volunteer for a study on personality structure. Participants were then asked by a second experimenter to write an essay arguing against funding for handicapped services at their university, under conditions of high or low choice. Participants returned to the first experimenter and read a paragraph that described an aspect of their personality that was identified by the computerized personality inventory. Some participants received positive, relevant feedback: They were told that they had scored highly in the trait of compassion. Other participants received positive, irrelevant feedback: They were told that they scored highly in the trait of creativity. A control group received no feedback at all.

A knock on the door brought the return of the out-of-breath, embarrassed second experimenter. As in the J. Aronson et al. (1995) procedure, he explained that he had forgotten to administer the questionnaire that the university wanted all participants to complete. This questionnaire included the major dependent measure: the assessment of attitudes toward handicapped funding.

The results showed strong evidence for our predictions. As can be seen in Figure 3, we found a main effect for choice and an interaction between choice and affirmation. In keeping with dissonance theory predictions, the results for the control (no-feedback) conditions showed a significant simple effect for choice: High-choice participants expressed attitudes that were more in line with the position of their essay than did low-choice participants. When participants read information that showed how positively compassionate they were (relevant-affirmation conditions), dissonance was increased. The same simple effect between high and low choice that had been found in the control condition was also found in the relevant-affirmation condition, but the effect was larger. Finally, the 2 × 3 factorial resulted in a significant interaction between choice and affirmation, aided by the lack of any difference between choice conditions when the affirming information was irrelevant to the topic of the essay. Thus, facing directly affirming information drives people further toward the need for dissonance re-

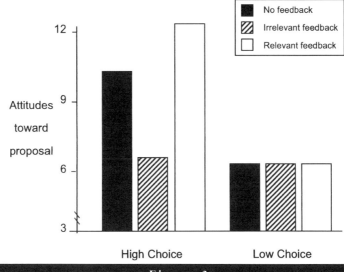

Figure 3

Attitudes toward proposal of withdrawing funding for the handicapped after receiving relevant and irrelevant affirming information. Higher numbers indicate more favorable attitudes toward the proposal. From "When Bad Things Happen to Good Feedback: Exacerbating the Need for Self-Justification With Self-Affirmations," by H. Blanton, J. Cooper, I. Skurnik, and J. Aronson, 1997, *Personality and Social Psychology Bulletin, 23*, p. 689. Copyright 1997 by Sage. Adapted with permission.

duction and increases, rather than decreases, dissonance-produced attitude change.

The Fuzzy (but Temporary), Good Feeling of Self-Affirmation

There is evidence in the Blanton et al. (1997) study that suggests that positive information people receive about themselves does seem to reduce the need for attitude change, provided that the information is not relevant to the self-attribute threatened by the counterattitudinal behavior. Note the lack of attitude change in the high-choice, irrelevant-feedback condition depicted in Figure 3. If direct self-affirmations result in increased dissonance, why does the indirect affirmation lead to less dissonance?

We think that the reason people show less dissonance motivation when receiving positive, but irrelevant, information is that they are literally distracted from the task at hand. They are distracted from the behavioral consequence by the fuzzy, good feeling of learning about a good attribute they possess. As we have argued, responsibly creating an aversive consequence creates arousal that is experienced as negative affect. When people add to that hedonic equation some positive news about themselves, their discomfort is reduced, and the exigent need to change their attitude is diminished.

However, such positive affect is fragile. We already know, from the results of the research presented here, that positive information will not lead to distracting, positive affect if it serves to make accessible a personal standard that has been directly violated by the attitude-discrepant behavior. We suspect that even irrelevant information (i.e., information that does not make the violated personal standard salient) will reduce negative affect only temporarily. It can fail: People can cease paying attention to it, or the information might be shown to be wrong. In such cases, we predict that the dissonance will return with a magnitude at least as great as that which existed before the positive, irrelevant information was introduced.

Galinsky, Stone, and Cooper (1997) conducted a study to examine the latter hypothesis. We allowed participants in a dissonance experiment to think of some of their positive self-values. Similar to previous affirmation experiments, we facilitated participants' basking in this information and feeling good about its implications by giving them the AVL. Then, for some participants, we negated the information by providing information that questioned whether they indeed possessed these positive values. We predicted that the participants would no longer have their fuzzy, good feeling. Instead, they would need to reconfront their psychological discomfort, and the need to change their attitude would reemerge.

There is a tradition at Princeton University that is generally supported by undergraduate students and opposed by the town police and university officials. It occurs on the day of the first snowfall of the season and is euphemistically known as the Nude Olympics. In a typical induced-compliance procedure, we asked (or told) students to make speeches arguing for an end to their treasured Nude Olympics. Then, in keeping with the procedure of Steele and Liu (1983), participants filled out the AVL, which gave them the opportunity to express themselves on valued dimensions of their personality.

Some participants immediately filled out an attitude survey that asked their positions on a number of campus issues, including the degree to which they supported the Nude Olympics. Other participants were given the opportunity to affirm the self by expressing their values on the AVL. Two other conditions, one that performed the dissonant behavior under conditions of high choice and the other under conditions of low choice, were randomly assigned to the negation condition. These participants received alleged feedback based on their responses to the AVL. They were shown graphs that placed their scores in the context of other university students. The graphs showed them that the positive values they thought characterized their personalities were, in fact, not characteristic of them at all. Essentially, their affirmations were negated. Following the viewing of the graphs, participants in the affirmation and negation conditions filled out attitude scales and other measures.

The results of the attitude measure are depicted in Figure 4. We found that participants who were distracted by the positive information about their values did not manifest attitude change toward the Nude Olympics and differed significantly from the high-choice–no-feedback participants. However, when the participants learned that they had scored low on those treasured values that they thought characterized their personalities, their attitudes reverted to those expressed by the high-choice–no feedback participants. In other words, the relief from needing to deal with the aversive consequences of their behavior was short-lived. As soon as the positive information was negated, the need to deal with the reality of the aversive event returned, and so did dissonance-produced attitude change.

Low-choice–negation participants did not show justification of their dissonant behavior. This result indicates that it was not negative feedback per se that caused attitude change. Rather, discrediting partic-

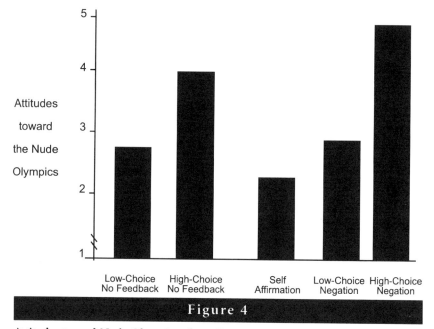

Figure 4

Attitudes toward Nude Olympics after affirmation and negation. Higher numbers indicate more favorable attitudes toward the proposal.

ipants' values produced attitude change only for those participants who initially experienced dissonance and who had attempted to deal with the situation by focusing on their positive values.

In a separate experiment, using a very similar procedure, we examined the effect of affirming or negating positive, self-relevant information on the participants' emotional experience. Using a measure developed by Elliot and Devine (1994), participants were asked to rate their affect after producing a counterattitudinal speech, after self-affirming on the AVL, or after receiving information that negated their affirmation, depending on the experimental condition to which they had been assigned. They were asked to rate their psychological discomfort by indicating the degree to which they felt uncomfortable, uneasy, and bothered.

In keeping with the attitude data presented in Figure 4, participants in the high-choice–no-feedback condition who did not have the opportunity to think about their favorite values showed a high degree of psychological discomfort, as dissonance theory predicts. On the other hand, participants who contemplated their positive values expressed a very low level of psychological discomfort, as predicted by self-affirmation. However, when the positive thoughts were negated by information showing that participants did not possess a high degree of those values, the psychological discomfort reemerged at a level similar to that of the high-choice—no-feedback participants. As in the previous experiment, low-choice—negative feedback participants did not experience discomfort. This demonstrates that the negation information per se did not have a negative impact on the participants' discomfort level. Rather, writing a counterattitudinal essay under high-choice conditions appears to be necessary to invoke the feeling of discomfort, a feeling state akin to Festinger's (1957) original conceptualization of dissonance. Writing under low choice produced no psychological discomfort, even when it was accompanied by information showing people that the degree to which they held certain treasured values was not very high. Allowing people to bask in the belief that they did have treasured values reduced psychological discomfort, but the relief was fragile and fleeting. Discomfort reemerged in full force when the participants' belief in their values was negated by the computerized feedback.

Putting the Pieces Together

In summary, the current portion of my argument is that dissonance reduction is not a strategy to make the self feel better or affirmed. Rather, it is the result of an unpleasant arousal state and is designed to render the consequence of a behavior nonaversive. Our data have shown that (a) people do not wish to find out about positive features of the self that have been threatened by attitude-discrepant behaviors, even though such information could directly repair the integrity of the compromised self; (b) people who are induced to confront affirming information directly manifest an increased need to reduce dissonance through attitude change; and (c) people who receive positive information that is not related to the compromised part of the self may show less of a need for attitude change after counterattitudinal behavior, but such reduction is temporary and fragile, with attitude change re-emerging if the affirmations fail. I am not arguing that people do not have an independent motive to feel good about themselves or to direct their actions toward restoring self-integrity. However, I am arguing that in situations in which people responsibly produce unwanted consequences, they must deal directly with the cognitive representation of those consequences—usually by changing their attitudes. Attempts to deal with their compromised self-integrity must wait until they have dealt with the unwanted consequences of their behavior.

SPECULATIONS ON A NEW ROLE FOR THE SELF IN DISSONANCE

Earlier, I indicated that there was no necessary role played by the self in dissonance reduction. That statement is now qualified to mean that dissonance is not confined to people with a particular self view or to people with a particular level of self-esteem or to people with a particular personality trait. Much of the data presented in this chapter has focused on whether dissonance is merely one of many possible strategies to make a shattered self feel better and concluded that that was not a proper role for the self in dissonance theory.

However, the self is very much involved in dissonance if one takes a somewhat broader perspective. First, the self plays a role as a standard against which a consequence can be considered wanted or unwanted. When self-standards are made highly accessible by environmental events or, in what I suspect are rare circumstances, by chronic accessibility, then they supersede normative standards in determining the aversiveness of a behavioral outcome. Second, and somewhat more speculatively, the self may be intimately connected to the ontogeny of dissonance.

In the original new look paper (1984), Fazio and I suggested that dissonance developed as a learned drive. Think about how children may learn to anticipate negative events in their lives. They learn that certain behaviors are followed by punishments and threats. Soon, children learn to anticipate the connection between behaviors and negative outcomes, and they avoid behaving in ways that bring such outcomes. Sullivan

(1953), in his social psychiatric theory of personality development, discussed the creation of the self-system as a way of bringing about security while avoiding anxiety. The key to the system is that the self develops as a complex system of cognitions and behaviors, all designed to anticipate and cope with anxiety-producing reactions from people in the environment. It seems reasonable that one such negative, painful reaction from the environment occurs when a child brings about a consensually agreed, negative outcome. Hurting one's mother, or a baby sister, or even knocking over a lamp may qualify as normatively defined negative events. Children thus learn to anticipate that such events lead to profound negative responses and are to be avoided. So an uncomfortable emotional reaction may develop at any hint or anticipation of responsibly bringing about an aversive event. If children do bring about an aversive event, then they need to develop ways to cope. One way might be to deny responsibility; if that fails, they may need to change what was once aversive into something nonaversive. What may develop as a response to the anxiety reactions and sanctions of significant people in the environment may eventually develop its own autonomy and become the tension state known as dissonance.

The gist of the analysis is to speculate that the development of ways to cope with producing aversive behavioral outcomes may be intimately related to the development of the entire self-system. Avoiding dissonance situations is learned as part of the self-system, as are coping mechanisms, should unwanted, aversive events occur. Dealing with significant others in the environment helps us form our self-systems, and, part and parcel of that development, is the development of cognitive dissonance.

Dissonance theory, throughout its long history, has been marked by extensions and applications into new and uncharted territory. Examining the role of the self in dissonance theory may provide another new opportunity. Although I have taken issue with the precise way that theories of self-consistency and self-affirmation view the involvement of self in dissonance, examining dissonance within the context of the self-system may prove a fertile area for future theory and research.

REFERENCES

Allport, G. W., Vernon, P. E., and Lindzey, G. (1960). *Allport-Vernon-Lindzey Study of Values.* Chicago: Riverside.

Aronson, E. (1968). Dissonance theory: Progress and problems. In R. Abelson, E. Aronson, W. McGuire, T. Newcomb, M. Rosenberg, & P. Tannnenbaum (Eds.), *Theories of cognitive consistency: A sourcebook* (pp. 5–27). Chicago: Rand McNally.

Aronson, E. (1992). The return of the repressed: Dissonance theory makes a comeback. *Psychological Inquiry, 3,* 303–311.

Aronson, J., Blanton, H., & Cooper, J. (1995). From dissonance to disidentification: Selectivity in the self-affirmation process. *Journal of Personality and Social Psychology, 68,* 986–996.

Blanton, H., Cooper, J., Skurnik, I., & Aronson, J. (1997). When bad things happen to good feedback: Exacerbating the need for self-justification with self-affirmations. *Personality and Social Psychology Bulletin, 23,* 684–692.

Brehm, J. W. (1956). Post-decision changes in desirability of alternatives. *Journal of Abnormal and Social Psychology, 52,* 384–389.

Briggs, K. C., & Myers, I. B. (1958). *Myers-Briggs Type Indicator. Form F.* Palo Alto: Consulting Psychologist Press.

Cooper, J. (1997, May). *On the motivational engines that drive dissonance: Is dissonance one motive or many?* Paper presented at the annual meeting of the Society of Personality and Social Psychology, Washington, DC.

Cooper, J., & Fazio, R. H. (1984). A new look at dissonance theory. In L. Berkowitz (Ed.), *Advances in experimental social psychology* (Vol. 17, pp. 229–266). New York: Academic Press.

Cooper, J., & Scalise, C. (1974). Dissonance produced by deviations from life styles: The interaction of Jungian typology and conformity. *Journal of Personality and Social Psychology, 29,* 566–571.

Cooper, J., & Worchel, S. (1970). Role of undesired consequences in arousing cognitive dissonance. *Journal of Personality and Social Psychology, 16,* 199–206.

Cooper, J., Zanna, M. P., & Goethals, G. R. (1974). Mistreatment of an esteemed other as a consequence affecting dissonance reduction. *Journal of Experimental Social Psychology, 10,* 224–233.

Elliot, A., & Devine, P. (1994). On the motivational nature of cognitive dissonance: Dissonance as psychological discomfort. *Journal of Personality and Social Psychology, 67*, 382–394.

Festinger, L. (1957). *A theory of cognitive dissonance.* Stanford, CA: Stanford University Press.

Festinger, L., & Carlsmith, J. M. (1959). Cognitive consequences of forced compliance. *Journal of Abnormal and Social Psychology, 59*, 203–210.

Galinsky, A., Stone, J., & Cooper, J. (1997). *The reinstatement of dissonance and psychological discomfort following failed affirmations.* Unpublished manuscript, Princeton University, Princeton, NJ.

Hoyt, M. F., Henley, M. D., & Collins, B. E. (1972). Studies in forced compliance: The confluence of choice and consequences on attitude change. *Journal of Personality and Social Psychology, 23*, 205–210.

Kunda, Z. (1990). The case for motivated reasoning. *Psychological Bulletin, 108*, 480–498.

Scher, S. J., & Cooper, J. (1989). Motivational basis of dissonance: The singular role of behavioral consequences. *Journal of Personality and Social Psychology, 56*, 899–906.

Steele, C. M. (1988). The psychology of self-affirmation: Sustaining the integrity of the self. In L. Berkowitz (Ed.), *Advances in experimental social psychology* (pp. 261–302). Hillsdale, NJ: Erlbaum.

Steele, C. M., & Liu, T. J. (1983). Dissonance processes as self-affirmation. *Journal of Personality and Social Psychology, 41*, 831–846.

Steele, C. M., Spencer, S. J., & Lynch, M. (1993). Self-image resilience and dissonance: The role of affirmational resources. *Journal of Personality and Social Psychology, 64*, 885–896.

Sullivan, H. S. (1953). *Interpersonal theory of psychiatry.* New York: Norton.

8

What Exactly Have I Done? The Role of Self-Attribute Accessibility in Dissonance

Jeff Stone

The publication of *A Theory of Cognitive Dissonance* (Festinger, 1957) introduced a rich and fascinating interplay between cognition and motivation to generations of social psychologists. As is illustrated in this volume, contemporary researchers still explore Festinger's original monograph and pull from it important insights into the human mind. At age 40, the tenets of cognitive dissonance continue to inspire new research, stir controversy, and provide a useful framework from which to understand a variety of social behavior.

This chapter focuses on what role is played by cognitions about the self in dissonance processes. In the decades since the original publication, dissonance researchers have identified at least two ways in which self-relevant thought influences responses to discrepancies between behavior and belief. The early theories proposed that cognitions about the self operated as standards or expectancies in the dissonance process (e.g., E. Aronson, 1968; E. Aronson & Carlsmith, 1962; Duval & Wick-

This chapter was prepared while I was a postdoctoral fellow at Princeton University and was supported by a Postdoctoral Award from the National Institute of Mental Health. I am now at the Department of Psychology, University of Arizona.

lund, 1972). As such, cognitions about the self were thought to serve as a measuring stick for determining the psychological meaning and significance of a given behavior. In contrast, the recent theories maintain that cognitions about the self operate as a resource for dissonance reduction. Research on self-affirmation theory (Steele, 1988) and self-evaluation maintenance (see Tesser, 1988) has shown that if people can focus on positive attributes or accomplishments, self-reflective thought will reduce the need to justify behavior (e.g., Steele & Liu, 1983; Tesser & Cornell, 1991). Thus, according to previous theory and research, cognitions about the self may serve more than one function in the process of dissonance arousal and reduction.

Less clear, however, are the conditions under which different self-functions operate in the dissonance process. Some theorists argue that the resource function of the self holds primacy over the expectancy function (e.g., Steele & Spencer, 1992). Alternatively, research indicates that there are limitations to how cognitions about the self reduce dissonance (e.g., J. Aronson, Blanton, & Cooper, 1995), and under some conditions of dissonance arousal, people may prefer to maintain specific self-attributes even when the opportunity to affirm the global self is available (e.g., Stone, Wiegand, Cooper, & Aronson, 1997). Nevertheless, the specific antecedents for these self-functions in dissonance continue to be a contemporary matter of some debate.

The research presented here was designed to shed light on the conditions under which cognitions about the self serve an expectancy versus a resource function. It seems likely that under some conditions of dissonance arousal, people can be motivated by a desire to maintain important beliefs they have about themselves (i.e., focus on *self-expectancies*). In other circumstances, people may choose to think about other positive self-attributes rather than face the implications of their behavior (i.e., focus on *self-resources*). It also seems likely that under some conditions, idiosyncratic cognitions about the self may not enter into the processing of a discrepant behavior (e.g., Cooper, 1992; Cooper & Fazio, 1984). The specific role played by the self in dissonance may depend on when and how people think about themselves in the context of having committed a discrepant act.

THE SELF AS AN EXPECTANCY IN DISSONANCE

The expectancy role of the self in dissonance derives from the self-consistency revision of dissonance theory (e.g., E. Aronson, 1968; E. Aronson & Carlsmith, 1962; see Thibodeau & Aronson, 1992). According to self-consistency theory, people hold standards for competent and moral behavior that are based on the conventional morals and prevailing values of society (Thibodeau & Aronson, 1992, p. 592). Dissonance is aroused when people perceive a discrepancy between their behavior and their personal standards for competence and morality. The reduction of dissonance is aimed at maintaining these important self-beliefs through justification of the behavior (Thibodeau & Aronson, 1992).

Self-consistency theory further proposes that dissonance is a function of what a person expects his or her behavior to reflect about the standards for competence and morality. For example, if a person did not hold very high expectations for upholding these standards, would misleading another person about the dullness of a task arouse dissonance (e.g., Festinger & Carlsmith, 1959)? From the self-consistency perspective, it would not; if a person did not expect to behave in a competent or moral fashion, misleading another person would be consistent with his or her negative expectations for competent and moral behavior. Thus, people with negative expectancies will not experience dissonance under the same conditions as people with positive expectancies for behavior. Although the consistency effect for those with negative expectancies has been difficult to replicate (e.g., Cooper & Duncan, 1971; Ward & Sandvold, 1963; see Shrauger, 1975, for a review), self-consistency theory maintains that people with negative expectancies or low self-esteem may not experience dissonance when their behavior is discrepant from socially accepted standards for conduct (e.g., E. Aronson & Carlsmith, 1962; Glass, 1964; Maracek & Mettee, 1972).

THE SELF AS A RESOURCE IN DISSONANCE

The resource role of the self derives from research on *self-affirmation* theory (Steele, 1988; see also Spencer, Josephs, & Steele, 1993) and *self-evaluation maintenance* (Tesser, 1988; Tesser & Cornell, 1991), both of which maintain that dissonance experiments typically induce participants to engage in actions that pose a threat to the self. However, unlike self-consistency theory, self-affirmation and self-evaluation maintenance theory hold that the primary goal of a dissonance-reduction strategy is to restore the positive integrity of the overall self-system. Self-reflective thought accomplishes this goal when other cherished aspects of the self become accessible (e.g., important values, Steele & Liu, 1983; positive social comparisons, Tesser & Cornell, 1991), thereby reducing psychological discomfort without addressing directly the discrepant cognitions (e.g., Stone et al., 1997).

One tenet of the self-resource function concerns the dispositional availability of positive self-attributes. For self-relevant thought to attenuate justification, people must think about more positive than negative self-attributes. This prediction was supported in an experiment by Steele, Spencer, and Lynch (1993, Experiment 2), in which participants with high and low self-esteem participated in the *free-choice* dissonance paradigm (e.g., Brehm, 1956). For some of the participants, self-attributes were brought "on-line" (i.e., primed) when they completed the Rosenberg (1979) Self-Esteem Scale before making a difficult decision between two desirable alternatives; the other participants made their decision without having their self-attributes primed. The results showed that when self-attributes were primed before the dissonant act, participants with high self-esteem did not justify their decision, whereas participants with low self-esteem showed significant justification of their decision. In the no-prime control, both groups showed similar levels of significant postdecision justification.

These data indicate that when people with high self-esteem are made to focus on their dispositional wealth of positive attributes, they may be able to avoid justification of a discrepant behavior. In comparison, people with low self-esteem, who presumably have less positive attributes available, have to justify the act to reduce their discomfort. This finding contradicts the prediction made by the expectancy theory of the self in dissonance (Thibodeau & Aronson, 1992), which maintains that people with high self-esteem are precisely the people who will be motivated to justify a discrepant act.

THE ROLE OF SELF-FOCUSED ATTENTION

What mechanisms determine whether the self serves as an expectancy versus a resource in dissonance? One important factor may be *self-focused attention*. Recall that in the decision-only control condition reported in Steele et al. (1993, Experiment 2), both self-esteem groups showed equal evidence of dissonance reduction. This suggests that when no explicit reference to the self is made in the context, most people will focus on the characteristics of the choice alternatives (e.g., Brehm, 1956; Festinger, 1957) or on the unwanted outcome produced by their decision (Cooper & Fazio, 1984). As a result, individual differences in the content and structure of the self-concept may not moderate systematically the dissonance process.

In contrast, when made to focus on the self, idiosyncratic self-attributes can become accessible and influence the way in which people perceive their behavior. In the research by Steele et al. (1993), self-esteem differences moderated postdecision justification only when idiosyncratic self-attributes were primed during the experiment. This suggests that self-focused attention may be a necessary condition for self-concept differences to moderate the dissonance that follows a difficult decision (e.g., Spencer et al., 1993).

Furthermore, once attention is directed toward the self, there may be a variety of factors that determine how self-relevant thought influences dissonance arousal and reduction. One factor suggested by the Steele et al. (1993, Experiment 2) procedure concerns the *timing* of self-focused attention, the point at which cognitions about the self enter into the dissonance process. Recall that participants in Steele et al. were asked to complete the self-prime just before the free-choice task: Self-attributes were made accessible before the difficult decision was made. However, in considering the meaning of their data, Steele et al. did not take into account the timing of the self-prime. Steele et al. (1993) concluded that because the observed self-esteem differences were opposite of the self-consistency prediction, "the cognition-to-self image inconsistency that Aronson (1968) proposed ... is not enough to arouse dissonance.... The motive for self-consistency may be absent from mental life altogether" (p. 894–895).

Another interpretation of this finding is that a cognition-to-self-image inconsistency did not occur because the procedures induced self-focused attention before participants committed the dissonant act. That is, by making self-attributes accessible before the difficult decision, the Steele et al. (1993) procedure manipulated a self-image-to-cognition temporal processing sequence. This sequence, in my view, reversed the cognition-to-self-image processing sequence implicit to the expectancy model, which assumes that the motive for self-consistency follows when people make a difficult decision, write a counterattitudinal essay, or harm an innocent victim, and then think about their personal standards for competence and morality (e.g., E. Aronson, 1992). In the Steele et al. (1993) procedure, with self-attributes accessible before behavior, it is difficult to predict what other competing dissonance processes, including the expectancy process, might have operated after dissonance arousal.

The self-expectancy approach, however, makes clear predictions about how self-attributes function when self-focused attention is induced after, rather than before, a dissonant act. According to self-affirmation theory (e.g., Steele, 1988), and based on the *self-resource flexibility* hypothesis (e.g., Steele et al., 1993), people with high self-esteem bring to mind more positive self-resources with which to reaffirm their global self-integrity. Their moment of positive self-reflection reduces dissonance and the need to justify the discrepant behavior. In contrast, for people with low self-esteem, self-focused attention brings to mind more negative self-attributes. Having fewer positive attributes available means that those with low self-esteem should be more likely to justify a discrepant act. Note that if the attributes in working self-knowledge (e.g., Markus & Wurf, 1987) serve systematically as resources for the reduction of dissonance, then making self-attributes accessible after behavior will have the same effect as when self-attributes are made accessible before behavior (e.g., Steele et al., 1993).

From the self-expectancy viewpoint, however, self-focused attention after a dissonant act could backfire on a person with high self-esteem. Specifically, if self-focused attention made self-expectancies for behavior accessible, it might increase awareness of the incompetence or immorality of the behavior (Thibodeau & Aronson, 1992). Accordingly, people with high self-esteem, having higher expectations for competent and prudent behavior, would seek more justification of their behavior. In contrast, people with low self-esteem, having less positive expectations for competent and prudent behavior, would be less likely to justify their behavior. The questionable decision would be consistent with their moderate expectancies, which would reduce the need to justify the discrepant act.

EXPERIMENT 1: THE TIMING OF SELF-FOCUSED ATTENTION

In an experiment designed to test how the timing of self-focused attention influences the role of the self in dissonance, I (see Stone, 1994) replicated the free-choice procedures reported by Steele et al. (1993, Experiment 2). The experimental design was a 2 × 3 factorial, which crossed participants' level of self-esteem (high vs. low) with the sequence of self-focused attention (before decision vs. after decision vs. a decision-only control group). The participants were 50 undergraduates, whose level of self-esteem had been measured with the Rosenberg (1979) Self-Esteem Scale during a mass pretest session. Those whose self-esteem scores fell above or below the upper (i.e., ≥ 34) and lower (i.e., ≤ 29) 30th percentile of the pretest distribution were invited to participate.

Method

Participants completed the free-choice procedures ostensibly as part of a study about the relationship between personality and preference for music. Participants examined 10 compact discs (CDs) and rated each for desirability, after which they were asked to rank order the CDs based on their preferences. After collecting their rankings, the experimenter announced that the marketing company who was sponsoring the research had decided to give participants one of the popular CDs as a bonus for participating in the research. Participants then made a choice between the two CDs they had ranked as their 4th and 5th preference.

To manipulate the timing of self-focused attention, some of the participants completed the Rosenberg Self-Esteem Scale before their initial rating of the CDs (before decision); in another condition, participants completed the Self-Esteem Scale immediately after they had made their choice (after decision); and in the no-prime control condition, participants did not complete the Self-Esteem Scale during the procedures. After the decision task and self-focus manipulation, participants completed a filler task, after which they were asked to rerate the 10 CDs for desirability. The primary dependent measure was the *spread* of alternatives, or the difference between the first and second desirability ratings for the two items offered as a bonus for participation in the study.

Results

The analysis of the postdecision ratings revealed, after I controlled for the prechoice ratings, a marginally significant Self-Esteem $\times$ Self-Focus interaction, $F(2, 44) = 2.76$, $p < .07$. First, as seen in Figure 1, the basic spreading-of-alternatives effect (e.g., Brehm, 1956) was replicated in the decision-only control condition, as participants with low self-esteem and high self-esteem showed significant justification of their decision, combined $t(44) = 3.32$, $p < .001$. In contrast, when self-focused attention was induced before the decision, participants with low self-esteem showed significantly more justification of their choice compared with participants with high self-esteem, $t(44) = 2.33$, $p < .02$, who did not alter their ratings significantly ($t < 1$). Also contributing to the interaction was the difference in the opposite direction for participants who focused on the self after the choice. Although the difference between the two self-esteem groups was not significant in itself, $t(44) < 1$, participants with high self-esteem showed significant justification of their decision, $t(44) = 2.16$, $p < .03$, whereas participants with low self-esteem did not show significant justification of their decision ($t < 1$).

The pattern of data from Experiment 1 showed support for the hypotheses that self-focused attention, and the point at which it enters into the dissonance process, can influence how cognitions about the self operate in dissonance. As predicted, self-attributes did not function

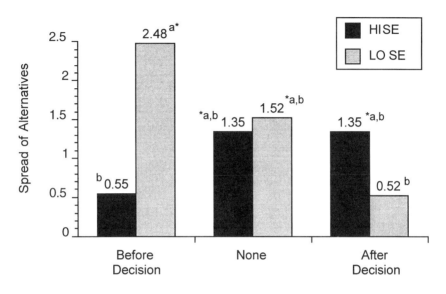

Self-focused attention

Figure 1

The effect of self-esteem and the timing of self-focused attention on the postdecision spread of alternatives. HI SE = high self-esteem; LO SE = low self-esteem. Means with different superscripts differ significantly from each other at $p < .05$. Means marked by an asterisk indicate that the spread of alternatives is significantly greater than zero at $p < .05$ for that group.

as a resource or as an expectancy unless something drew attention to them in the context of the difficult decision. In the present decision-only condition, in which self-focused attention was not induced directly, participants with high and low self-esteem showed similar levels of significant postdecision justification. This replicated the findings reported by Steele et al. (1993) and suggested that in the absence of something to focus their attention on the self, people with high and low self-esteem focused on the inconsistency inherent in the choice (e.g., Festinger, 1957) or on how their decision may have produced an unwanted outcome (Cooper & Fazio, 1984).

Under conditions of self-focused attention, self-concept differences did moderate the dissonance process, the nature of which depended on when attention was drawn to the self relative to behavior. When primed for self-attributes before the decision, participants with high self-esteem showed significantly less postdecision justification compared to those with low self-esteem. This self-concept difference also replicated that reported by Steele et al. (1993), and it suggested that when people can reflect on positive attributes before dissonance is aroused, self-focused attention may provide dispositional resources with which to buffer the onslaught of psychological discomfort.

In contrast, self-focused attention after the dissonant act did not serve a self-resource function: There was a tendency for participants with high self-esteem to show more justification of their decision compared to participants with low self-esteem. This pattern suggested that once the dissonant act occurred, self-focused attention brought self-expectancies on-line and caused participants to consider how the undesirable aspects of the decision (e.g., turning down the positive attributes of the unchosen alternative) were discrepant from their personal standards for competent and prudent behavior. These data replicated partially the pattern of self-concept differences reported in early research on the role of the self in dissonance (e.g., E. Aronson & Carlsmith, 1962; Glass, 1964; Maracek & Mettee, 1972).

Discussion

The overall pattern of data from Experiment 1 suggests that the timing of self-focused attention may be an important factor in how cognitions about the self operate in dissonance. Another factor that may influence how the self functions in dissonance is the type of self-relevant thought engaged by self-focused attention. For example, previous research on the resource function of the self shows that once dissonance is aroused, justification is attenuated when people are provided the opportunity to reflect on important values (Steele & Liu, 1983) or are provided with positive social comparisons (Tesser & Cornell, 1991). Thus, self-focused attention may induce different self-processes by way of how people think about themselves, by the nature of the self-attributes that become accessible, after a discrepant behavior. The next experiment was designed to investigate directly how different types of self-relevant thought influence the self-processes that underlie dissonance phenomena.

The Role of Self-Standards

According to the self-consistency perspective, self-expectancies operate when people perceive that their behavior is discrepant from their own personal standards for conduct (Thibodeau & Aronson, 1992). This assumption about the type of self-relevant thought necessary to invoke the self-expectancy function, however, has never been tested directly. That is, there is no direct evidence that focus on personal self-standards (as opposed to other types of standards), or focus on the specific attributes of competence and morality (as opposed to other positive self-attributes), promotes systematically the self-esteem differences predicted by the self-consistency revision of dissonance.

For example, with respect to the representation of self-standards, it may be important to consider the degree to which personal standards also represent the norms for behavior. According to the self-consistency perspective, the personal standards to which people subscribe are "culturally derived, and largely shared, by most people within a given society or subculture" (Thibodeau & Aronson, 1992, p. 596). As such, these standards may represent the expectations held by important social groups (e.g., Miller & Prentice, 1996). But if personal standards are derived from and subscribed to by most who live within a particular subculture, how can their use as a measuring stick for behavior promote subjectivity and self-concept differences in dissonance?

One answer may be that in addition to thinking about the norms for behavior, people also think about how well they typically uphold normative standards—their actual self-attribute (e.g., Higgins, 1989). Extrapolating from the tenets of self-consistency theory (e.g., E. Aronson, 1992; Thibodeau & Aronson, 1992), my colleagues and I (Stone, Cooper, Galinsky, & Kelly, 1998) proposed that self-expectancies may be represented cognitively by two elements: (a) the self-concept, an actual self-attribute for competence or morality, and (b) the normative social standards for these dimensions. Together, the representation of an actual self-attribute and normative standard form a self-expectancy, in that people expect their behavior to confirm or verify the chronic relationship between the actual self and the normative standards for competence and morality. For example, once induced to tell someone a boring task is really interesting (e.g., Festinger & Carlsmith, 1959), people may assess the competence or morality of the act by comparing their behavior (e.g., "I just said something stupid and immoral") against an idiosyncratic representation of how well they typically uphold the normative standards for these attributes (e.g., "I am usually a smart and decent person, relative to the norm for competence and morality"). The magnitude of dissonance should be a function of the perceived discrepancy between the behavioral outcome and how well people believe they uphold the norms for competent and prudent behavior.

What might distinguish people with positive versus negative expectancies for their behavior is the size of the chronic discrepancy between their actual self and the normative standards for competence and morality. The self-consistency perspective proposes that people with positive self-expectancies will experience dissonance after acts that involve deviations from the norms for "lying, advocating a position contrary to their own beliefs, or otherwise acting against one's principles" (Thibodeau & Aronson, 1992, p. 592). In our view, these actions fall outside the latitude of what people with high self-esteem are willing to accept as an accurate reflection of the self. In contrast, because their actual self lies much further from the norm, the same behavior is within the realm of what people with low self-esteem accept as self-descriptive. Consequently, the same behavior may promote different reactions from those with high and low self-esteem when it is perceived to fall within the latitude of rejection for those with high self-esteem but within the latitude of acceptance for those with low self-esteem (cf. Fazio, Zanna, & Cooper, 1977; Rhodewalt & Agustsdottir, 1986).

The key to the activation of self-expectancies, however, lies in the way in which people think about themselves after a dissonant act. The proposed model suggests that for chronic self-expectancies to moderate dissonance, the normative standard cannot be the only accessible criterion by which people determine the meaning of their behavior. In addition to the norms, an idiographically based, unique conception of the self-concept must also become accessible during the evaluation of behavior (e.g., actual self-attributes). Otherwise, if they simply focus on the norms for behavior, people with different self-expectancies may perceive the same discrepancy between their behavior and the normative standard. If idiosyncratic actual self-attributes are not also made accessible, then most people, regardless of their self-expectancies, should perceive the behavior as discrepant from the norm, and dissonance should manifest itself without self-concept moderation of the process.

It was hypothesized then that the role of the self as an expectancy in dissonance depends on the type of self-standards made salient in the context of an induced behavior. It was predicted that if self-focused attention made personal standards for behavior accessible, idiosyncratic self-expectancies would be activated, and self-esteem differences would moderate dissonance reduction. In contrast, if participants focused on normative standards for behavior after a dissonant act, it was predicted that self-concept differences would not moderate dissonance arousal and that both self-esteem groups would show evidence of dissonance reduction.

The Role of Attribute Framing

A second type of self-relevant thought that might influence the activation of different self-processes concerns how specific self-attributes frame a discrepant act. Recent work suggests that people will avoid thinking about positive self-attributes that frame an act as a negative outcome (e.g., J. Aronson et al., 1995), and when they cannot avoid exposure to self-attributes that cast a negative light on behavior, self-focused attention will increase self-justification (Blanton, Cooper, Skurnik, & Aronson, 1997). Together, these studies indicate that focus on positive aspects of the self that frame a behavior as a discrepancy exacerbates dissonance, presumably because it makes expectancies salient, whereas focus on attributes that frame the act as a positive outcome reduces dissonance, presumably through the self-resource process.

In the present decision context, if participants focus on standards for behavior that framed a difficult choice as a positive reflection of the self, the need to justify the decision might be reduced. For example, if after a difficult choice, people think about the standards for creative and flexible behavior and they perceive their decision as a reflection of these positive qualities, they may feel self-affirmed and have less need to justify their decision. In contrast, if after a difficult choice, people think about the standards for competent and rational behavior and they perceive their choice as a failure to uphold these positive attributes, dissonance will manifest itself, and they will be motivated to justify their decision. Thus, the effect of making self-standards accessible on dissonance processes may depend on the way in which the standards frame the outcome of an induced behavior.

EXPERIMENT 2: THE ACCESSIBILITY OF SELF-STANDARDS

We tested these predictions by manipulating the type of self-standards made accessible after participants had made a decision in the free-choice paradigm (Stone et al., 1998). The overall design of this experiment was a 2 (self-esteem: high vs. low) × 2 (standards perspective: personal vs. normative) × 2 (attribute frame: positive vs. negative) factorial, with a decision-only external-control condition that included both self-esteem groups. Participants were 89 undergraduates, 45 with low and 44 with high self-esteem, as determined by the same percentile scores on the Rosenberg Self-Esteem Scale as used in the previous experiment.

Method

The free-choice procedures were also a conceptual replication of the first experiment, with two important exceptions. First, instead of music CDs, participants were asked to make a choice between two psychology studies to participate in for partial course credit. Participants were told that to get a full hour of credit for participation, they would have to participate in two short but unrelated studies. The first study was described as a survey for the psychology department, who were interested in the types of studies in which students liked to participate. The experimenter noted that they were also interested in the relationship between personality and preference for certain types of psychology research. Participants were told that once they had completed the survey, the experimenter would make arrangements for them to participate in another short study, which set the stage for the decision they would make during the experiment.

Second, instead of using their rankings of the alternatives, participants were offered a choice between alternatives that they had rated as similar in desirability on the first rating task (e.g., Brehm, 1956). Participants read a short description of 10 different psychology studies and were instructed to rate the desirability of participating in each type of research. After the ratings, participants ranked their preferences, during which the experimenter covertly examined their initial ratings to identify two studies rated similar in desirability (i.e., approximately 7 on a 9-point scale). Once the ranking task was complete, the experimenter announced that there were two other studies currently under way, either of which participants could use to finish their hour of credit. He then presented participants with the descriptions of the two studies they had rated as similar in desirability. Once they had indicated their preference, the experimenter introduced them to the personality measure, which served as the self-standard priming manipulations.

To measure self-understanding, the experimenter explained that he was collecting people's perceptions of various attributes. To measure their perceptions, participants were asked to write a short paragraph describing a target person on two trait dimensions. To manipulate the framing of the standards, participants in the negative-frame condition wrote about a person who exemplified the attributes of *competent* and *rational*; participants in the positive-frame condition wrote about a person who exemplified the attributes of *creative* and *flexible*.

To manipulate the perspective for each standard, participants in the personal-standpoint condition were instructed to describe the target person using their own personal standards for each trait. Participants in the normative-standpoint condition were directed to think about the standards from a societal perspective and to describe the target using the standards that most people apply to the target attributes. Once they had completed the self-standard priming task, participants were asked to complete a filler task, after which the experimenter asked them to rate the psychology studies again for desirability. The difference between the first and second ratings of the choice alternatives served as the primary dependent measure.

Results

As seen in Figure 2, a simple effects analysis of the decision-only external-control condition revealed that participants with high and low self-esteem showed significant levels of postdecision justification, combined $t(62) = 3.38$, $p < .001$, and the difference between these groups was not significant ($t < 1$). This indicates that by itself, the choice

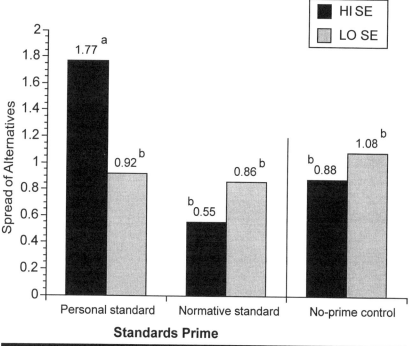

Figure 2

The means for the decision-only control group and the interaction between self-esteem and the perspective from which participants viewed their behavior on the postdecision spread of alternatives. HI SE = high self-esteem; LO SE = low self-esteem. Means with different superscripts differ significantly at $p < .05$. Note that all spread scores are significantly greater than zero at $p < .05$.

between psychology studies induced postdecision dissonance for participants in both self-esteem groups.

Analysis of the self-standard priming conditions revealed a significant main effect for the perspective prime, $F(1, 62) = 5.30$, $p < .02$, and a significant Self-Esteem × Perspective Prime interaction, $F(1, 62) = 4.48$, $p < .03$. The means in Figure 2 show that when primed to consider how their decision was discrepant from their own personal standards, participants with high self-esteem reported significantly more postdecision justification compared to the justification reported by participants with low self-esteem, $t(62) = 2.21$, $p < 03$. The level of justification was significant for both high and low self-esteem groups, test for significance from zero, $t(62) = 6.32$, $p < .0001$, and $t(62) = 3.41$, $p < .001$, respectively. In contrast, when primed to consider how their decision was discrepant from normative standards, participants with high and low self-esteem showed significant levels of postdecision justification, combined $t(62) = 3.50$, $p < .001$, and there was no difference between the groups ($t < 1$). Thus, as predicted, the accessibility of personal self-standards after the choice promoted a self-expectancy effect, whereas the accessibility of normative standards did not promote self-esteem differences in the level of postdecision dissonance.

The three-way interaction did not approach significance, $F(1, 62) < 1$, ns, indicating that the predicted effect of self-standards was not moderated by the specific type of self-attributes made accessible after the difficult decision. The Perspective × Relevance interaction, however, was marginally significant, $F(1, 62) = 2.97$, $p < .09$, revealing that when participants with high and low self-esteem viewed their decision from a normative perspective and thought of it as reflecting creativity and flexibility, they did not show significant justification of their choices ($M = 0.25$, test for significance from zero), $t(62) < 1$. Although the interaction did not reach conventional levels of significance, it might have implications for the type of self-relevant thought that is necessary for affirmation processes to operate (e.g., J. Aronson et al., 1995; Blanton et al., 1997). Specifically, it suggests that focus on irrelevant self-standards may reduce the need to justify behavior, but perhaps only if the standards are viewed from a normative perspective.

GENERAL DISCUSSION

The results of these experiments begin to shed light on the circumstances under which cognitions about the self function as an expectancy versus a resource in the dissonance process. It is clear from these data that there is not one master role for the self in the dissonance process. Instead, the specific role played by the self in dissonance depends on when self-focused attention occurs in temporal relation to behavior and also on the type of self-attributes that become accessible when attention is focused on the self.

When Does the Self Function as an Expectancy in Dissonance?

Both experiments produced self-esteem differences that reflected the self-expectancy function of the self in dissonance, a phenomenon that has proved difficult to replicate (e.g., Ward & Sandvold, 1963; see Shrauger, 1975). When attention was focused on the self after the difficult choice and, specifically, when attention was focused on personal self-standards, participants with high self-esteem showed more decision justification compared with participants with low self-esteem. This form of self-esteem moderation supports the predictions made by the self-consistency revision of dissonance (Thibodeau & Aronson, 1992), which maintains that having high self-esteem promotes *fragility*, or more need to justify behavior, whereas having low self-esteem promotes *flexibility*, or less need to resolve dissonance.

One caveat to a self-consistency interpretation of the self-esteem difference observed in the personal-standards priming condition of the second experiment is that relative to the effect for self-focused attention after behavior in Experiment 1, it did not completely attenuate self-justification among participants with low self-esteem. Relative to other types of self-focused attention, focus on self-standards in the context of a dissonant act may generally maintain the salience of the discrepancy and the magnitude of the psychological discomfort for most people (e.g., Blanton et al., 1997). However, the data indicate that when the standards were framed as personal, participants also engaged their idiosyncratic expectancies, which produced an increase in dissonance for those with high self-esteem but no increase for those with low self-esteem. Thus, focus on self-standards in the context of a dissonant act may promote dissonance for most people, but in addition, idiosyncratic expectancies can moderate the magnitude of dissonance when people view the standards from their own personal standpoint.

This interpretation suggests that when people focus on personal self-attributes that do not represent self-standards, self-focused attention could engage the expectancy function without increasing the overall magnitude of dissonance. Some evidence for this hypothesis comes from a pilot experiment (Kelly, Stone, & Cooper, 1996) in which participants with high and low self-esteem made a difficult decision and were then induced to list traits that described their actual self-attributes (see, e.g., Higgins, Klein, & Strauman, 1985). The effect of this actual self-prime replicated the self-expectancy pattern observed for self-focused attention after behavior in Experiment 1. Specifically, participants with high self-esteem showed significant justification of the decision ($M = 1.99$), whereas participants with low self-esteem did not show significant justification of their decision ($M = 0.29$), and the difference in the postdecision justification between these groups was significant, $t(12) = 2.53$, $p < 01$. Moreover, analysis of the valence of the actual self-attributes (e.g., Anderson, 1968) showed that the traits listed by participants with high self-esteem were significantly more positive ($M = 3.93$) than the traits listed by participants with low self-esteem ($M = 3.43$), $t(12) = 2.14$, $p < .05$. Together, the justification and valence data provide preliminary but encouraging support for the model presented earlier to account for the self-expectancy effect. Specifically, they show relatively direct evidence that the accessibility of dispositionally positive actual self-attributes facilitates dissonance for people with high self-esteem, whereas the accessibility of dispositionally less positive self-attributes reduces dissonance among people with low self-esteem.

In summary, the research presented here provides sufficient evidence to suggest that under some conditions of dissonance arousal, possessing high self-esteem creates more fragility than flexibility in response to discrepancies between behavior and belief (e.g., Thibodeau

& Aronson, 1992). The role of the self as an expectancy appears to be an important aspect of dissonance phenomena, and it may play a more important role in mental life than has been suggested elsewhere (e.g., Steele et al., 1993).

When Does the Self Function as a Resource?

Recent work on self-affirmation theory (Steele, 1988) and self-evaluation maintenance processes (e.g., Tesser & Cornell, 1991) shows that self-focused attention can provide people with resources by which to reduce dissonance. It is therefore somewhat striking that in the current research, despite the number of conditions in which people focused on self-attributes, the self-resource flexibility hypothesis (e.g., Steele et al., 1993) was supported only when self-focused attention occurred before the dissonant act in the first experiment. This indicates that self-focused attention before committing a dissonant behavior promotes flexibility among people with high self-esteem, but it is unclear how self-focused attention affects the dissonance process in this way. For example, bringing to mind positive self-attributes, such as through feedback from others (e.g., Heine & Lehman, 1997; Steele et al., 1993) or through the completion of a self-evaluative scale, may motivate people with high self-esteem to bias their perceptions and attributions about the outcome of subsequent behavior (see, e.g., Blaine & Crocker, 1993). If so, then focusing on positive self-attributes before a dissonant act may prevent the arousal of dissonance rather than assisting in its reduction (e.g., Steele et al., 1993). In the light of the recent work suggesting that affirmation effects may operate through trivialization processes (e.g., Simon, Greenberg, & Brehm, 1995) or through the reduction of negative affect (e.g., Galinsky, Stone, & Cooper, 1998), more research is needed to understand how the accessibility of self-attributes, before and after behavior, attenuates cognitive dissonance processes.

Taking a Fresh Look at an Old Debate

Finally, the current set of studies may have implications for the debate between two contemporary revisions of dissonance theory, the self-consistency revision (E. Aronson, 1968; Thibodeau & Aronson, 1992) and the new look, or aversive-consequences, revision (Cooper & Fazio, 1984). These two perspectives on dissonance share many common assumptions, for example, both accept that dissonance is a state of psychological discomfort that follows from a discrepancy between behavior and a preexisting set of cognitions. Where they appear to differ most is in their assumptions about the role played by idiosyncratic views of the self. Specifically, whereas self-consistency has argued that dissonance is a subjective matter and depends on the idiosyncratic content of the actor's self-concept (Thibodeau & Aronson, 1992), the new look has argued that idiosyncratic representations of the self are not relevant to the assessment of an aversive outcome (e.g., Cooper & Fazio, 1984; see Cooper, 1992). The current set of studies may offer one means by which to synthesize these perspectives on cognitive dissonance phenomena (e.g., Berkowitz & Devine, 1989).

First, as noted above, when people commit a discrepant act, they may not systematically engage idiosyncratic views of the self in the process. In the decision-only control conditions from both experiments, participants with different self-concepts were equally motivated to justify their behavior, perhaps because both groups were focused on the inconsistency inherent in the decision itself (e.g., Festinger, 1957) or on the unwanted consequences of giving up the positive aspects of the unchosen alternative (e.g., Cooper & Fazio, 1984). The significant dissonance reduction observed in both self-esteem groups suggests that for idiosyncratic self-knowledge to moderate dissonance, something in the context may need to draw attention to the self. Otherwise, people with different underlying self-knowledge appear to operate on the same information and draw the same conclusion about the psychological meaning of their behavior (cf. Cooper, 1992; Cooper & Fazio, 1984).

However, if something in the context makes salient the relevance of a decision to self-evaluation, then people may bring their personal self-attributes on-line. According to the self-consistency revision of dissonance, people determine the meaning of their behavior by comparing it against idiosyncratic self-standards for competent and moral conduct (e.g., Thibodeau & Aronson, 1992). To the degree the behavior is perceived as inconsistent, or as falling outside of what they had expected, dissonance is aroused. It appears that self-concept differences can moderate the dissonance process, but perhaps only when people use their own, personal self-expectancies to determine the psychological meaning and significance of their behavior.

The new look model (Cooper & Fazio, 1984), on the other hand, suggests a more shared or normative view of the information people rely on to assess a behavioral outcome. Although Cooper and Fazio (1984) did not discuss directly the process by which people judge the aversiveness of a behavioral outcome, they did suggest that dissonance arousal can be viewed as a conditioned emotional response learned early in childhood: "Being responsible for some negative consequences leaves [a child] open to some form of negative sanctions from parents and/or peers.... Given a sufficient number of such experiences, an association is apt to develop between personally producing negative effects and arousal" (p. 244). According to the new look model then, dissonance is aroused when assessment of an unwanted behavioral outcome implies negative sanctions from others.

In the second experiment reported above, when they focused on self-standards from a normative perspective, participants with both high and low self-esteem showed significant decision justification. This finding supports the new look assumption that if the outcome of a behavior is viewed from the standpoint of others (e.g., one's parents or peers), most people, regardless of their idiosyncratic expectancies, will perceive a discrepancy and be motivated to justify their actions. Self-concept differences, then, may not moderate the dissonance process when people rely on normative or shared standards to determine the quality of a behavioral outcome.

If we view the role of the self in dissonance as a function of the context, it is no longer a question of whether personal self-attributes or normative sanctions are the predominant cognitions. Instead, we should ask, how are people thinking about what they have done? To the degree that self-attributes are accessible, differences in the content and structure of the self may cause them to interpret their behavior in terms of personal expectancies for behavior. This may lead different people to different conclusions about what they have done. The accessibility of more shared or normative information, in contrast, may cause people to think about what they have done from the perspective of others. This, in turn, may lead different people to the same conclusion about what they have done. Thus, how people evaluate and interpret a discrepant act, and the specific nature of dissonance motivation, can be a function of qualitatively different processes, the activation of which may depend on the information made accessible in the context of an unwanted behavior.

REFERENCES

Anderson, N. H. (1968). Likableness ratings of 555 personality-trait words. *Journal of Personality and Social Psychology, 9,* 272–279.

Aronson, E. (1968). Dissonance theory: Progress and problems. In R. Abelson, E. Aronson, W. McGuire, T. Newcomb, M. Rosenberg, & P. Tannenbaum (Eds.), *Theories of cognitive consistency: A sourcebook* (pp. 5–27). Chicago: Rand McNally.

Aronson, E. (1992). The return of the repressed: Dissonance theory makes a comeback. *Psychological Inquiry, 3,* 303–311.

Aronson, E., & Carlsmith, J. M. (1962). Performance expectancy as a determinant of actual performance. *Journal of Abnormal and Social Psychology, 65,* 178–182.

Aronson, J., Blanton, H., & Cooper, J. (1995). From dissonance to disidentification: Selectivity in the self-affirmation process. *Journal of Personality and Social Psychology, 68,* 986–996.

Berkowitz, L., & Devine, P. G. (1989). Research traditions, analysis, and synthesis in social psychological theories: The case of dissonance theory. *Personality and Social Psychology Bulletin, 15,* 493–507.

Blaine, B., & Crocker, J. (1993). Self-esteem and self-serving biases in reactions to positive and negative events: An integrative review. In R. F. Baumeister (Ed.), *The puzzle of low self-regard* (pp. 55–85). New York: Plenum.

Blanton, H., Cooper, J., Skurnik, I., & Aronson, J. (1997). When bad things happen to good feedback: Exacerbating the need for self-justification with self-affirmations. *Personality and Social Psychology Bulletin, 23,* 684–692.

Brehm, J. W. (1956). Postdecision changes in the desirability of alternatives. *Journal of Abnormal and Social Psychology, 52,* 384–389.

Cooper, J. (1992). Dissonance and the return of the self-concept. *Psychological Inquiry, 3,* 320–323.

Cooper, J., & Duncan, B. L. (1971). Cognitive dissonance as a function of self-esteem and logical inconsistency. *Journal of Personality, 39,* 289–302.

Cooper, J., & Fazio, R. H. (1984). A new look at dissonance theory. In L. Berkowitz (Ed.), *Advances in experimental social psychology* (Vol. 17, pp. 229–262). Hillsdale, NJ: Erlbaum.

Duval, S., & Wicklund, R. A. (1972). *A theory of objective self-awareness.* New York: Academic Press.

Fazio, R. H., Zanna, M. P., & Cooper, J. (1977). Dissonance and self-perception: An integrative view of each theory's proper domain of application. *Journal of Experimental Social Psychology, 13,* 464–479.

Festinger, L. (1957). *A theory of cognitive dissonance.* Stanford, CA: Stanford University Press.

Festinger, L., & Carlsmith, J. M. (1959). Cognitive consequences of forced compliance. *Journal of Abnormal and Social Psychology, 58,* 203–210.

Galinsky, A., Stone, J., & Cooper, J. (1998). *The reinstatement of dissonance and psychological discomfort following failed affirmations.* Manuscript submitted for publication.

Glass, D. (1964). Changes in liking as a means of reducing cognitive discrepancies between self-esteem and aggression. *Journal of Personality, 32,* 531–549.

Heine, S. J., & Lehman, D. R. (1997). Culture, dissonance, and self-affirmation. *Personality and Social Psychology Bulletin, 23,* 389–400.

Higgins, E. T. (1989). Self-discrepancy theory: What patterns of self-beliefs cause people to suffer? In L. Berkowitz (Ed.), *Advances in experimental social psychology* (pp. 93–136). Hillsdale, NJ: Erlbaum.

Higgins, E. T., Klein, R., & Strauman, T. (1985). Self-concept discrepancy theory: A psychological model for distinguishing among different aspects of depression and anxiety. *Social Cognition, 3,* 51–76.

Kelly, K. A., Stone, J., & Cooper, J. (1996, March). *The role of self-attributes in dissonance arousal and reduction.* Paper presented at the 67th Eastern Psychological Association Conference, Philadelphia.

Maracek, J., & Mettee, D. (1972). Avoidance of continued success as a function of self-esteem, level of esteem certainty, and responsibility for success. *Journal of Personality and Social Psychology, 22*, 98–107.

Markus, H., & Wurf, E. (1987). The dynamic self-concept: A social-psychological perspective. In M. R. Rosenberg & L. W. Porter (Eds.), *Annual review of psychology* (pp. 299–337). Palo Alto, CA: Annual Reviews.

Miller, D. T., & Prentice, D. A. (1996). The construction of social norms and standards. In E. T. Higgins & A. W. Kruglanski (Eds.), *Social psychology: Handbook of basic principles* (pp. 799–829). New York: Guilford Press.

Rhodewalt, F., & Agustsdottir, S. (1986). Effects of self-presentation on the phenomenal self. *Journal of Personality and Social Psychology, 50*, 47–55.

Rosenberg, M. (1979). *Conceiving the self.* New York: Basic Books.

Shrauger, J. S. (1975). Responses to evaluation as a function of initial self-perceptions. *Psychological Bulletin, 82*, 581–596.

Simon, L., Greenberg, J., & Brehm, J. (1995). Trivialization: The forgotten mode of dissonance reduction. *Journal of Personality and Social Psychology, 68*, 247–260.

Spencer, S. J., Josephs, R. A., & Steele, C. M. (1993). Low self-esteem: The uphill struggle for self-integrity. In R. Baumeister (Ed.), *Self-esteem: The puzzle of low self-regard* (pp. 21–36). New York: Plenum.

Steele, C. M. (1988). The psychology of self-affirmation: Sustaining the integrity of the self. In L. Berkowitz (Ed.), *Advances in experimental social psychology* (Vol. 21, pp. 261–302). Hillsdale, NJ: Erlbaum.

Steele, C. M., & Liu, T. J. (1983). Dissonance processes as self-affirmation. *Journal of Personality and Social Psychology, 45*, 5–19.

Steele, C. M., & Spencer, S. J. (1992). The primacy of self-integrity. *Psychological Inquiry, 3*, 345–346.

Steele, C. M., Spencer, S. J., & Lynch, M. (1993). Dissonance and affirmational resources: Resilience against self-image threats. *Journal of Personality and Social Psychology, 64*, 885–896.

Stone, J. (1994). *Self-esteem, self-accessibility, and reconsidering one's alternatives: Examining the temporal sequences in post-decision dissonance.* Unpublished doctoral dissertation, University of California, Santa Cruz.

Stone, J., Cooper, J., Galinsky, A., & Kelly, K. (1998). *Self-attribute accessibility in dissonance: The mirror has many faces.* Manuscript in preparation.

Stone, J., Wiegand, A. W., Cooper, J., & Aronson, E. (1997). When exemplification fails: Hypocrisy and the motive for self-integrity. *Journal of Personality and Social Psychology, 72,* 54–65.

Tesser, A. (1988). Toward a self-evaluation maintenance model of social behavior. In L. Berkowitz (Ed.), *Advances in experimental social psychology* (pp. 181–228). New York: Academic Press.

Tesser, A., & Cornell, D. P. (1991). On the confluence of self processes. *Journal of Experimental Social Psychology, 27,* 501–526.

Thibodeau, R., & Aronson, E. (1992). Taking a closer look: Reasserting the role of the self-concept in dissonance theory. *Personality and Social Psychology Bulletin, 18,* 591–602.

Ward, W. D., & Sandvold, K. D. (1963). Performance expectancy as a determinant of actual performance: A partial replication. *Journal of Abnormal and Social Psychology, 67,* 293–295.

9

A Self-Accountability Model of Dissonance Reduction: Multiple Modes on a Continuum of Elaboration

Michael R. Leippe and Donna Eisenstadt

A ttitude-discrepant behavior and the cognitive dissonance aroused by it are common, daily experiences (cf. E. Aronson, 1968). It is important, therefore, to reach a fuller understanding of how people deal with the dissonance aroused under the varying conditions in their day-to-day lives while maintaining stable identities and attitude systems. What modes of dissonance reduction are used, and what qualities of the person and the situation determine which mode is used when? Curiously, 40 years of cognitive dissonance research has shed relatively little light on these questions of dissonance reduction, largely because, until recently, researchers have been occupied primarily with identifying the conditions necessary for dissonance arousal (cf. Elliot & Devine, 1994; Kunda, 1990). In this chapter, we describe a model that focuses on the situational and intrapsychic factors that promote certain cognitive processes over others in the service of dissonance reduction. We then describe several experiments that have examined dissonance reduction and attempt to integrate relevant findings from the dissonance experiments of other investigators.

DISSONANCE AND DISSONANCE REDUCTION: A SELF-ACCOUNTABILITY MODEL

Festinger's (1957) original formulation has been modified a number of times (e.g., E. Aronson, 1969; Brehm & Cohen, 1962; Cooper & Fazio, 1984; Greenwald & Ronis, 1978; Tedeschi, Schlenker, & Bonoma, 1971). The present model of dissonance is a variant of reformulations that emphasize the centrality of the self (E. Aronson, 1969; Schlenker, 1982, 1986; Steele, 1988). Specifically, we define *dissonance* as the psychological distress that occurs when some aspect of one's behavior threatens one's sense of self-integrity. Inconsistencies, such as those entailed in the counterattitudinal behavior associated with induced compliance, normally arouse dissonance because they implicate the self. In keeping with Schlenker's (1982) identity-analytic model, self-inconsistencies draw the individual's attention to some aspect of the self that may be seen as undesirable by either oneself (private self) or others (public self). In turn, genuine cognitive and attitudinal changes may occur that allow the individual to restore an internal perception of self-integrity. In effect, our perspective is that dissonance is created whenever an individual feels *accountable* for a self-discrepant behavior, either to internal standards (private self-accountability, e.g., as aroused by the perception that one freely chose to engage in the behavior or by its aversive consequences) or to others (public self-accountability, e.g., as aroused by the perception that one's reputation with an identifiable public might be damaged). To feel accountable, following Tetlock (1983), is to believe that one's actions (attitude-discrepant actions, in this case) require explanation.

The Magnitude of Dissonance

Festinger (1957) maintained that the magnitude of dissonance is a function of (a) the importance of the dissonant cognitive elements and (b) the number of dissonant (vs. consonant) elements. Both factors can be defined in terms of self-accountability. Most contemporary conceptualizations of attitude importance at least partly define it in terms of connectedness to some aspect of self-definition: self-interest, reference-group identification (i.e., the collective self), or self-defining values (Boninger, Krosnick, Berent, & Fabrigar, 1995). Thus, a cognitive element is important to the extent that it is relevant, critical, or central to one's self-definition, so that removing it or challenging it threatens that self-definition and creates self-accountability. The more self-relevant a cognitive element is, moreover, the more likely it is to have ties to personal values and worldviews, to knowledge about oneself, and to numerous related attitudes (see, e.g, Higgins & King, 1981; Judd & Krosnick, 1989). It follows that a dissonant cognition will be dissonant with a greater number of other cognitive elements, the more relevant it is to the self.

Modes of Dissonance Reduction

Consider the induced-compliance situation in which people behave in a fashion that contradicts their specific attitude. For example, a college student who opposes a tuition increase might comply with a request to write an essay endorsing an increase, ostensibly to be submitted to a university office considering tuition matters. Festinger (1957) identified three modes of reducing the dissonance this counterattitudinal behavior would create. One mode of dissonance reduction is to change one of the two conflicting cognitions (i.e., the original attitude and knowledge of the behavior). Attitude is the more likely to be altered (e.g., the student becomes more in favor of a tuition hike), as reality constraints usually preclude denying the behavior. A second mode is to add cognitions (e.g., perceptions of low choice or high reward) that allow the self-discrepancy to be seen as consistent within a larger framework (e.g., the student claims he or she was coerced to write the essay). Finally, the subjective importance of either the behavior or the attitude can be reduced (e.g., the student believes any tuition hike will be small), a *trivialization* mode of reduction (Simon, Greenberg, & Brehm, 1995).

Each of these three modes of dissonance reduction, under some circumstances, could suffice by itself to reduce dissonance. Furthermore, each, under some circumstances, could involve simply a clean *categorical change* of a single cognitive element. One could, for example, change one's attitude after induced compliance and be done with it. In some situations, however, a single cognitive alteration might not suffice to reduce dissonance. Instead, dissonance might be reduced by a more complicated *cognitive restructuring* (Hardyck & Kardush, 1968), which refers to changing at least one cognition other than the immediately conflicting ones. Restructuring could involve bringing a number of related cognitive elements into a new integration by altering each of them slightly. Or it could involve applying multiple modes of dissonance reduction to the same self-discrepancy (e.g., trivialization and attitude change). Cognitive restructuring could be compelled by any of several factors. First, the focal cognitive elements might both be sufficiently important to self-image that the person can let neither element go or render them consonant by any single rationalization. Second, a categorical change in one cognition may make that element inconsistent, in a self-threatening way, with a cognition that was not initially implicated in the focal inconsistency. Festinger recognized that "that in the process of trying to reduce dissonance, it might even be increased" (1957, pp. 23–24). Finally, although superficially specific and seemingly unimportant, many attitudes are plugged in to large, complex, and possibly self-defining attitude and belief systems (cf. Pratkanis & Greenwald, 1989). Accordingly, under some circumstances, cognitive activity in the service of dissonance reduction may *spontaneously activate* related cognitions within the attitude system, which might then require adjustment if they proved dissonant with the new order.

Hardyck and Kardush (1968) saw multiple-adjustment cognitive restructuring as especially likely when the inconsistent cognitions are sufficiently important that one cannot be abandoned or changed in a superficial way. They made the reasonable assumption that restructuring requires more effort, thus more dissonance motivation, than categorical change. Hardyck and Kardush noted also that dissonance might be reduced, or at least removed, with less effort than that required for categorical change. People simply might *passively forget* about or cease attending to a dissonance-arousing inconsistency.

Arranged in order from passive forgetting to categorical change to cognitive restructuring, these summary modes of dissonance reduction fall on a dimension of *amount of elaboration* much like Petty and Cacioppo (1986) have described in their elaboration-likelihood model of persuasion. When exposed to a persuasive communication, recipients may give it little thought and base their attitude response on some cue such as source credibility. At the other extreme, they may carefully scrutinize the message's arguments and relate them to their own ideas and knowledge. Research indicates that amount of elaboration depends on the recipient's motivation and ability to elaborate (Chaiken, Liberman, & Eagly, 1989; Petty & Cacioppo, 1986). These same factors also may determine how elaborate a dissonance-reduction strategy is used by a "recipient" of induced compliance.

Motivation to elaborate is a positive function of the personal relevance and importance of a message issue (e.g., Petty & Cacioppo, 1986; Thomsen, Borgida, & Lavine, 1995). Similarly with dissonance, the importance of the dissonant cognitions, a prime determinant of the magnitude of dissonance, may also be positively related to the elaborateness of dissonance reduction. This relationship also follows from consideration of the proposed basis of dissonance, namely, self-accountability. There is strong evidence that accountability (e.g., expecting to explain one's attitude publicly) increases cognitive effort, compelling people to think more complexly and hence to develop more sophisticated and integrative attitude positions (e.g., Tetlock, 1983). And when people feel accountable to themselves (on personal matters), their close scrutiny is engaged (cf. Greenwald, 1982).

In persuasion, ability to elaborate can be reduced or enhanced by person (e.g., knowledgeability) and situational (e.g., distraction) factors. The research presented in this chapter is concerned mainly with motivational influences on dissonance reduction. Note, however, that akin to the magnitude of persuasive-message processing, ability-relevant qualities may influence the magnitude of cognitive elaboration in the service of dissonance reduction. Intrapsychically, elaborate cognitive restructuring seems more likely when the issue surrounded by dissonance is embedded in a large network of knowledge, beliefs, and feelings. Situationally, distraction (Zanna & Aziza, 1976) and time pressure may limit ability for dissonance reduction to extend beyond a categorical shift.

The motivation-relevant (e.g., importance) and ability-relevant (e.g., connectedness to knowledge–belief structures) factors that influence mode of dissonance reduction are, in some cases, the same factors postulated to influence the magnitude of dissonance. In part because of this, the magnitude of dissonance and the elaborateness of reduction mode typically will be positively related, but not necessarily so. For example, a tremendous amount of dissonance could be created if individuals were induced to support a counterattitudinal policy that was personally costly and thus objectionable but essentially unconnected to many other cognitions of any significance. Considerable attitude change might occur (because the magnitude of dissonance was great), but there would be little cognitive restructuring beyond that (because the attitude and the behavioral endorsement were isolated from the larger cognitive system).

Alternatively, individuals could be induced to endorse a counterattitudinal policy that was not especially personally important, yet something in the situation made the self-discrepancy salient and encouraged rumination that activated normally weak connections to other cognitions. Here, despite the low dissonance magnitude, some cognitive restructuring might occur.

Intrapsychic and Situational Determinants of Dissonance-Reduction Mode

The preceding discussion highlights intrapsychic qualities such as issue importance, self-definition, and the connectedness of the larger attitude system. What are the situational factors that influence dissonance reduction? The social context during and after induced compliance may heighten the salience of the attitude-discrepant behavior's implications for self-integrity and thus increase the sense of accountability. Accountability to self should be heightened by a direct query about one's attitude relevant to induced behavior. An attitude query, which is almost always present in induced-compliance research, should bring to mind the fact that one's most recent behavior does not jibe with preexisting beliefs or ideas. The magnitude of dissonance should increase. At the same time, the attitude query may also make salient a specific mode of dissonance reduction: categorical attitude change. Confronted with both opportunity and pressure to reduce dissonance through attitude change, people may do so. If they can fully or sufficiently do so, there is little likelihood of further cognitive restructuring. In general, any stimulus that reminds people of their attitude-discrepant behavior should increase accountability to self and hence dissonance. If the stimulus also suggests a categorical, one-change mode of dissonance reduction, the likelihood of that categorical change should increase, with a corresponding decrease in restructuring.

A factor that should enhance accountability to others is the publicity of the attitude-discrepant act (Baumeister & Tice, 1984). If the "glare of publicity" is ongoing (e.g., the audience continues to be implicitly or explicitly present), cognitive restructuring is likely to the extent that the publicity keeps the person in a state of self-awareness that encourages rumination involving comparisons of the current self with public-self and private-self standards (e.g., Eisenstadt & Leippe, 1994; Hass & Eisenstadt, 1990; Wicklund, 1975).

STUDIES OF DISSONANCE REDUCTION (AND OTHER MATTERS)

Experiment 1: Situational Influences on Dissonance Reduction Regarding a Trivial Matter

The effect of two situational variables, publicity and the immediacy of an attitude query, on how dissonance is reduced were examined in an experiment by Leippe and Elkin (1992). In this experiment, the likelihood of internal motivation to put effort into elaborate dissonance reduction was kept low by inducing counterattitudinal behavior relevant to a rather trivial attitude issue.

Method

College students ($n = 75$) wrote a counterattitudinal essay supporting the imposition of a small student parking fee at their university. Before doing so, these students had completed a campus issues survey, in which a question was embedded regarding their attitude toward a campus parking fee. Responses to this question confirmed that the parking fee was extremely counterattitudinal ($M = 2.08$ on a 31-point scale ranging from 1 [*disagree*] to 31 [*agree*]. Participants were informed that the study involved a survey for the university administration, which was considering the parking fee and collecting arguments (essays) from students on both sides of the issue. Participants in a low-choice control condition were told they had been assigned to write a pro-parking fee essay. (As noted earlier, dissonance and the sense of self-accountability are assumed to be relatively weak when people perceive they have little choice but to do a behavior.) The rest were told that enough anti essays had been collected. While asserting the voluntary nature of their choice of which side to endorse, the experimenter noted that the administration committee now needed "strong, forceful essays in support of parking fees." In addition, high-choice participants signed (or checkmarked) a release form attesting to their free will in choosing their essay endorsement and knowledge of possible aversive consequences (i.e., their essay would go to a policymaking committee).

Publicity was manipulated by a series of directed behaviors. Participants randomly assigned to the high-publicity condition were asked to sign and place their phone numbers on the release form. Later, they also signed their essays and handed them (and also their postessay attitude responses) unconcealed to the experimenter. In contrast, participants in the low-publicity condition merely checked a space on the release form, were explicitly asked not to write their names anywhere, and sealed their essays and attitude responses in envelopes. Crossed with publicity was the timing of the attitude query. After writing their essay, participants indicated their agreement with the parking fee proposal (on a 31-point scale that was identical to the embedded preessay attitude item). Participants in the immediate-assessment condition responded to the attitude query immediately after completion of their essay. Then they had a 15-min break, during which they sat in their cubicle while the experimenter was ostensibly attending to another participant. After this break, immediate-assessment participants wrote a second essay concerning parking fees. Delayed-assessment participants, in contrast, first (after their initial essay) took a 15-min break. Half of the delayed-assessment participants then wrote a second essay before responding to the attitude query, whereas the other half went directly to the attitude query after their break.

By means of procedures described by Tetlock (1983), the second essays were scored for cognitive complexity. In general, cognitive complexity is defined as a positive function of differentiation (essentially, the number of characteristics of the issue taken into account) and integration (essentially, the extent of connections made among considered characteristics). We assumed that a more cognitively complex post-dissonance-arousal essay about parking fees would be the end result of rumination involving cognitive restructuring activities such as forming, modifying, and integrating multiple issue-related ideas, beliefs, and attitudes. Raters trained to identify differentiation and integration read and scored the second essays on a descriptively anchored scale that ranged from 1 (low differentiation and low integration) to 7 (high differentiation and high integration) with intervening points referring to combinations of the two properties in low, moderate, or high amounts.

Results and Discussion

It was expected that there would be more cognitive restructuring when publicity was high, especially when attitude assessment, the cue to the "easy" dissonance-reduction mode of attitude change, was withheld for 15 min. When publicity was low, less restructuring was expected regardless of assessment timing. Delayed assessment, instead, was expected to make it less likely that any active dissonance reduction would occur. For the most part, these predictions were confirmed. As can be seen in Figure 1, whereas high-publicity participants evinced significant and considerable attitude change whether assessment was immediate or delayed, low-publicity participants changed their attitude only if their attitude was immediately assessed. In addition, high-publicity participants' second essays revealed significantly greater cognitive complexity than those of their low-publicity counterparts, especially when attitude assessment was delayed.

Thus, it seems that the publicity of a counterattitudinal act and its aftermath compels active, elaborate cogitation about the self-discrepancy, leading not only to a change of attitude but to additional

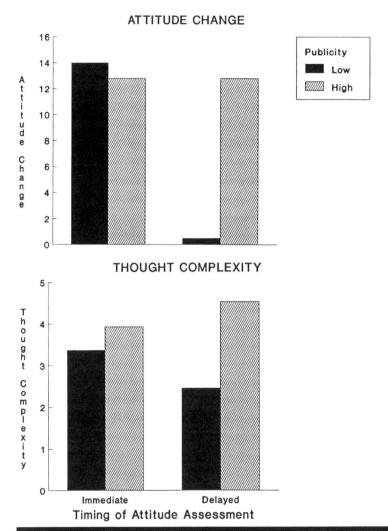

Results of Experiment 1 (low-choice control attitude-change $M = 0.00$). Attitude change is the difference between preessay attitudes and postessay attitudes, which were measured on a 31-point scale ranging from 1 (*disagree*) to 31 (*agree*). Thought-complexity scores could range from 1 to 7, with 1 indicating low differentiation and low integration of issue-relevant thoughts (as judged by raters) and 7 indicating high differentiation and high integration of thoughts (as judged by raters).

adjustments of relevant beliefs and ideas. The most elaboration seemed to occur when participants did not immediately encounter an explicit attitude-change opportunity. This was an expected outcome, because reducing dissonance by the made-available attitude-change option would lessen motivation to consider the issue further. By contrast, whereas cogitation about the dissonance seemed to carry on over time under high publicity, it seemed to quickly cease under low publicity. Unless queried immediately, low-publicity participants showed no evidence that they ever experienced dissonance. They seem to have forgotten all about it.

Additional evidence for these conclusions came from responses to a postexperimental request for participants to recall their preessay attitude. When postessay attitude assessment had been immediate, both high- and low-publicity participants showed considerable evidence of *biased misrecall*. On average, they remembered their prior attitudes to be about 8 scale points less negative than they actually had been (low-choice controls, by contrast, had near-perfect recall; see Brehm & Cohen, 1962, and Bem & McConnell, 1970, for other examples of biased memory after dissonance). Possibly, active dissonance reduction involving attitude change might be accomplished, in part, by selective distortion in remembering one's personal history with the dissonance issue.

If attitude assessment was delayed, however, the memory picture was entirely different. Low-publicity participants, on average, still erred in recalling their prior attitude by about 6 scale points, but these errors were rather well distributed in both directions. The misrecall seemed almost random (vs. biased) and, thus, indicative of mere passive forgetting. High-publicity, delayed-assessment participants, in marked contrast, had excellent memory of their preessay attitudes, erring, on average, by less than 2 scale points. One interpretation of this is that if allowed to "stew" in their public dissonance, participants engaged in an integrative cognitive restructuring in which preexisting positions were confronted and incorporated into a new attitude with a different point value but more broadly integrated cognitive and behavior (at least as remembered) components. In other words, if not influenced to reduce dissonance quickly and categorically, individuals were free to engage in a cognitive restructuring that did not require suppression of inconsistent cognitions.

In conclusion, the results of the Leippe and Elkin (1992) study suggest that when the situation enhances accountability for self-discrepancy, people engage in more elaborate dissonance reduction (cognitive restructuring), especially if a less effortful, elaborative option (categorical attitude change) is not made salient. When self-integrity is less threatened and no "quick fix" dissonance-reduction option is situationally salient, the dissonance simply may be forgotten.

The restructuring conclusion resonates well with other findings that dissonance reduction involves rumination and cogitation beyond attitude change. J. Aronson, Blanton, and Cooper (1995) found that after a counterattitudinal behavior that compromised their self-view on a personal dimension (compassion), people changed (in a positive, compensating direction) their self-view on a different dimension (independence) that lent integrity to their behavior. In addition to this complex act of rationalization, participants also changed their attitude toward greater agreement with their now-self-justified essay, suggesting even further restructuring.

Elaborate dissonance-reducing strategies also were in evidence in a pair of studies by Monteith (1993), who induced participants to inadvertently discriminate against a member of a stigmatized group. When this behavior was inconsistent with an important aspect of self-definition (i.e., being egalitarian and unprejudiced), individuals spent more time reading an essay that described the difficulty of avoiding discriminatory behavior, had better recall of the essay, and, in listing their thoughts about the essay, focused more on the whys and hows of their own self-discrepancies. In short, dissonance reduction involved multiple efforts to restructure the self.

The idea that people may ruminate about their dissonance and reduce it over time is supported by a number of studies. These include research on postdecisional dissonance (Festinger, 1964). Within the induced-compliance paradigm, Goethals and Cooper (1975) told some participants that an aversive consequence was possible and that they would find out soon whether it would indeed occur. Whereas participants who found out that the aversive consequence would occur changed their attitude, those who found out the aversive consequence would not occur did not. Goethals and Cooper (1975) suggested that these participants did not immediately reduce their dissonance, but, instead, opted to "live with it ... waiting to find out whether other routes of dissonance reduction will open up" (p. 366). Conceivably, participants ruminated as they waited, exploring their options and what it would mean to change an attitude. At the very least, this research strongly implies that categorical change is not spontaneous.

Beauvois, Joule, and Brunetti (1993) induced cigarette smokers to make a dissonance-producing commitment to an aversive act (an 18-hr abstinence from smoking) either immediately or several hours before requesting a more costly related act (a 6-day abstinence). Verbal acceptance of the second request was quite likely in the immediate condition but significantly less likely in the delayed condition. Apparently, people immediately confronted with the second request accepted it as a means of rationalizing the initial, dissonance-producing commitment. In the absence of this situational cue to expensive dissonance reduction, participants "had the necessary time to rationalize in another way, most likely by a cognitive rationalization" (Beauvois et al., 1993, p. 3). In other words, the delay effect implies that dissonance reduction may occur gradually and involve multiple cognitions.

Experiment 2: Restructuring Beyond Attitude Change on a Socially Significant Matter of Prejudice

Our subsequent studies of dissonance reduction after induced compliance retained the essential features of the essay-writing paradigm. The essay issues, however, involved policies relevant to the potentially prejudiced beliefs of the White participants toward Blacks. Owing to their linkage with race, prejudice, and associated values (e.g., fairness, equity; see Katz, 1981; Katz & Hass, 1988), however, the issues had considerable relevance to self-definition. Thus, a self-discrepancy concerning the issue carried the capacity to arouse considerable self-accountability. Moreover, the linkage of the attitude issues to a larger network of racial attitudes, beliefs, and values provided a "mental forum," in which we could observe a cognitive restructuring process incited by counteratti-tudinal behavior. Because the essay issue was plugged into this larger, self-relevant network, we expected that cognitive restructuring, a gen-eralization of attitude change to related cognitions, would be a natural product of any dissonance created by induced compliance.

Method

In Leippe and Eisenstadt (1994, Experiment 1), choice (high vs. low) and publicity (high vs. low) were manipulated as previously. Because there was no preessay assessment, a no-essay control condition was included. White college students ($n = 64$) were asked or told to write an essay endorsing a policy proposal that "of the total amount of money the university has available for scholarships, the percentage committed to deserving Black students should be at least doubled." After writing the essay, participants indicated their attitude toward this policy (on a 31-point scale ranging from *disagree* [1] to *agree* [31]). After a 5-min wait, a second experimenter was introduced, who administered some questionnaires for an ostensibly unrelated study.

Embedded in the first of these questionnaires were 10 items each of two racial beliefs scales developed by Katz and Hass (1988). The Pro-Black Scale assesses positive, sympathetic beliefs ("pro-Black beliefs") about Blacks, based especially on perceptions of the unfairness and disadvantages of past and current discrimination against Blacks. The Anti-Black Scale assesses negative sentiment ("anti-Black beliefs") about Blacks, based mainly on the belief that they have done too little to help themselves. Items were responded to on a 6-point scale ranging from -3 (*disagree strongly*) to 3 (*agree strongly*), so scores on each scale could range from -30 to 30.

Results and Discussion

The upper panel of Figure 2 contains attitude scores for participants who wrote essays that unequivocally endorsed the scholarships policy. Relative to the no-essay control condition, attitudes were more favorable toward the proposal endorsed in the essay in all conditions except that in which both choice and publicity were low. Thus, either high choice or high publicity was sufficient for attitude change. Moreover, attitudes

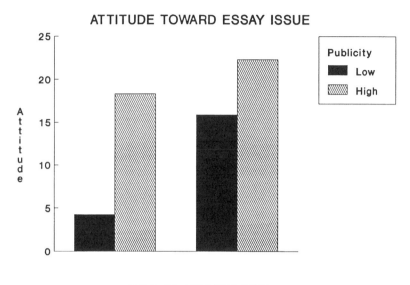

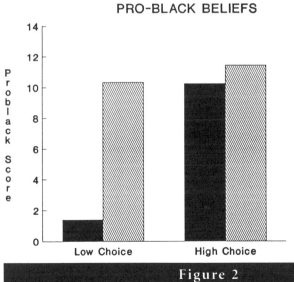

Figure 2

Results of Experiment 2 (no-essay control $Ms = 11.40$ [attitude] and 3.10 [beliefs]). Attitude was assessed on a 31-point scale ranging from 1 (*disagree* [with policy endorsed in essay]) to 31 (*agree* [with policy endorsed in essay]). Pro-Black scores could range from -30 to $+30$, with higher numbers indicating greater positivity toward Blacks.

were most favorable when both choice and publicity were high, suggesting these variables may combine additively to increase dissonance.

The attitude change under low choice is interesting in the light of the traditional assumption that perceived decision freedom is necessary for dissonance (e.g., Brehm & Cohen, 1962). This finding is not unprecedented (e.g., Baumeister & Tice, 1984). Perhaps even low-choice behaviors arouse dissonance if the cognition "I was assigned to do it" is not sufficient justification when weighed against other, negative-to-self, aspects of the behavior. In the present case, the self-symbolic meaning and possible negative consequences of considerable social significance may have pushed the attitude-discrepant behavior into this difficult-to-justify category.[1]

As seen in the lower panel of Figure 2, dissonance-reduction efforts extended beyond attitude change into related beliefs about Blacks. Like attitudes, pro-Black beliefs were significantly more positive relative to the no-essay control condition in all experimental conditions except the low-choice–low-publicity condition. This generalization of dissonance-driven change suggests, in keeping with our theorizing, that attitude–behavior inconsistency can implicate more aspects of the person and his or her beliefs than just the immediately "grating" cognitions and thus compel change among those aspects.[2]

In contrast to pro-Black beliefs, anti-Black beliefs were completely unaffected by induced compliance. This is important evidence that restructuring is not a random or arbitrary process. Katz and Hass

---

[1]Two considerations suggest that the attitude change under low choice did not simply reflect impression management. First, although attitude change when choice was low occurred only when publicity was high in Experiment 2, other experiments observed attitude change under low-choice when attitude responses were completely private within the experimental context (i.e., Baumeister & Tice, 1984; Eisenstadt & Leippe, 1997; Leippe & Eisenstadt, 1994, Experiment 3). Second, in the next experiment reported here, attitude change occurred under low choice only when assessment was immediate, not when it was delayed. It is unclear why a 15-minute delay would remove impression-management concerns when the experimenter had the same access to both essay and attitude responses whether assessment was immediate or delayed.

[2]In Experiments 2 and 3, about 45% of the high-choice participants did not fully comply with the request to write an essay endorsing the scholarships policy. Instead, they argued that it was good to increase scholarships for Blacks and acknowledged their special needs but lamented that it was unfair to take scholarship funds away from deserving Whites. Most semicompliers, that is, endorsed the proposal's spirit but not its implementation. Although semicompliers did not become

(1988) have demonstrated that pro-Black and anti-Black beliefs are pretty much independent. And pro-Black beliefs were more highly correlated with the scholarship essay issue, an issue more related to the egalitarian—humanitarian themes of pro-Black beliefs than to the work ethic—family-values themes of anti-Black beliefs. Thus, resolving the specific self-discrepancy of the other cognitive elements within a participant's race-relevant attitude—belief system involving the scholarship issue apparently was most likely to bring to mind, or have implications for, pro-Black beliefs concerning egalitarian values and themes. Indeed, research on communication-mediated indirect attitude change suggests just such a process of directional generalization, in that change in a specific attitude tends to spread to those attitudes most logically and psychologically related to it (see, e.g., McGuire, 1960; Wyer & Goldberg, 1970).

It is interesting to compare this changing of only beliefs that bore some thematic similarity to the focal attitude to recent studies by Stone, Wiegand, Cooper, and Aronson (1997), who created dissonance by making salient to participants their hypocrisy. For example, after publicly advocating the safe-sex practice of condom use, individuals were led to examine their own failures to practice what they had preached. Afterward, participants showed a clear preference, from among equally self-affirming prosocial acts, for engaging in the act most relevant to their dissonance (e.g., supporting AIDs research vs. a food drive for the homeless). Both Stone et al.'s studies and Experiment 2 suggest that when dissonance is aroused, the primary preoccupation concerns diminishing the focal discrepancy and that unless directed elsewhere (e.g., by a salient opportunity for global self-affirmation), change will occur among those cognitions most related to the discrepancy.

---

more positive toward the scholarship policy, they did evince significant positive change in pro-Black beliefs. In fact, their postessay pro-Black beliefs were just as positive as those of full compliers in dissonance-arousing conditions. As we discussed in more detail elsewhere (see Leippe & Eisenstadt, 1994), this appeared to be because, in bending over backwards to avoid sounding prejudiced, most semicompliers added statements that probably were more strongly positive toward Blacks than their typical opinion stances. This created dissonance that could be reduced by adjusting pro-Black beliefs up to the same level of positivity.

Experiment 3: More Prejudice Reduction Through Dissonance Reduction

Our next experiment (Leippe & Eisenstadt, 1994, Experiment 2) explored whether delaying attitude assessment while the participants sat in the glare of publicity would serve to increase the amount of change (restructuring) in related race-relevant beliefs, as the results of Experiment 1, the parking-fee study, suggest it might.

Method

All of the White, college student participants ($n = 118$) experienced the high-publicity conditions of Experiment 1. Choice (high or low) was crossed with timing of attitude assessment (immediate vs. 15-min after the counterattitudinal essay). A no-essay control condition also was included. After the experimenter collected their essays, participants were administered the attitude scale (followed by the "separate study" racial belief scales) either immediately or after 15 min.

Results and Discussion

Figure 3 displays condition means for participants who wrote fully in favor of the scholarships proposal. Attitudes were significantly more favorable when choice was high (vs. low) and when assessment was immediate (vs. delayed). Although attitudes were less favorable in the low-choice–immediate-assessment condition than in high-choice conditions, they were nonetheless significantly more favorable than attitudes in the no-essay condition. This suggests, again, that dissonance can be aroused when choice is low and that choice and high publicity (a constant in this study) increase the magnitude of dissonance. The only essay-writing condition in which attitudes were not reliably more positive than no-essay control attitudes was the low-choice–delayed-assessment condition.

As in Experiment 2, heightened positivity of pro-Black beliefs was observed in every condition in which attitude change occurred. Only participants in the low-choice–delayed-assessment condition failed to evince more positive pro-Black beliefs. Anti-Black beliefs again did not differ from no-essay controls in any conditions.

The main focus of Experiment 3 was on whether a delay in attitude

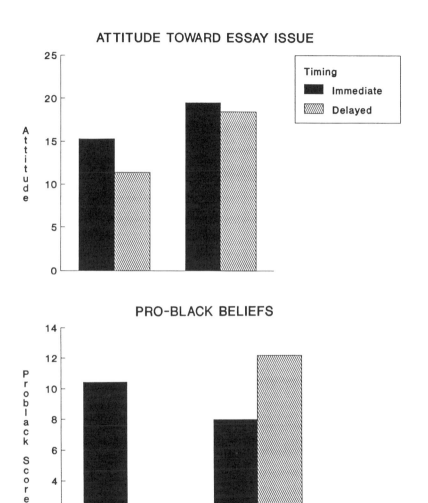

Figure 3

Results of Experiment 3 (no-essay control Ms = 11.53 [attitude] and 5.05 [beliefs]). Attitude was assessed on a 31-point scale ranging from 1 (*disagree* [with policy endorsed in essay]) to 31 (*agree* [with policy endorsed in essay]). Pro-Black scores could range from −30 to +30, with higher numbers indicating greater positivity toward Blacks.

assessment would serve to increase the amount of change in attitude-related beliefs when dissonance was intense (i.e., choice was high), thereby suggesting that cognitive restructuring continued until some explicit closure occurred. No such delayed increase in beliefs was observed, however. The absence of this delay effect does not necessarily rule out that such ongoing rumination might occur in some situations. In a situation such as that created in Experiment 3, however, perhaps it is more likely that dissonance-related rumination will attenuate soon after the dissonance-producing act unless some situational cue keeps people attentive to their dissonance. Or, instead of ever-increasing polarization of beliefs toward the counterattitudinal behavior, restructuring might involve achieving an integrative balance among beliefs, attitudes, and behaviors at some asymptotic level of overall change.

There was one effect of assessment delay, corresponding to the flip side of an increase with delay of elaborate dissonance reduction under strong dissonance. That is, when dissonance was weak, owing to low choice, neither attitudes nor beliefs changed when assessment was delayed. This outcome resembled the assessment-delay effect in the low-publicity condition of Experiment 1. There, as well, no signs of attitude change or any form of dissonance reduction were apparent. It is reasonable to assume that the amount of dissonance created in the high-choice–low-publicity–trivial-issue circumstances of Experiment 1 was at about the same low level as that created in the low-choice–high-publicity–somewhat-significant-issue circumstances of Experiment 3. In these circumstances, people might experience only a weak undercurrent of dissonance that translates into active, mind-altering dissonance reduction only if it is pounced on by some query that makes accountability salient.

When dissonance is aroused only weakly, and no reminder of the self-discrepancy or cue to reduce it comes quickly along, dissonance might not be reduced, but simply forgotten. This would help explain the "don't remind me" effect reported by Elkin and Leippe (1986), who observed that physiological arousal persisted throughout a 6-min recording time that followed attitude assessment. When attitudes were not immediately assessed, however, physiological arousal dissipated well within the 6-min span. Although choice and consequences were high, publicity was relatively low, and the essay issue was rather trivial. Accordingly, forgetting, as Elkin and Leippe speculated, seems tenable in the light of the current results.

Harmon-Jones, Brehm, Greenberg, Simon, and Nelson (1996) showed that induced compliance might lead to dissonance and attitude change even under very austere conditions of self-accountability (i.e., no aversive consequences, virtually total privacy, and a trivial opinion issue). If only slight self-indiscretions created a ripple of dissonance arousal, it would be highly functional that the slighter ones would go away through a simple shift of attention. This forgetting route to dissonance reduction not only provides a tenable account of the delayed-assessment effects in Experiments 1 and 3 but also suggests a fundamental mechanism that facilitates escape from dissonance through misattribution (e.g., Zanna & Cooper, 1974) and distraction (e.g., Zanna & Aziza, 1976).

Experiment 4: Dissonance Meets Racial Ambivalence, and Restructuring Extends Further

In Experiment 4 (Eisenstadt & Leippe, 1997), we created an opportunity to see if the repercussive effects of dissonance reduction might be even deeper and more elaborate when the focal attitude issue assumed yet greater importance. In the preceding experiments, there was no change in anti-Black beliefs, apparently because anti-Black beliefs were less relevant than pro-Black beliefs to the scholarship issue. Yet both types of beliefs do exist about Black Americans. Moreover, for many Whites, their positions on the two belief dimensions are evaluatively discordant, yielding a chronic state of racial ambivalence (Katz & Hass, 1988). According to Katz (1981), each side of this ambivalence supports self-defining values. Pro-Black beliefs define the person as egalitarian and humane, whereas anti-Black beliefs reflect one's work ethic and self-image as discerning in helping only deserving others. Normally, because the cognitive contents of the two sides are not logically contradictory, the ambivalent attitude–belief system is stable and something one can and does live with. However, if sufficient expression or change occurs on only one side of the duality, instability and emotional tension develop because of the threat to the self-values associated with the other side. This should force change or action on this other side, most likely in the form of bolstering that side. Possibly, participants in the preceding experiments were able to fully reduce their dissonance with changes in pro-Black beliefs small enough not to pose a threat to the self-defining values reflected in anti-Black beliefs. If so, perhaps a more personally costly race-relevant counterattitudinal act would implicate change in pro-Black beliefs beyond some tolerable limit and thereby foster restructuring that bridges the duality.

Experiment 4 tested also whether either the symbolic or personal-relevance importance, or both, of the counterattitudinal act increases dissonance and attitude change. We varied whether a costly tuition-hike policy was to help only Black students or all deserving students. We hypothesized that dissonance would be greater when essays promoted a policy that helped only Blacks (high racial symbolism), because, as a result of the complexity and extensiveness of race-related attitude systems, writing for a racially biased policy would bring more dissonant cognitions into play. We also varied the likelihood that the tuition hike would be personally experienced. High personal relevance is positively correlated with perceived importance and number of self-implications (see, e.g., Krosnick, 1988). As such, we hypothesized that personal relevance would increase dissonance.

Method

White college students ($n = 171$) participated in the basic induced-compliance procedure. Essay-writing participants were either asked (high choice) or instructed (low choice) to write in support of a university proposal to increase tuition by $2,000 per year as a means of providing more scholarship funds to either "deserving Black students" (high racial symbolism) or "deserving students" (low racial symbolism). If approved, the tuition hike would occur either the next year (high personal relevance) or in 6 years (low personal relevance). Postessay attitudes and racial beliefs were obtained as in previous experiments. Finally, there were four no-essay control groups corresponding to each condition of the 2 (symbolism) $\times$ 2 (relevance) design.

Results and Discussion

Both attitude and beliefs scores were converted to pseudo-change scores by subtracting from a participant's score the mean score on that measure in the no-essay control group corresponding to that participant's symbolism and relevance condition (cf. Liberman & Chaiken, 1996). Among full compliers (see Footnote 2), greater attitude change occurred when choice was high as opposed to low (Ms = 4.82 vs 1.68). Looking specifically within the high-choice conditions, there was a significant interaction of symbolism and relevance. As seen in Figure 4, in the high-relevance condition, attitude change was nonsignificantly less when symbolism was high (vs. low). In contrast, in the low-relevance condition, attitude change was significantly greater when symbolism was high (vs. low).

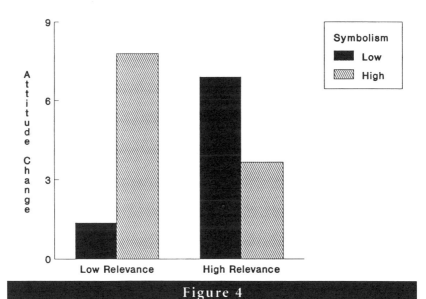

Figure 4

Attitude results in the high-choice conditions of Experiment 4. Attitude was assessed on a 31-point scale ranging from 1 (*disagree* [with policy endorsed in essay]) to 31 (*agree* [with policy endorsed in essay]). Attitude change corresponds to the difference between attitude scores in a condition and the mean attitude score in the no-essay control condition having the same level of relevance and symbolism as that condition.

The latter relationship—that greater symbolism yielded greater attitude change under low relevance—may be combined with another outcome apparent in Figure 4: Greater relevance produced greater attitude change under low (vs. high) symbolism. Taken together, these patterns indicate that either heightened symbolism or heightened personal relevance increase attitude change. This is consistent with the idea that both symbolism and personal relevance serve to engage more cognitive elements in the dissonance process and to increase the importance of those elements.

Yet, unexpectedly, higher levels of symbolism and relevance did not combine additively to produce even more attitude change. In fact, no significant attitude change occurred when both symbolism and relevance were high. This intriguing result actually concurs with other evidence that categorical change on the focal issue is not a likely route of dissonance reduction when the issue implicates self-identity in especially important ways (see, e.g., Gotz-Marchand, Gotz, & Irle, 1974; Hardyck & Kardush, 1968). High-symbolism–high-relevance participants must have felt great self-accountability, having endorsed a steep increase in the costs of their education and compromised some of their beliefs relevant to equity and equality. Thus, these participants may have been highly motivated to find avenues of dissonance reduction other than accommodating their attitude (and, thus, their self-image) to the behavior. Such avenues might include cognitive restructuring that preserved the attitude in an altered cognitive context, suppression (cf. Hardyck & Kardush, 1968), or self-distraction (cf. Zanna & Aziza, 1976).

This interplay of relevance and symbolism did not occur with racial beliefs. Rather, there were main effects of racial symbolism regardless of relevance, choice, and degree of attitude change. Both pro-Black and anti-Black beliefs (pseudo-change Ms = 2.57 and 2.95) tended to increase when symbolism was high (but not when symbolism was low, Ms = −0.56 and −1.78). Thus, individuals expressed both more positive and more negative sentiments about Blacks, that is, heightened ambivalence. Analyses of racial ambivalence scores created using a conversion metric developed by Katz and Hass (1988) revealed that high-symbolism essay writers had significantly greater ambivalence than either low-symbolism essay writers or high-symbolism no-essay control participants.

The changes in pro-Black and anti-Black beliefs, yielding increased ambivalence, suggest that the counterattitudinal act unsettled one side of an ambivalent attitude system enough to require adjustment of the other side. In helping well beyond their extant pro-Black sentiments, endorsers of the racially biased policy needed not only to increase their pro-Black beliefs but also to increase their anti-Black beliefs, to protect aspects of self-identity tied up with this negative side of the ambivalence. Dissonance again spread beyond the focal self-discrepancy into the surrounding cognitive landscape, this time even further than in the preceding studies.

CONCLUSION

The original dissonance theory can be seen as short on specificity, especially in two areas: the concept of importance and modes of dissonance reduction. These areas are critically interrelated. Our self-accountability account defines the importance of dissonant cognitive elements in terms of how strongly related the elements are to self-definitions, including the private self (e.g., values), the public self (e.g., integrity within a situation as a "person of one's word"), and the collective self (e.g., attitudes, beliefs, lifestyles associated with reference groups). A cognitive element can be related to self-definition because it is central to that definition, or, as in the case of race-relevant attitudes, because it is embedded within an attitude system or network with self-defining values and worldviews at the core. With this definition of importance in hand, it becomes possible to specify, and thus to manipulate, situational variables that have a direct effect on importance and, in turn, the magnitude of dissonance.

According to the self-accountability model, importance is relevant not only to magnitude of dissonance but also to how dissonance is reduced. There now is extensive knowledge of how importance is positively related to both the amount of cognitive elaboration regarding an attitude issue and number of cognitive elements potentially implicated in this elaboration. Accordingly, as our experiments demonstrate, cogitation associated with dissonance reduction is more likely to transcend categorical attitude change, the more the initiating self-discrepancy is itself important or is linked to important cognitions.

Our research, we believe, makes three important inroads in the area of dissonance reduction. First, it provides a conceptual framework, the self-accountability model, for investigating this topic. Second, it provides evidence that triggered by essentially the same attitude-discrepant behavior, the mode of dissonance reduction can run the gamut from forgetting to categorical attitude change to cognitive restructuring involving changes in beliefs related to the focal attitude. Third, it indicates that the immediate situation can channel dissonance reduction through a specific mode. Making and keeping a self-discrepancy public, for example, make restructuring more likely, whereas making an attitude query may compel attitude change that may have not occurred in the absence of the query.

Situational channeling is evident in some extant research. Focusing people on their initial attitude, for example, makes attitude change less likely and encourages misremembering of the dissonance-inducing behavior as not particularly attitude discrepant (Scheier & Carver, 1980). In a similar fashion, having people judge the importance, in the grand scheme of things, of their counterattitudinal espousal results in diminished attitude change, as individuals trivialize their self-discrepancy (Simon et al., 1995). Our research extends this evidence of situational determination of reduction mode by showing that situations can influence not only which cognitive elements change but also the effort and elaboration involved in the change.

Despite these advances, our work leaves many questions unanswered and points up several issues. One issue concerns the forgetting of dissonance. When dissonance is weak, our data suggest it simply may be forgotten. However, demonstrating this empirically is difficult because dissonance may be reduced in some active, but unmeasured, mental manner. And what about the possibility of forgetting at the other end of the magnitude-of-dissonance spectrum? Some theorists (e.g., Hardyck & Kardush, 1968) have speculated that extremely high dissonance may be actively suppressed. Bolstering of a betrayed attitude (e.g., Sherman & Gorkin, 1980) and the use of alcohol (which eliminates attitude change after induced compliance; Steele, Southwick, & Critchlow, 1981) may be examples of behaviors that support thought suppression.

The self-affirmation effect (Steele, 1988), in which affirming one's self-worth after induced compliance eliminates attitude change, may be related to forgetting. A self-esteem-enhancing event may grab attention as a means of escaping an exceptionally self-threatening dissonance and also facilitate forgetting a trivial dissonance.

On another issue, Simon et al. (1995) have contrasted an *on−off switch* model of dissonance reduction, in which a single change fully eliminates dissonance, and a *hydraulic* model, in which dissonance reduction may flow into multiple paths of change. These researchers favor the on−off model on the basis of their research, which found that induced-compliance participants used whatever path of dissonance reduction was made available to them first and then showed no change at all when the second route also was offered (see also Gotz-Marchand et al., 1974). Yet other research has shown multiple changes even when dissonance-reduction options are presented sequentially (e.g., J. Aronson et al., 1995). Our research, of course, is entirely indicative of hydraulic, multiple-change dissonance reduction. Most likely, a single change may eliminate dissonance under some circumstances but not under others. A single change may not suffice when more important self-discrepancies are involved and in situations that maintain the salience of the self-discrepancy.

A final issue is the process by which people come to actively reduce dissonance through cognitive restructuring. One possibility is a resolution-motivated process, in which self-accountability pressure motivates people to work through the self-systemic implications of their self-transgression. As a result, related cognitive elements get pulled into the change process, and there is restructuring. Alternatively, or in addition, an availability-cued process may be involved. Important self-discrepancies that are well connected to a large attitude−belief network may automatically activate many cognitive elements, which then are naturally elaborated systematically. Most likely, both processes are at work in cognitive restructuring. Further research on this would yield greater understanding of the intrapsychic processes (vs. products) of dissonance reduction.

REFERENCES

Aronson, E. (1968). Dissonance theory: Progress and problems. In R. P. Abelson, E. Aronson, W. T. McGuire, T. M. Newcomb, M. J. Rosenberg, & P. H. Tannenbaum (Eds.), *Theories of cognitive consistency: A sourcebook* (pp. 5–27). Chicago: Rand McNally.

Aronson, E. (1969). The theory of cognitive dissonance: A current perspective. In L. Berkowitz (Ed.), *Advances in experimental social psychology* (Vol. 4, pp. 1–34). New York: Academic Press.

Aronson, J., Blanton, H., & Cooper, J. (1995). From dissonance to disidentification: Selectivity in the self-affirmation process. *Journal of Personality and Social Psychology, 68*, 986–996.

Baumeister, R. F., & Tice, D. M. (1984). Role of self-presentation and choice in cognitive dissonance under forced compliance: Necessary or sufficient causes? *Journal of Personality and Social Psychology, 46*, 5–13.

Beauvois, J. L., Joule, R. V., & Brunetti, F. (1993). Cognitive rationalization and act rationalization in the escalation of commitment. *Basic and Applied Social Psychology, 14*, 1–17.

Bem, D. J., & McConnell, H. K. (1970). Testing the self-perception explanation of dissonance phenomena: On the salience of premanipulation attitudes. *Journal of Personality and Social Psychology, 14*, 23–31.

Boninger, D. S., Krosnick, J. A., Berent, M. K., & Fabrigar, L. R. (1995). The causes and consequences of attitude importance. In R. E. Petty & J. A. Krosnick (Eds.), *Attitude strength: Antecedents and consequences* (pp. 159–189). Mahwah, NJ: Erlbaum.

Brehm, J. W., & Cohen, A. R. (1962). *Explorations in cognitive dissonance.* New York: Wiley.

Chaiken, S., Liberman, A., & Eagly, A. H. (1989). Heuristic and systematic information processing within and beyond the persuasion context. In J. S. Uleman & J. A. Bargh (Eds.), *Unintended thought: Limits of awareness, intention, and control* (pp. 212–252). New York: Guilford Press.

Cooper, J., & Fazio, R. H. (1984). A new look at dissonance theory. In L. Berkowitz (Ed.), *Advances in experimental social psychology* (Vol. 17, pp. 229–266). New York: Academic Press.

Eisenstadt, D., & Leippe, M. R. (1994). The self-comparison process and self-discrepant feedback: Consequences of learning you are what you thought you were not. *Journal of Personality and Social Psychology, 67,* 611–626.

Eisenstadt, D., & Leippe, M. R. (1997). *Dissonance and ambivalence as factors in induced compliance in the domain of prejudice.* Manuscript submitted for publication.

Elkin, R. A., & Leippe, M. R. (1986). Physiological arousal, dissonance, and attitude change: Evidence for a dissonance–arousal link and a "don't remind me" effect. *Journal of Personality and Social Psychology, 51,* 55–65.

Elliot, A. J., & Devine, P. G. (1994). On the motivational nature of cognitive dissonance: Dissonance as psychological discomfort. *Journal of Personality and Social Psychology, 67,* 382–394.

Festinger, L. (1957). *A theory of cognitive dissonance.* Stanford, CA: Stanford University Press.

Festinger, L. (1964). *Conflict, decision, and dissonance.* Stanford, CA: Stanford University Press.

Goethals, G. R., & Cooper, J. (1975). When dissonance is reduced: The timing of self-justificatory attitude change. *Journal of Personality and Social Psychology, 32,* 361–367.

Gotz-Marchand, B., Gotz, J., & Irle, M. (1974). Preference of dissonance reduction modes as a function of their order, familiarity, and reversibility. *European Journal of Social Psychology, 4,* 201–228.

Greenwald, A. G. (1982). Ego-task analysis: An integration of research on ego-involvement and self-awareness. In A. H. Hastorf & A. M. Isen (Eds.), *Cognitive social psychology* (pp. 109–147). New York: Elsevier/North-Holland.

Greenwald, A. G., & Ronis, D. L. (1978). Twenty years of cognitive dissonance: Case study of the evolution of a theory. *Psychological Review, 85,* 53–57.

Hardyck, J. A., & Kardush, M. (1968). A modest modish model for dissonance reduction. In R. P. Abelson, E. Aronson, W. T. McGuire, T. M. Newcomb, M. J. Rosenberg, & P. H. Tannenbaum (Eds.), *Theories of cognitive consistency: A sourcebook* (pp. 684–692). Chicago: Rand McNally.

Harmon-Jones, E., Brehm, J. W., Greenberg, J., Simon, L., & Nelson, D. E. (1996). Evidence that the production of aversive consequences is not necessary to create cognitive dissonance. *Journal of Personality and Social Psychology, 70,* 5–16.

Hass, R. G., & Eisenstadt, D. (1990). The effects of self-focused attention on perspective-taking and anxiety. *Anxiety Research, 2,* 165–176.

Higgins, E. T., & King, G. (1981). Accessibility of social constructs: Information-processing consequences of individual and contextual variability. In N. Cantor & J. Kihlstrom (Eds.), *Personality, cognition, and social interaction* (pp. 69–121). Hillsdale, NJ: Erlbaum.

Judd, C. M., & Krosnick, J. A. (1989). The structural bases of consistency among political attitudes: Effects of political expertise and attitude importance. In A. R. Pratkanis, S. J. Breckler, & A. G. Greenwald (Eds.), *Attitude structure and function* (pp. 99–128). Hillsdale, NJ: Erlbaum.

Katz, I. (1981). *Stigma: A social psychological analysis.* Hillsdale, NJ: Erlbaum.

Katz, I., & Hass, R. G. (1988). Racial ambivalence and American value conflict: Correlational and priming studies of dual cognitive structures. *Journal of Personality and Social Psychology, 55,* 893–905.

Krosnick, J. A. (1988). Attitude importance and attitude change. *Journal of Experimental Social Psychology, 24,* 240–255.

Kunda, Z. (1990). The case for motivated reasoning. *Psychological Bulletin, 108,* 480–498.

Leippe, M. R., & Eisenstadt, D. (1994). The generalization of dissonance reduction: Decreasing prejudice through induced compliance. *Journal of Personality and Social Psychology, 67,* 395–413.

Leippe, M. R., & Elkin, R. A. (1992). *Dissonance reduction and accountability: Effects of assessment and self-presentational concern on mode of inconsistency resolution.* Unpublished manuscript, Adelphi University, Garden City, NY.

Liberman, A., & Chaiken, S. (1996). The direct effect of personal relevance on attitudes. *Personality and Social Psychology Bulletin, 22,* 269–279.

McGuire, W. (1960). Direct and indirect effects of dissonance-producing messages. *Journal of Abnormal and Social Psychology, 60,* 354–358.

Monteith, M. J. (1993). Self-regulation of prejudiced responses: Implications for progress in prejudice-reduction efforts. *Journal of Personality and Social Psychology, 65,* 469–485.

Petty, R. E., & Cacioppo, J. T. (1986). The elaboration likelihood model of persuasion. In L. Berkowitz (Ed.), *Advances in experimental social psychology* (Vol. 19, pp. 123–205). New York: Academic Press.

Pratkanis, A. R., & Greenwald, A. G. (1989). A sociocognitive model of attitude structure and function. In L. Berkowitz (Ed.), *Advances in experimental social psychology* (Vol. 10, pp. 173–220). New York: Academic Press.

Scheier, M. F., & Carver, C. S. (1980). Private and public self-attention, resistance to change, and dissonance reduction. *Journal of Personality and Social Psychology, 39*, 390–405.

Schlenker, B. R. (1982). Translating actions into attitudes: An identity-analytic approach to the explanation of social conduct. In L. Berkowitz (Ed.), *Advances in experimental social psychology* (Vol. 15, pp 193–247). New York: Academic Press.

Schlenker, B. R. (1986). Self-identification: Toward an integration of the private and public self. In R. F. Baumeister (Ed.), *Public and private self* (pp. 21–62). New York: Springer-Verlag.

Sherman, S. J., & Gorkin, L. (1980). Attitude bolstering when behavior is inconsistent with central attitudes. *Journal of Experimental Social Psychology, 16*, 388–403.

Simon, L., Greenberg, J., & Brehm, J. (1995). Trivialization: The forgotten mode of dissonance reduction. *Journal of Personality and Social Psychology, 68*, 247–260.

Steele, C. M. (1988). The psychology of self-affirmation: Sustaining the integrity of the self. In L. Berkowitz (Ed.), *Advances in experimental social psychology* (Vol. 21, pp. 261–302). New York: Academic Press.

Steele, C. M., Southwick, L. L., & Critchlow, B. (1981). Dissonance and alcohol: Drinking your troubles away. *Journal of Personality and Social Psychology, 41*, 831–846.

Stone, J., Wiegand, A. W., Cooper, J., & Aronson, E. (1997). When exemplification fails: Hypocrisy and the motive for self-integrity. *Journal of Personality and Social Psychology, 72*, 54–65.

Tedeschi, J. T., Schlenker, B. R., & Bonoma, T. V. (1971). Cognitive dissonance: Private ratiocination or public spectacle. *American Psychologist, 26*, 685–695.

Tetlock, P. E. (1983). Accountability and complexity of thought. *Journal of Personality and Social Psychology, 45,* 74–83.

Thomsen, C. J., Borgida, E., & Lavine, H. (1995). The causes and consequences of personal involvement. In R. E. Petty & J. A. Krosnick (Eds.), *Attitude strength: Antecedents and consequences* (pp. 191–214). Mahwah, NJ: Erlbaum.

Wicklund, R. A. (1975). Objective self-awareness. In L. Berkowitz (Ed.), *Advances in experimental social psychology* (Vol. 8, pp. 233–275). New York: Academic Press.

Wyer, R. S., & Goldberg, L. A. (1970). A probabilistic analysis of the relationships between beliefs and attitudes. *Psychological Review, 77,* 100–120.

Zanna, M. P., & Aziza, C. (1976). On the interaction of repression–sensitization and attention in resolving cognitive dissonance. *Journal of Personality, 44,* 577–593.

Zanna, M. P., & Cooper, J. (1974). Dissonance and the pill: An attribution approach to studying the arousal properties of dissonance. *Journal of Personality and Social Psychology, 29,* 703–709.

PART THREE

Mathematical Models
of Dissonance

10

Computer Simulation of Cognitive Dissonance Reduction

Thomas R. Shultz and Mark R. Lepper

Cognitive-dissonance phenomena have often been considered "exotic" and quite different from less counterintuitive psychological phenomena. Dissonance effects, particularly those involving insufficient justification, are frequently considered to contradict both common sense and other established psychological principles. When people change their attitudes more after being paid less to engage in counterattitudinal behavior (Festinger & Carlsmith, 1959), this strikes both the ordinary observer and the professional psychologist as surprising, or even wrong. Conventional theories of conflict, decision, reinforcement, and rational choice often seem to generate different predictions than does dissonance theory. Thus, when the first dissonance experiments appeared, they were greeted by suspicion, disbelief, and alternative explanations.

In our recent efforts to simulate dissonance phenomena, we have discovered that the reduction of cognitive dissonance can be modeled

This research was supported by a grant from the Social Sciences and Humanities Research Council of Canada and by National Institute of Mental Health Grant MH-44321. Readers interested in obtaining the consonance program may contact Thomas R. Shultz.

according to established principles of constraint satisfaction (Shultz & Lepper, 1996). Activations of neuronlike units change to increase consonance in a network of these units, satisfying as many of the constraints imposed by initial activations and connections among units as well as possible. This is interesting not only because simulations can generate precise predictions for a wide range of dissonant situations but also because it suggests that dissonance reduction may be more like a variety of other psychological processes known to operate in constraint-satisfaction terms (e.g., memory retrieval, belief revision, schema completion, analogical reasoning, and causal explanation and attribution) than is currently imagined. All of these processes appear to operate by the progressive application of constraints supplied by personal attitudes, beliefs, and memory traces.

In this chapter, we explore this recent work on the modeling of dissonance reduction, by (a) discussing the nature of constraint-satisfaction processes, (b) presenting our own consonance model, which applies constraint-satisfaction ideas to dissonance reduction, (c) showing in detail how such simulations are conducted and presenting a tool that others can use to work with this model, and (d) reviewing the specific dissonance simulations that we have already conducted with this model.

CONSTRAINT SATISFACTION

Problems typically entail constraints of various kinds and often can be solved by satisfying these constraints. For example, designs must be created by a particular time, under a specified cost, making use of certain materials. Committee schedulers, similarly, must find a time to meet before the report is needed, when everyone is free and a suitable room is available. Constraint-satisfaction methods try to find a problem state in which all of the various constraints are satisfied. In general, this can be done by applying whatever constraints are known and then propagating these to generate other parts of the solution. Such procedures are relevant to a wide array of problems in areas from design and scheduling to vision and memory. Knowing that one part of a visual image has a certain characteristic can allow propagation of constraints to neighboring parts (Waltz, 1975). For example, in a fork-shaped intersection of three planes, the fact that one line of the fork is a convex edge implies that the other two lines also are convex. If on a box, this configuration defines the intersection of these three planes as the nearest corner of the box. Likewise with the retrieval of information from memory. Think of the name of a Japanese automobile manufacturer whose name begins with the letter *T*. In such cases, some memory contents serve as cues to the rest of the memory. Such memories are said to be content addressable (i.e., addressable from any of their contents). Because only memories containing the cues constitute an acceptable response, the cues can be considered as constraints on the retrieval process.

Constraint satisfaction is not confined to psychology, but is characteristic of many physical processes. Consider, for example, the water that results from snow melt on the top of a mountain. Due to the constraint of gravitational forces, the water runs downhill but not straight into the ocean—it meanders around local barriers (i.e., constraints) on the mountain, and at least some of it remains in locally minimal elevations in the form of mountain lakes. All of these events can be described in terms of so-called relaxation mathematics, which explains how systems settle into low-energy states, subject to the various constraints that impinge on the system. The physical principle of entropy embodies this idea.

One convenient way to implement such ideas for modeling psychological phenomena is in terms of artificial neural networks. These are brainlike devices, run on a computer, that contain units similar to neurons and connection weights similar to synapses. Activations (activity levels) of the units can change, subject to the constraints supplied by the connection weights, initial activations of the units, and external input to those units. As activation is passed around inside such a network, the network settles into a locally optimal state, in which as many constraints are satisfied as well as possible. Constraints that do not need to be completely satisfied are called soft constraints. Softness is important because it is common for constraints to be incompatible to varying degrees, and thus global minima are difficult to achieve. The importance of particular constraints, conveyed by magnitudes of activations, connections, and inputs, also is taken into account, with more important constraints receiving more attention in the satisfaction process. Recently, a large number of phenomena in social psychology, in addition to dissonance, have been successfully modeled with constraint-satisfaction networks—including attitude change, impression formation, and cognitive balance (reviewed in Read & Miller, 1998).

THE CONSONANCE MODEL

In our own work, we have used an artificial neural network model—which we call the *consonance* model because it attempts to increase consonance or consistency—to simulate various phenomena in the cognitive dissonance literature (Shultz & Lepper, 1996). In this model, the motivation to increase cognitive consonance, and thus to reduce dissonance, results from the various constraints on the beliefs and attitudes that a person holds at a given point in time. Our basic procedure is to create consonance networks corresponding to participants' representations of the various conditions of a cognitive dissonance experiment.

Variations across a number of parameters may help to model differences among different experimental conditions. Thus, units in a network can be variously active, representing the direction and strength of a person's cognitions (i.e., attitudes and beliefs). Units can also vary in their resistance to change, reflecting differences in the extent to which particular cognitions may be supported by other cognitions or anchored in reality. Connection weights between cognitions represent perceived causal implications between the cognitions. The connections between any two units in a network can be excitatory, inhibitory, or nonexistent. Different conditions of a particular dissonance experiment are implemented by particular patterns of initial unit activations and connection weights.

We define *consonance* as the degree to which similarly active units are linked by excitatory (+) weights and differently active units or inactive units are linked by inhibitory $(-)$ weights. Unit activations change over time, to satisfy the various constraints and thus increase consonance. Somewhat more formally, the consonance contributed by a particular unit i is

$$\text{consonance}_i = \sum_j w_{ij} a_i a_j, \tag{1}$$

where w_{ij} is the connection weight between units i and j, a_i is the activation of the receiving unit i, and a_j is the activation of the sending unit j. The summation sign indicates that the triple products of sending-unit activation, connection weight, and receiving-unit activation are summed across the various incoming connections, indexed by j. An illustrative computation for a hypothetical, four-unit network is shown in Figure 1.

Consonance over an entire network is defined as the values given by Equation 1 summed over all receiving units in the network:

$$\text{consonance}_n = \sum_i \sum_j w_{ij} a_i a_j. \tag{2}$$

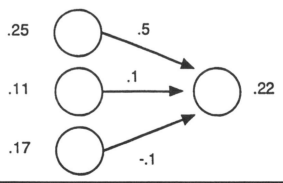

Figure 1

The consonance contributed by one particular unit is computed as the sum of sending-unit activations, connection weights, and receiving-unit activation. In this case, the unit on the right contributes a consonance value of $(.25 \times .5 \times .22) + (.11 \times .1 \times .22) + (.17 \times -.1 \times .22) = .0275 + .00242 - .00374 = .02618$.

Because units in our consonance networks have connection weights going in both directions, each unit serves both sending and receiving roles in these equations.

Activation is propagated over time around the network, in conformity with two rules that update the activation of units:

$$a_i(t + 1) = a_i(t) + \text{net}_i[\text{ceiling} - a_i(t)], \text{ when net}_i \geq 0, \quad (3)$$

$$a_i(t + 1) = a_i(t) + \text{net}_i[a_i(t) - \text{floor}], \text{ when net}_i < 0, \quad (4)$$

where $a_i(t + 1)$ is the activation of receiving unit i at time $t + 1$, $a_i(t)$ is the activation of unit i at time t, ceiling is the maximal level of unit activation, floor is the minimal level of unit activation, and net_i is the scaled net input to unit i, defined as

$$\text{net}_i = \text{resist}_i \sum_j w_{ij} a_j. \quad (5)$$

The parameter resist_i indicates the resistance of receiving-unit i to having its activation changed. Smaller values of this parameter indicate greater resistance because smaller values mean less impact of the net input. Thus, the net input to a unit whose activation is being updated is the sum of the products of connection weight and activations of their respective sending units. These products are summed over the various sending units, indexed by j. A sample computation of net input is shown in Figure 2 for a hypothetical four-unit network.

In the case shown in Figure 2, the net input equals $-.083$, so Equation 4 applies. Equation 4 says to scale the net input by the distance from the current activation to the activation floor. In our simulations, activation floor has a default value of 0.0, and in this example, the current activation is .12, so the distance to the floor is .12. The scaled net input is $.12 \times -.083 = -.00996$. Then Equation 4 says to add this scaled net input to the current activation, to obtain the updated activation, $-.00996 + .12 = .11004$. More generally, Equations 3 and 4 say to scale the net input to the unit being updated by the distance to the floor (for negative net input) or to the ceiling (for positive net input) and to add this scaled net input to the current activation. The idea of scaling the net input by the distance to the floor or ceiling is to keep

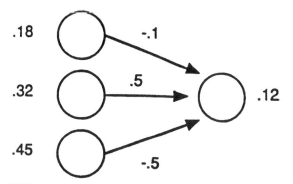

Figure 2

Net input to a receiving unit is computed as the sum of the products of sending-unit activation and connection weights. In this case, the receiving unit on the right has a net input of (.18 × −.1) + (.32 × .5) + (.45 × −.5) = −.018 + .16 − .225 = −.083. The text explains how to convert this net input into an updated activation for the receiving unit.

unit activations between floor and ceiling. This type of nonlinearity in activation functions is characteristic of biological neurons and has important implications for computations in artificial neural networks. For one thing, it keeps networks from overheating by cumulative increases in activation.

At each time step, n units are randomly selected and updated according to Equations 3–5, where n is the number of units in the network. The update rules in Equations 3–5 ensure that consonance either increases or remains the same across time cycles. When overall consonance reaches its asymptote, the updating process is stopped because the network has settled into a stable, low-energy state with most of the constraints pretty well satisfied.

MAPPING THE CONSONANCE MODEL TO DISSONANCE PHENOMENA

Six theoretical principles are used to map the consonance model onto dissonance theory. These principles constrain the design of networks representing the conditions of each experiment being simulated. Each condition in an experiment is represented by a separate network containing a set of cognitions arranged with a particular set of relations and initial activations.

Principle 1: Representation of Cognitions

Each cognition is implemented by the net activation of a pair of negatively connected units, one to represent the positive end (in which something is believed to be true or is highly valued) and the other to represent the negative end (in which something is believed to be false or is disliked). *Net* activation for the cognition is the difference between activation of the positive unit and activation of the negative unit. Activations can range between a floor and a ceiling. By default, the floor parameter is 0. The default ceiling parameter is 1 for positive units and 0.5 for negative units. The use of two different default ceilings is based partly on neurological and computational considerations (neurons that represent positive information have a larger activation range than those representing negative information; Anderson, 1995) and partly on the fact that it works well in the domain of cognitive-consistency seeking (Shultz & Lepper, 1996). This bipolar representation scheme allows for some degree of ambivalence in cognitions, although the inhibitory connections between the two poles tend to discourage such ambivalence.

Principle 2: Relationships Among Cognitions

Cognitions are connected to each other on the basis of their causal implications. If quantitative increases in Cognition 1 would cause quantitative increases in Cognition 2, then Cognition 1 is considered a facilitatory cause of Cognition 2; if quantitative increases in Cognition 1 would cause quantitative decreases in Cognition 2, then Cognition 1 is considered a inhibitory cause of Cognition 2. These relations are implemented in a network by connection weights between the units.

Connection weights range from -1 to 1, with 0 representing a lack of causal relation. When two cognitions are positively related, their positive poles are connected with excitatory $(+)$ weights, as are their negative poles. Inhibitory $(-)$ weights connect the positive pole of one cognition with the negative pole of the other cognition and vice versa.

Such connections are reversed for two cognitions that are negatively related. In addition, each unit has an inhibitory self-connection (to keep its activation from growing too large). Finally, all connection weights are bidirectional, meaning that there is a connection weight from Unit 1 to Unit 2 and another from Unit 2 to Unit 1. Connection weights have a default value of 0.5, representing a strong connection, but occasionally our simulations require weak connections, which have a default value of 0.1. These weight values are somewhat arbitrary, but it is important that strong connections are noticeably stronger than weak ones.

Principle 3: Magnitude of Dissonance

Total dissonance in a network is defined as the negative of total consonance divided by r, the number of nonzero relations among cognitions:

$$\text{dissonance} = \frac{-\text{consonance}_n}{r}. \qquad (6)$$

We divide by r to standardize dissonance across networks of different size and connection density by controlling for the number of relevant relations. Self-connections to units are excluded from this computation of dissonance, so that dissonance will not be an artifact of the amount of activation. This definition of *dissonance* offers some advantages over that of Festinger (1957) because it is mathematically formalized, can easily be applied to complex belief structures, permits measures of the amount of dissonance in each intercognition relation, includes within-cognition ambivalence if there is any, and varies even when all individual relations are dissonant or consonant.

This definition of *dissonance* is analogous to Hopfield's (1982, 1984) definition of *energy* in neural networks, and the definition of *consonance* is analogous to Rumelhart, Smolensky, McClelland, and Hinton's (1986) definition of *goodness* in neural networks. In our networks, energy (dissonance) decreases as goodness (consonance) increases.

Principle 4: Dissonance Reduction

Networks settle into more stable, less dissonant states as unit activations are updated according to Equations 3–5. There are two parameters that affect the process of dissonance reduction, *cap* and *rand%*. A cap parameter, with a default of -0.5, corresponds to the connection between each unit and itself, w_{ii}, and prevents activations from reaching the activation ceiling. This activation limitation is appropriate for most dissonance experiments, because they typically do not deal with highly important situations.

The rand% parameter provides a means of globally testing the robustness of results obtained in simulations in the face of variations in the specific numerical values used to instantiate key variables. At the start of each network run, connection weights, resistances, and initial activations all are randomized by adding or subtracting a random proportion of their initial amounts. The rand% parameter specifies the proportion range in which these additions and subtractions are selected under a random uniform distribution. Ordinarily, we use small (.1), medium (.5), and large (1.0) levels of rand%. Randomizing network values in this way increases psychological realism, because not everyone can be expected to share exactly the same parameter values. Randomizing of weight values also violates the symmetry of connection weights, so that $w_{ij} \neq w_{ji}$, and thus makes network solutions less stable, meaning that outcomes are more variable. Comparisons of the solutions obtained from networks at high levels of randomization indicate the robustness of results.

Principle 5: Changes in Cognitions

Although connection weights are not allowed to change in our dissonance simulations, cognition unit activations do change over time as dissonance is reduced. Some cognitions are more resistant to change than others, as implemented in Equation 5. *Beliefs* (i.e., cognitions regarding behaviors and justifications) are more resistant to change than are *evaluations* (i.e., attitudes). Although participants in dissonance experiments are usually well aware of what just happened to them and what they just did (and these factors are more difficult to alter in reality), they may not be confident about how they feel about aspects of the somewhat novel situation characterizing the experiment. The *resist* parameter has default values of 0.5 for low resistance and 0.01 for high resistance. This may seem the wrong way around, but according to Equation 5, the larger the resistance multiplier, the more readily the unit changes its activation.

Principle 6: Importance of Dissonance

An *importance* parameter multiplies all connection weights and unit activations at the start of each run, before the initial randomizations described under Principle 4. Typically, we use values of 1.0 in control conditions, 0.5 for conditions that lessen the importance of a dissonant situation, and 1.5 for conditions that enhance the importance of a dissonant situation. Again, the precise values used are somewhat arbitrary, but it is important that they differ substantially to generate different results. Factors that lessen the importance of dissonance might include tranquilizing drugs and information that affirms other aspects of the self-concept; factors that enhance the importance of dissonance might include stimulant drugs and physical exercise or other activities that may heighten general arousal. Later, we examine how such factors account for a variety of arousal and self-concept phenomena in the dissonance literature.

These six mapping principles convey the basics of designing consonance networks, but additional details can be found in Shultz and Lepper (1996, 1998a).

AN ILLUSTRATIVE SIMULATION

To make these issues more concrete, in this section, we present a detailed example of our consonance modeling. We first describe the experiment to be simulated, then the conceptual design of the networks representing the different experimental conditions, the implementation of these networks in a computer simulation, and finally, the results of that simulation.

Insufficient Justification Through Forced Compliance

The example focuses on perhaps the most influential paradigm generated from dissonance theory—namely, *insufficient justification*. The insufficient-justification paradigm deals with situations in which participants are induced to engage in some counterattitudinal action, with either rather little or with considerably greater justification for that action. For these situations, classical dissonance theory predicts that the less the justification for the behavior, the greater the dissonance and, at least when the action cannot be retracted, the more people will be motivated to change their attitudes to provide additional justification for their actions.

In the popular subparadigm called *forced compliance*, participants are paid to do something that is discrepant with their own attitudes. Somewhat paradoxically, smaller inducements to engage in the counterattitudinal action lead to larger changes in attitude than do large inducements. In the first experiment of this type, Festinger and Carlsmith (1959) found that being paid $1 to describe a boring task as interesting led to higher subsequent evaluations of the task itself than did being paid $20 to tell this lie. Because being paid to lie is consonant with telling the lie, it should be more dissonant to lie for a small reward than for a large reward.

Like many other results in the insufficient-justification paradigm, this finding was considered to be counterintuitive. For one thing, it seemed to contradict the idea that behavior strength would increase with the degree of reinforcement for the behavior. In this case, payment might have reinforced giving a positive description of the task. As with other early insufficient-justification results, alternative explanations quickly appeared in the literature. One such explanation was based on *evaluation apprehension*, the idea that participants in psychology experiments might suspect that they are being evaluated by the experimenter. In the Festinger and Carlsmith (1959) experiment, participants might have felt that their honesty was being evaluated. Perhaps resisting the temptation to "be bought" would result in a more favorable evaluation by the experimenter, and perhaps evaluation apprehension was higher with a larger payment than with a smaller payment. Another alternative explanation was based on deception. Participants might have suspected that they were being deceived and, as a result, resisted confirming what they perceived to be a test of the reinforcement hypothesis. Participants in the $20 condition might have found the payment to be too large for the situation and guessed that the payment was actually designed, instead, to alter their beliefs.

To rule out these and other alternative explanations, a subsequent study by Linder, Cooper, and Jones (1967) added conditions in which participants were not given a choice about writing the counterattitudinal essay. Linder et al. found that the dissonance effect obtained only when participants had a choice about whether to write the counterattitudinal essay; without a choice, the opposite effect was found, with higher payment leading to more attitude change in the direction of the view supported in the essay. We decided, in this and other cases of insufficient justification, to simulate this second-generation experiment (Shultz & Lepper, 1996). In addition to ruling out alternative explanations, second-generation experiments like Linder et al. would present a greater challenge for simulations than would the original experiments, in which simple main effects were observed.

Network specifications for this simulation (Shultz & Lepper, 1996) are shown in Tables 1 and 2. Table 1 contains specifications of the cognitions in the four conditions of the Linder et al. (1967) experiment, and Table 2 contains specifications of the relations among these cognitions. As in most insufficient-justification experiments, there were three relevant cognitions in each condition: attitude, writing the essay, and payment. Each of these three cognitions was represented with two negatively connected units, as specified in Mapping Principle 1. Initial activations for the cognitions were based on the ways in which the experiment was set up. Initial attitude was highly negative, reflecting these liberal college students' negative views of banning controversial speakers on campus. Writing the essay was set to highly positive because the essay was indeed written. And payment for writing was either high or low, depending on the payment condition.

Relations among the three cognitions reflect assumed causal implications, as specified in Mapping Principle 2 and shown in Table 2. In

Table 1

Specification of Cognitions in the Simulation of Linder, Cooper, and Jones (1967)

Condition	Initial activations	
	Positive	Negative
Choice, low pay		
Attitude	0	high
Essay	high	0
Pay	low	0
Choice, high pay		
Attitude	0	high
Essay	high	0
Pay	high	0
No choice, low pay		
Attitude	0	high
Essay	high	0
Pay	low	0
No choice, high pay		
Attitude	0	high
Essay	high	0
Pay	high	0

Note. Types of cognitions were evaluation (for attitude), behavior (for essay), and justification (for pay).

the choice conditions, the more one supports the position in the essay, the more likely it is that one would write the essay, so the relation between the attitude and essay cognitions is high and positive. The more one is paid, the more one would agree to write the essay, so the relation between the payment and essay cognitions is also high and positive. Finally, the more favorable one's attitude, the less one would need to be paid to write an essay at some particular level of support;

Table 2

Specification of Relations in the Simulation of Linder, Cooper, and Jones (1967)

Cause	Effect	Relation
Choice, low-pay condition		
Attitude	Essay	Highly positive
Pay	Essay	Highly positive
Attitude	Pay	Highly negative
Choice, high-pay condition		
Attitude	Essay	Highly positive
Pay	Essay	Highly positive
Attitude	Pay	Highly positive
No-choice, low-pay condition		
Attitude	Essay	None
Pay	Essay	Highly positive
Attitude	Pay	Highly positive
No-choice, high-pay condition		
Attitude	Essay	None
Pay	Essay	Highly positive
Attitude	Pay	Highly positive

therefore, the relation between the attitude and payment cognitions is high and negative.

Relations among the cognitions are the same in the no-choice conditions, except that the relation between attitude and essay is zero because without a choice, there is no causal connection between the two, and the relation between attitude and payment is positive, reflecting a better mood with higher pay.

Designing and Running a Simulation

Recent changes to our computer program for designing and running consonance networks implement a graphical interface in which users no longer need to write programming code. Instead, the program can interface with the user entirely through dialog boxes. Dialog boxes are so called because they enable a dialog between the program and the user. If users do not want to write program code (in the LISP programming language), they can design and run simulations merely by pointing and clicking the mouse and occasionally typing in a name.

If a user opts to run the program by means of dialog, the main dialog box appears on the screen. There are options to clear all of the global variables (which is like starting with a clean slate), change parameter values, show the current parameter values, show the current network, make a network, run a simulation with the current network, and exit. As with all such selection dialogs, the user selects one of these actions by pointing and clicking the mouse and then either clicking the OK button or pressing the return key.

If the selection is to change parameters, then another dialog box appears on the screen. Because there are so many parameters, there is a scrolling bar on the right side to scroll down to additional parameters. Because simulation results are much more impressive when incidental parameters remain constant across different procedures, for most simulations, the only parameters that typically need to be set are path (to ensure that results are saved in the right folder), *ncycles* (to ensure that simulations stop after a particular number of update cycles, typically when the networks settle into stable states from which activations no longer change), and rand% (to test robustness of the simulation results against variation in parameters). If a parameter is selected for changing, then a dialog box appears asking for the new entry for that parameter.

A user who is ready to build a network would select the "make-network" option from the main dialog box. The main things to do from the "make-network" dialog box are first to enter the cognitions of interest and then to enter the relations among these cognitions. Relations cannot be established until the cognitions are in place. Along the way, the user may be interested in viewing the network that is being made. There are also options for deleting either a cognition or a relation; if a cognition is deleted, then all of the relations in which it participates also are deleted automatically. After a simulation has been run, the generic network is saved along with the rest of the results. There is an option in the "make-network" dialog box for restoring a previously saved network; this would obviate having to reenter all of the network information.

If a user opts to enter a new cognition, a dialog box appears that allows the user to enter the name of the new cognition. Such names are arbitrary, but it is recommended that semantically appropriate, mnemonic names be used. For example, the participant's attitude toward banning controversial speakers on campus for the simulation of Linder et al. (1967) might be labeled *attitude*. After a new cognition has been named, a dialog box appears that asks the user to select the type of the new cognition. There are three types available that cover all of the cognitions in dissonance experiments that we know about: evaluation, behavior, or justification. The attitude cognition is of the evaluation type and thus has a low resistance to change.

The next step in creating a cognition is to give it initial activation values on its positive and negative poles. There is a choice between using default values and entering particular numeric values. In either case, two values are entered, one for the positive and one for the negative pole of the cognition. Default values can be low, high, or zero. At any time, the current network may be displayed from the "make-network" dialog box.

When a user decides to run a network (by selecting "run" in the main dialog box), there is an opportunity to enter the number of networks to be run. Because of the randomization of connection weights and initial activations using the rand% parameter and the random selection of units to be updated, each network settles into a somewhat different stable state by a different route. Thus, it may be interesting to run a number of networks to assess variability in network performance.

Results

Our simulation of the four conditions of the Linder et al. (1967) study was reported in Shultz and Lepper (1996). The networks were designed as specified in Tables 1 and 2. We ran 20 networks (to assess variation in results) for 20 cycles (by which time dissonance values had reached asymptote) at each of three levels of parameter randomization (0.1, 0.5, and 1.0). The cognition predicted to change most was attitude toward banning controversial speakers. This was computed as the difference between activations on the positive and negative ends of the attitude cognition and was automatically saved in a file. Of primary interest were the attitude scores at the end of 20 cycles when dissonance reduction was completed. At this point, the networks showed the same crossover interaction found by Linder et al. with college students—that is, a dissonance effect under choice, with more attitude change after low payment than after high payment, and the reverse effect under no choice, with more attitude change after high payment than after low payment—as shown in Figure 3.

Just as with our other simulations of insufficient justification, the results for this experiment held up at every level of parameter randomization but were sharper at small and moderate levels than at high levels. The results plotted in Figure 3 are for moderate randomization (rand% = 0.5). These attitude scores were subjected to a factorial analysis of variance (ANOVA), in which the presence of choice and amount of payment were the factors. The predicted interaction between choice and payment was reliable, $F(1, 76) = 57.71$, $p < .0001$. Note that the consonance model covers the full interaction obtained by Linder et al. (1967), whereas classical dissonance theory covers only the dissonance effect under choice.

It is also possible to examine the scores for the other two cognitions in the experiment, namely, essay and pay. Because these two cognitions are relatively resistant to change, they are not expected to show much movement over time. Ratings on these two cognitions are not ordinarily assessed in psychological experiments and were not included in the reports of our simulations (Shultz & Lepper, 1996), but it is worth noting how they change over the course of dissonance reduction in the simulations. Data on these two cognitions are automatically saved in files named for the respective cognitions. The essay cognition concerns the belief that one did write the counterattitudinal essay. It starts out with a net value of about .5 and does not change much with time. There are no significant effects in the Choice

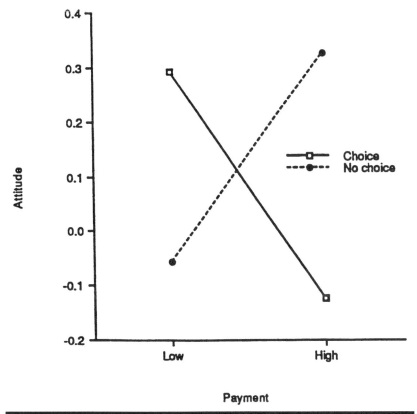

Figure 3

Mean attitude after dissonance reduction in the four conditions of the simulation of Linder, Cooper, and Jones (1967), with moderate parameter randomization (from Shultz & Lepper, 1996, adapted with permission).

× Amount of Payment ANOVA, confirming that there is nothing systematic happening with this cognition. The story is slightly different for the cognition concerning the payment received for writing the essay, because of the amount-of-payment manipulation. This cognition begins with a net value of about .1 in the low-payment condition and .5 in the high-payment condition, and these values do not change much over time. The Choice × Amount of Payment ANOVA reveals only a strong main effect of payment, $F(1, 76) = 195$, $p < .0001$, reflecting the obvious fact that payment is seen as higher when it is indeed higher.

An additional variable that is automatically recorded during consonance network simulations is dissonance, as specified in Equation 6. Mean dissonance is plotted over time for the four conditions of the simulation of Linder et al. (1967) in Figure 4. This plot reveals relatively high dissonance in the choice–low-pay condition, which is substantially reduced over time.

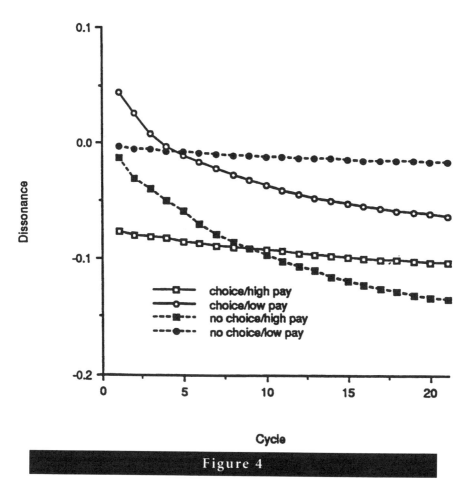

Cycle

Figure 4

Mean dissonance in the four conditions of the simulation of Linder, Cooper, and Jones (1967), with moderate parameter randomization.

| | Table 3 | | | | | |

First 10-Unit Activation Updates of a Network Run at Moderate
Parameter Randomization in the Choice–Low-Payment Condition
of the Simulation of Linder, Cooper, and Jones (1967)

Update	Unit (cognition and pole)	Current activation	Net input	Scaled net input	Distance from floor or ceiling	Updated activation
1	Essay—positive	0.473	−0.379	−0.005	0.473	0.471
2	Essay—negative	0.0	−0.029	0.0	0.0	0.0
3	Essay—negative	0.0	−0.029	0.0	0.0	0.0
4	Pay—negative	0.0	−0.524	−0.005	0.0	0.0
5	Essay—positive	0.471	−0.378	−0.005	0.471	0.469
6	Pay—positive	0.059	0.536	0.003	0.941	0.062
7	Attitude—positive	0.456	−0.251	−0.108	0.456	0.407
8	Pay—negative	0.0	−0.497	−0.005	0.0	0.0
9	Attitude—positive	0.0	−0.06	−0.041	0.0	0.0
10	Pay—positive	0.062	0.499	0.003	0.938	0.064

There is an option in the consonance program to record all unit-activation updates in the order they occur. It is assumed that users would do this only for a single network because it is too much detail for routine simulation. Each update is recorded by saving the number of the randomly selected unit to be updated, current activation of the unit, raw net input to the unit, scaled net input (net input × resistance, as in Equation 5), distance of scaled net input from ceiling (for positive scaled net input) or from floor (for negative scaled net input), and updated activation of the unit (as in Equations 3 and 4). The first 10 activation updates for a network run at moderate parameter randomization in the choice–low-payment condition of the simulation of Linder et al. (1967) are shown in Table 3. Each entry in this table is rounded to three decimal places, but in an actual simulation, many more decimal places are used for greater accuracy. Examination of tables like this can provide a feeling for the course of constraint-satisfaction computations.

OTHER CONSONANCE SIMULATIONS

In addition to the simulations just detailed, we have conducted a variety of other simulations of cognitive-dissonance phenomena, covering all of the major paradigms except selective exposure.[1]

Other Insufficient-Justification Effects

Insufficient Justification Through Prohibition

In addition to insufficient justification through forced compliance, there are insufficient justification subparadigms based on prohibition and initiation. The classic study on prohibition was conducted by Aronson and Carlsmith (1963), who forbade nursery schoolers to play with an attractive toy under either mild or severe threat of punishment. They found that children devalued the forbidden toy more under mild than under severe threat, presumably because of greater dissonance under mild threat due to the additional justification provided by the severe threat. To rule out a number of alternative explanations of these initial results, Freedman (1965) added surveillance conditions to this experimental design. Under surveillance conditions, the experimenter stayed in the room during the "temptation" period. The presence of the experimenter was presumed to lessen dissonance by increasing the potency of the threats. Several weeks later, only children in the mild-threat, nonsurveillance condition showed significant devaluation of the forbidden toy.

It was this second-generation experiment by Freedman (1965) that we chose to simulate (Shultz & Lepper, 1996). After unit-activation changes reached asymptotic values, our networks showed more devaluation of the forbidden toy under mild than under severe threat, but

---

[1]Some of the difficulties of covering selective exposure phenomena are discussed in Shultz and Lepper (1998a). These effects have been among the most difficult to replicate in the dissonance literature (e.g., Freedman & Sears, 1965; Frey, 1986).

only in the nonsurveillance conditions, thus paralleling Freedman's data.

Insufficient Justification Through Initiation

A third insufficient-justification subparadigm concerns the consequences of suffering an initiation to join a group. The classic experiment found that people initiated into a boring group liked the group better after undergoing a severe than after undergoing a mild initiation (Aronson & Mills, 1959). The conventional dissonance explanation was that the relatively greater dissonance generated by a severe initiation could be reduced by increasing one's evaluation of the group. A subsequent experiment by Gerard and Mathewson (1966) eliminated various alternative explanations for these results, mainly by adding noninitiation conditions with the same severe and mild levels of unpleasantness. Gerard and Mathewson used two different levels of electric shock, administered as part of an initiation or as part of an unrelated experiment. After overhearing a boring discussion by a group they had volunteered to join, participants rated the group. As predicted by dissonance theory, participants liked this group better after having undergone a severe initiation than after a mild initiation. In contrast, in the noninitiation condition, participants liked the group better after receiving mild shock than after receiving severe shock, a finding not predicted by dissonance theory because dissonance theory only concerns the initiation conditions.

In our simulations, we found that when dissonance reduction reached asymptote, attitude results showed the interaction that Gerard and Mathewson (1966) found with humans: a dissonance-reduction effect under initiation conditions, with more liking for the group after severe than after mild initiation, and the reverse effect under noninitiation conditions (Shultz & Lepper, 1996). Thus, the consonance model covers the full interaction, whereas classical dissonance theory only covers the effects of shock under initiation conditions.

Free Choice and the Reevaluation of Alternatives

The *free-choice* paradigm concerns the consequences of making a choice among alternatives. Making such a decision is theorized to arouse dissonance because both the negative features of the chosen alternative and the positive features of the rejected alternative are inconsistent with one's action in making an irreversible choice. After an irrevocable choice has been made, dissonance can be reduced by seeing the chosen object as more desirable and the rejected object as less desirable. This dissonance reduction further separates the alternative choices in terms of desirability. In addition, the amount of dissonance is predicted to be greater the more difficult the decision, that is, the closer the alternatives are in desirability before the choice.

In the original free-choice experiment, Brehm (1956) found that the more the dissonance created by a choice, the more the separation between, or spreading apart of, the alternatives after the choice. That is, there was more separation between alternatives after a difficult choice between two highly evaluated alternatives than after an easy choice between a liked and a disliked alternative. In planning our simulations of the Brehm experiment, we created a third condition, in which participants could also be given a difficult choice, but this time between two disliked alternatives (Shultz & Lepper, 1996). We called this the *difficult–low* choice condition because evaluation of the alternatives began at a low level, in contrast to Brehm's difficult–high choice condition, which offered a choice between highly valued alternatives.

Following Brehm's (1956) procedure, we computed evaluation changes as final evaluation minus initial evaluation for each alternative. When simulated dissonance reduction reached asymptotic values, liking for the chosen object had increased, mostly in the difficult–low choice condition, and evaluation of the rejected object had decreased, mostly in the difficult–high choice condition. A new psychology experiment with 13-year-olds choosing among posters under these three conditions replicated Brehm's results in the difficult–high and easy choice conditions and confirmed the predictions of our consonance networks for the difficult–low choice condition (Shultz, Léveillé, & Lepper, in press). Once again, the consonance simulations fit the data better than did classical dissonance theory, which only predicted more separation after difficult than after easy choices.

The Role of Arousal

In recent years, increasing attention has been paid to the arousal properties of dissonance (Cooper & Fazio, 1984; Zanna & Cooper, 1974). A
key finding in this research has been that dissonance arousal can be
modulated by the administration of various drugs. One of the clearest
studies in this tradition had university students writing counterattitudinal essays under either high- or low-choice conditions (Cooper,
Zanna, & Taves, 1978). The students had just previously taken a pill
that they were told was a placebo. However, the pill actually contained
either phenobarbital, amphetamine, or a placebo in different conditions.
The usual dissonance effect was produced in the placebo condition—
more attitude change in the direction of the essay under high choice
than under low choice. This dissonance effect was eliminated in the
tranquilizer condition. In contrast, amphetamine enhanced attitude
change under both high- and low-choice conditions.

Our simulations focused on the Cooper et al. (1978) experiment
(Shultz & Lepper, 1998b). Arousal manipulations were implemented
with an importance parameter that scaled the initial activations and
connection weights before they were randomized. The importance scalar was 1.0 for the placebo condition, 0.5 for the tranquilizer condition,
and 1.5 for the amphetamine condition. We were guided here by evidence that drugs such as phenobarbital depress neural firing rates and
synaptic transmission, whereas drugs such as amphetamine enhance
neural firing rates and synaptic transmission. After the networks had
stabilized, the Drug × Choice interaction effects on attitude closely
simulated those shown in the Cooper et al. experiment. There was a
dissonance effect in the placebo condition, with more attitude change
under high than under low choice; no effect of choice and little attitude
change in the tranquilizer condition; and enhanced attitude change
along with the dissonance-choice effect in the amphetamine condition.

Self-Concept and Dissonance

Modern research has also highlighted the role of the self-concept in the
arousal of dissonance (Steele, 1988; Thibodeau & Aronson, 1992). It has
been argued that dissonance occurs primarily when behavior is incon-

sistent with one's self-concept. Because most people have a positive self-concept, such behaviors as lying or arguing for a position that is contrary to one's beliefs should arouse dissonance. In contrast, people with a negative self-concept who engage in such behaviors might not experience dissonance.

Dissonance and Machiavellianism

The first evidence supporting this idea came from a study examining differences in dissonance arousal among people scoring high or low on the trait of Machiavellianism (Epstein, 1969). It was argued that people scoring low on this trait would experience dissonance in a situation of forced compliance with insufficient justification but that those scoring high on the trait would not. For high Machiavellians, writing a counterattitudinal essay would not be inconsistent with their self-concept, because such behavior would be viewed as a legitimate social tactic.

Epstein's (1969) undergraduate participants all initially supported the fluoridation of water supplies. Those participants assigned to a dissonance condition were induced to give a speech against fluoridation and were paid $2 for doing it. Participants in a control condition gave no speech but read arguments against fluoridation and were paid $2 incidentally. Confirming dissonance-theory predictions, Epstein found that attitude change toward an antifluoridation position was higher for low Machiavellians who gave a speech than for low Machiavellians who did not. High Machiavellians showed the opposite trend, which Epstein explained by citing evidence that high Machiavellians are more susceptible to factual arguments than are low Machiavellians. In this case, the factual arguments were in the arguments read by participants in the control condition.

In our simulations, attitudes after network settling captured the crossover interaction found with Epstein's undergraduates (Shultz & Lepper, 1998b). Networks built with low Machiavellian parameters revealed a dissonance effect—more attitude change with a speech than without—whereas networks with high Machiavellian parameters showed the opposite effect. The reversal effect for high Machiavellians cannot be predicted within classical dissonance theory but is covered by the consonance networks.

Dissonance and Self-Affirmation

Still more subtle effects of self-concept on dissonance in a forced-compliance situation were obtained in studies on self-affirmation processes (Steele, 1988). If dissonance is generated when a one's actions threaten the self-concept, then anything that affirms an important aspect of the self-concept, even if irrelevant to the source of experimentally produced inconsistency, should minimize the need for dissonance reduction through attitude change. Steele's university students were selected for their strong opposition to a tuition rise. They were then induced to write essays in support of a large tuition increase, under either high-choice or low-choice conditions. Some of the students also had been previously assessed as having a strong economic–political value orientation. For such students, completing a political value scale would presumably affirm a valued part of their self-concept, but for others without this value orientation, this task would have little impact. Steele reported both a dissonance effect (more attitude change under high-choice than under low-choice conditions) and a self-affirmation effect (self-affirmation eliminated attitude change, even under high-choice conditions).

In our simulations of Steele's (1988) results, self-affirmation was implemented with an importance parameter of 0.5, as in the tranquilizer condition of the Cooper et al. (1978) simulation (Shultz & Lepper, 1998b). This effectively dampened all unit activations and connection weights before randomization of parameter values. After our networks settled, they showed the same pattern of results as Steele's undergraduate participants—more attitude change in the high-choice condition than in either the low-choice or the high-choice, self-affirmation conditions.

Steele (1988) also reported a free-choice experiment with self-affirmation effects. His participants ranked 10 record albums and were given a choice of keeping either their 5th- or 6th-ranked albums. Some of the participants had been selected for having a strong scientific value orientation and for indicating that a lab coat symbolized important values and goals. There were also other participants for whom science was not an important personal value. Within each of these two groups, one half of the participants were asked to wear a lab coat for the remainder of the experiment. Then all participants ranked the 10 albums once again.

Spread of alternatives after the choice was computed by adding the increase in liking for the chosen item and the decrease in liking for the rejected item. Spread was lower in the self-affirmation condition, in which scientifically oriented students wore lab coats, than in the other conditions, even though the affirmation procedure was irrelevant to the choice.

In our simulations of this experiment, an importance scalar of 0.5 was used to diminish all unit activations and connection weights in the self-affirmation condition (Shultz & Lepper, 1998b). Change in the value of one alternative was computed as the difference between its initial value and its final value. As in Steele (1988), spread of evaluation was the sum of the increase in the value of the chosen object and the decrease in the value of the rejected object. As with Steele's participants, there was a smaller spread of alternatives in the self-affirmation condition than in any of the other three conditions.

CONCLUSION

Dissonance researchers now have at their disposal computational modeling tools that are capable of simulating the results of a wide variety of dissonance experiments. Such simulations already have shown that dissonance reduction shares much in common with other psychological processes that operate in terms of constraint satisfaction. Some simulation predictions have been confirmed by psychological experimentation. The likelihood that the model could generate predictions for situations that have proved too complex for verbal dissonance formulations is particularly exciting. We hope that our computer program will become an integral part of the tool kit of other dissonance researchers.

REFERENCES

Anderson, J. A. (1995). *An introduction to neural networks.* Cambridge, MA: MIT Press.

Aronson, E., & Carlsmith, J. M. (1963). Effect of severity of threat on the devaluation of forbidden behavior. *Journal of Abnormal and Social Psychology, 66,* 584–588.

Aronson, E., & Mills, J. (1959). The effect of severity of initiation on liking for a group. *Journal of Abnormal and Social Psychology, 59,* 177–181.

Brehm, J. W. (1956). Post-decision changes in the desirability of choice alternatives. *Journal of Abnormal and Social Psychology, 52,* 384–389.

Cooper, J., & Fazio, R. H. (1984). A new look at dissonance theory. In L. Berkowitz (Ed.), *Advances in experimental social psychology* (Vol. 17, pp. 229–266). New York: Academic Press.

Cooper, J., Zanna, M. P., & Taves, P. A. (1978). Arousal as a necessary condition for attitude change following forced compliance. *Journal of Personality and Social Psychology, 36,* 1101–1106.

Epstein, G. F. (1969). Machiavelli and the devil's advocate. *Journal of Personality and Social Psychology, 11,* 38–41.

Festinger, L. (1957). *A theory of cognitive dissonance.* Stanford, CA: Stanford University Press.

Festinger, L., & Carlsmith, J. M. (1959). Cognitive consequences of forced compliance. *Journal of Abnormal and Social Psychology, 58,* 203–210.

Freedman, J. L. (1965). Long-term behavioral effects of cognitive dissonance. *Journal of Experimental Social Psychology, 1,* 145–155.

Freedman, J. L., & Sears, D. O. (1965). Selective exposure. In L. Berkowitz (Ed.), *Advances in experimental social psychology* (Vol. 2, pp. 57–97). New York: Academic Press.

Frey, D. (1986). Recent research on selective exposure to information. In L. Berkowitz (Ed.), *Advances in experimental social psychology* (Vol. 19, pp. 41–80). New York: Academic Press.

Gerard, H. B., & Mathewson, G. C. (1966). The effects of severity of initiation on liking for a group: A replication. *Journal of Experimental Social Psychology, 2,* 278–287.

Hopfield, J. J. (1982). Neural networks and physical systems with emergent collective computational abilities. *Proceedings of the National Academy of Sciences, USA, 79*, 2554–2558.

Hopfield, J. J. (1984). Neurons with graded responses have collective computational properties like those of two-state neurons. *Proceedings of the National Academy of Sciences, USA, 81*, 3008–3092.

Linder, D. E., Cooper, J., & Jones, E. E. (1967). Decision freedom as a determinant of the role of incentive magnitude in attitude change. *Journal of Personality and Social Psychology, 6*, 245–254.

Read, S. J., & Miller, L. C. (Eds.). (1998). *Connectionist models of social reasoning and social behavior.* Hillsdale, NJ: Erlbaum.

Rumelhart, D. E., Smolensky, P., McClelland, J. L., & Hinton, G. (1986). Schemata and sequential thought processes in PDP models. In D. E. Rumelhart & J. L. McClelland (Eds.), *Parallel distributed processing: Explorations in the microstructure of cognition* (Vol. 2, pp. 7–57). Cambridge, MA: MIT Press.

Shultz, T. R., & Lepper, M. R. (1996). Cognitive dissonance reduction as constraint satisfaction. *Psychological Review, 103*, 219–240.

Shultz, T. R., & Lepper, M. R. (1998a). The consonance model of dissonance reduction. In S. J. Read & L. C. Miller (Eds.), *Connectionist models of social reasoning and social behavior* (pp. 211–244). Hillsdale, NJ: Erlbaum.

Shultz, T. R., & Lepper, M. R. (1998b). *Consonance network simulations of arousal and self-concept phenomena in cognitive dissonance: The importance of psychological importance.* Manuscript submitted for publication.

Shultz, T. R., Léveillé, E., & Lepper, M. R. (in press). Free-choice and cognitive dissonance revisited: Choosing "lesser evils" vs. "greater goods." *Personality and Social Psychology Bulletin.*

Steele, C. M. (1988). The psychology of self-affirmation: Sustaining the integrity of the self. In L. Berkowitz (Ed.), *Advances in experimental social psychology* (Vol. 21, pp. 261–302). New York: Academic Press.

Thibodeau, R., & Aronson, E. (1992). Taking a closer look: Reasserting the role of the self-concept in dissonance theory. *Personality and Social Psychology Bulletin, 18*, 591–602.

Waltz, D. L. (1975). Understanding of line drawings of scenes with shadows. In P. H. Winston (Ed.), *The psychology of computer vision* (pp. 19–91). New York: McGraw-Hill.

Zanna, M. P., & Cooper, J. (1974). Dissonance and the pill: An attribution approach to studying the arousal properties of dissonance. *Journal of Personality and Social Psychology, 29*, 703–709.

11

A Multiplicative Power-Function Model of Cognitive Dissonance: Toward an Integrated Theory of Cognition, Emotion, and Behavior After Leon Festinger

Haruki Sakai

One of the most striking features of Festinger's (1957) theory of cognitive dissonance is that this theory does not draw sharp lines between cognition, emotion, motivation, and behavior. Every piece of knowledge that one holds constitutes a cognitive element. Thus, the term *cognitive element* refers not only to the knowledge about one's surroundings but also to the knowledge about what one believes, feels, wants, does, and is. In that, behavior becomes cognition. One's action is no longer regarded as a behavior but as a piece of knowledge about

Portions of this chapter were presented at the 48th Convention of the Japanese Psychological Association, Osaka, Japan, October 1984, and the 7th International Kurt Lewin Conference, Los Angeles, September 1996.

This research was in part supported by 1997 and 1998 research grants from Sapporo University, Sapporo, Japan. I express my sincere appreciation to the late Jun-ichi Shigeta, an excellent mathematician who died young, for his valuable comments on the initial version of my algebraic formulation of the magnitude of dissonance. I also greatly appreciate Miharu Honma's acting as the experimenter in my 1997 study, Gregg Gold at the University of California, Los Angeles, for his careful proofreading of my English manuscript, and Eddie Harmon-Jones and Judson Mills for their helpful suggestions and advice on drafts of this chapter. Special thanks are extended to my parents, Okuzaemon and Emiko Sakai, and wife, Kazue Sakai, for their help and encouragement throughout this research.

one's action. This special feature makes dissonance theory an integrated cognitive theory of behavior and cognition.

According to Festinger (1957), dissonance is typically created by decisions, forced-compliance, involuntary exposure to information, social disagreement, and discrepancy between reality and one's feeling or belief. Manifestations of dissonance reduction are behavior change, attitude change and cognitive reorganization, change of environment, perceptual and cognitive distortion, and selective exposure to persons, situations, and information. The evidence of dissonance reduction is a constellation of responses, not a single response, such as attitude change.

Festinger's (1957) theory stimulated numerous studies, both supportive and critical (for a review, see Aronson, 1968, 1992; Beauvois & Joule, 1996; Bem, 1972; Brehm & Cohen, 1962; Cooper & Fazio, 1984; Festinger, 1964; Frey, 1986; Steele, 1988; Takata, Shirai, & Hayashi, 1983; Tedeschi & Rosenfeld, 1981; Wicklund & Brehm, 1976). Although dissonance theory has wide applicability, most research, including Festinger (1964), has focused on the postdecision and the forced-compliance situations. Because of this attention to the postdecisional and the counterattitudinal behaviors, some researchers have suspected that dissonance theory may not be a cognitive but a behavioral theory (e.g., Abelson, 1983; Rosenberg, 1968).

The initial enthusiasm ended up in the mid-1970s as a general acceptance of the insights gained through dissonance-related research with low interest in further experimental research (cf. Jones, 1985). One obvious reason for the wane is that the innovative high-impact experimentation with deception produced serious ethical problems (for a history of the use of deception, see Korn, 1997). Indeed, it should be desirable not to deceive participants. However, are there any effective ways to create a "social illusion" (the term by J. Mills, personal communication, August 24, 1995) in the laboratory without any kind of deception? As Zajonc (1990) has suggested, experimental social psychology would not have emerged as a discipline if Leon Festinger and the innovative experimentation with deception had not appeared.

A MULTIPLICATIVE POWER-FUNCTION MODEL OF COGNITIVE DISSONANCE

Jones (1985) believed that main problems in dissonance theory were resolved before the mid-1970s. Thus, he inferred that the wane was in part due to the solution. Nevertheless, dissonance theory needs conceptual and quantitative specification so that it can be revived and expanded. This is why I propose a multiplicative power-function (MPF) model of cognitive dissonance.[1]

Conceptual Specification: Assumptions and Principles

The MPF model assumes the cognitive structure shown in Figure 1. Dissonance is associated with one particular key cognitive element. The cognitive structure consists of one key element K, m dissonant elements D_i ($i = 1$ to m), and n consonant elements. Each of the $m + n + 1$ cognitive elements is shown as a circle. The area of the circle denotes the importance of the cognitive element. The MPF model assumes that any change in the areas and relations in Figure 1 influences the state of dissonance. The process of dissonance reduction is in essence the process of change in the cognitive structure.

Any cognitive element is qualified to be a key element in the MPF model. If dissonance theory is to be a general theory of cognitive motivation, the key cognitive element must not be restricted to either an action-related or a behavior-related cognition. A belief-related cognition or a feeling-related cognition can be a key element. One of the crucial principles is that not only actors but also observers and perceivers experience dissonance.

---

[1]It seems quite natural for any scientific theory to evolve from verbal to mathematical formulation. However, Harris (1975, 1976) observed that social psychologists very much like verbally stated theories and very much dislike mathematical and computer-simulation models. He illustrated serious problems incurred by this attitude in his mathematical treatment of verbal theories. I can agree with his statement that Brehm and Cohen's (1962) prediction that "with the relative attractiveness of the alternatives held constant, the more attractive they both are, the greater is the magnitude of dissonance," (p. 6), is in fact one of the three predictions simultaneously derivable from Festinger's (1957) verbal statement. Harris (1975) concluded that the scientific status of social psychology is greatly threatened by the negative attitude toward mathematics, even if its subject matter is unique.

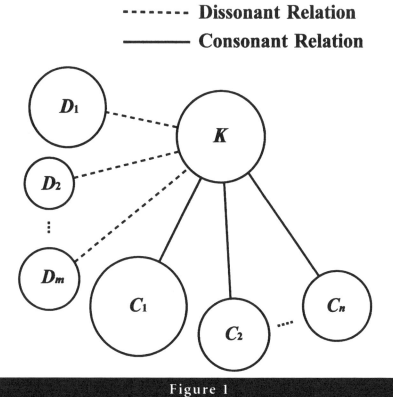

------- Dissonant Relation
——— Consonant Relation

Figure 1

A hypothetical cognitive system in which dissonance is associated with one particular key cognitive element. K denotes the key element, D_i denotes the ith element ($i = 1$ to m) dissonant with K, and C_j denotes the jth element ($j = 1$ to n) consonant with K. The area of each circle represents the importance of the element. From "On the Magnitude of Cognitive Dissonance: A Theoretical Note," by H. Sakai, 1980, *The Japanese Journal of Experimental Social Psychology, 20*, p. 82. Copyright 1980 by the Japanese Group Dynamics Association. Adapted with permission.

In the MPF model, the term *cognitive element* is redefined as a state of mind in a given situation. The state of mind can be cognitive, emotional, or motivational—or even unconscious. However, the state of mind must always be expressible in a sentence by the person in question, by the observer of this person, or by both. Any pair of cognitive elements that are verbalized as explicit sentences are in a dissonant relation if negation of one sentence follows from the other sentence. The importance of a cognitive element is defined as the importance of its verbalized sentence. This definition provides a measure of the importance of each cognitive element. A key cognitive element maintains its importance whether linked to or independent of the importance of the other relevant elements.

For example, each of the following sentences is a cognitive element in this model: P = "One day Mr. A woke up to find his beloved wife wearing a blue sweater," and Q = "Mr. A dislikes blue sweaters very much." Because negation of P follows from Q, Mr. A must have experienced dissonance in this situation. The magnitude of dissonance would have been less if sentence Q = "Mr. A does not like blue sweaters very much." This example also indicates a conceptual and quantitative transformation of the concept of balance (Heider, 1946, 1958) into the concept of dissonance in the MPF model. Festinger (1957) suggested that the state of imbalance is identical to dissonance, though he gave no conceptual bridge between them.

The greater the resistance to change of both the key element and the dissonant elements, the more lasting and easily observable are the manifestations of the dissonance associated with the key element. It is likely that the key element is the cognition that is most resistant to change at the very moment when dissonance arises in the mind. Nevertheless, it is not assumed that the key element must always be the cognition that is most resistant to change. This is because cognition about physical reality does not necessarily become a key element even though it is extremely resistant to change.

Quantitative Specification: Mathematical Formulation of the Magnitude of Dissonance

One of the most important concepts in dissonance theory is the magnitude of dissonance. Researchers must rely on the concept not only to determine the amount of existing dissonance in a given situation but also to examine the amount of remaining dissonance when various actions have been taken to reduce dissonance. Festinger (1957), however, merely presented verbal definitions of the magnitude of dissonance.

Let D, C, and K denote the sum of the m areas of the dissonant elements, the sum of the n areas of the consonant elements, and the one area of the key element itself, respectively (see also Figure 1). The magnitude of dissonance is formally defined as the following function:

$$d = [D/(D + C)]^{\theta_1} \times D^{\theta_2} \times K^{\theta_3}, \qquad (1)$$

where d represents the magnitude of dissonance associated with the key element, and θ_1, θ_2, and θ_3 represent exponents of the power functions. These three power parameters are theoretical constants. Each of the values holds positions between 0 and 1. All of the values of d, D, C, and K in Equation 1 are greater than or equal to zero (except that both D and C are simultaneously equal to zero).[2]

Equation 1 is a monotonically increasing function. However, it involves an important qualification due to the power parameters. That is, the increment in the magnitude of dissonance decreases as the value of each of the right-hand three variables increases (cf. Stevens's power law; Stevens, 1962). Estimation of the values of these parameters is helpful, in calculating the magnitude of dissonance more exactly (see Appendix).

Equation 1 shows that the key cognitive element is one of the crucial factors influencing the magnitude of dissonance. Festinger (1957) paid attention to the anxiety-provoking rumors following the Indian earthquake of 1934 that "predicted even worse disasters to come in the very near future" (p. vii). In his interpretation of the rumors, the key element must be the feeling of anxiety. The more important the key element, that is, the greater the anxiety, the more widely the rumors

---

[2]$D/(D + C)$ in Equation 1 does not represent the weighted proportion of the dissonant relations to the relevant relations in Festinger's (1957) verbal definition. Nevertheless, Equation 1 is congruent with his statement that each relevant relation must be weighted according to the importance of the elements involved in that relation. If researchers define the magnitude of dissonance as Festinger did, the weight through the importance of the key element disappears. This is because both the numerator, made up of the dissonant relations, and the denominator, made up of the dissonant and consonant relations, have the common weight through the importance of the key element. This common weight becomes canceled in the process of the reduction of the fraction. Therefore, it is crucial to introduce K in Equation 1.

will be accepted. Equation 1 algebraically makes it clear that the key element always can be a target for reducing dissonance. Festinger (1957) suggested that "divorcing himself psychologically from the action" (p. 29) and "revoking the decision psychologically" (p. 44) are rare but very effective ways to reduce dissonance. These responses reduce dissonance by decreasing the value of K in Equation 1. Simon, Greenberg, and Brehm (1995) found that decreasing the importance of counterattitudinal essay writing, which may be regarded as a key element, was a viable way to reduce dissonance. A mode of dissonance reduction aimed at the key element is referred to as the *K-aimed* mode in this MPF model.[3]

If the value of $[D/(D + C)]$ in Equation 1 is greater than .50, reversing the key element so as to become consonant with the existing dissonant elements is a most reasonable way to reduce dissonance. Even a habitual smoker can give up smoking if the value of this fraction continues to be greater than .50. In Festinger's (1957, pp. 162–176) gambling experiment, participants played a card game against the experimenter. Each participant had to make a choice as to which side he wanted to play on before the game. The experimenter told the participant that he would be allowed to switch once during the 30 trials but added that it would cost him $1 to do so. It is evident that the amount of winnings and the amount of losses corresponded to C and D, respectively. Thus, the value of $[D/(D + C)]$ for the losers would have been greater than .50. The results indicated that when the experimenter presented the dissonant graph after 12 trials, the percentage of participants who reversed their initial decision was significantly higher for the losers (40%) than for the winners (10%), although they had to pay money to change to the other side.

---

[3]Festinger (1957) mentioned a seemingly strange way to reduce dissonance: "compartmentalizing different cognitive clusters so that they, in effect, have nothing to do with one another" (p. 271). This also may be regarded as a special case of the K-aimed mode. The compartmentalization is a change of the state of the cognitive structure. No initially dissonant and consonant elements are related to the key element any longer. One effective way to isolate each element is either to eliminate the key element from the radial structure or to negate the existence of the key element in the structure. This is equivalent to decreasing the importance of the key element slowly or quickly until it reaches almost zero.

Equation 1 indicates that D has the greatest influence on the magnitude of dissonance. Thus, changing some or all of the dissonant elements into the consonant ones, decreasing the importance of the dissonant elements, or both are very effective ways to reduce dissonance. A mode of dissonance reduction aimed at the dissonant element is referred to as the *D-aimed* mode in the present model. On the other hand, C has far less influence on the magnitude of dissonance than D, because C merely constitutes a part of the fraction in Equation 1. Neither increasing the importance of the existing consonant elements nor adding new consonant elements is an effective way to reduce dissonance. This is because these ways reduce dissonance only by increasing the value of the denominator of the fraction. This fraction becomes zero if and only if C becomes positive infinity. A mode of dissonance reduction aimed at the consonant element is referred to as the *C-aimed* mode in the MPF model.

When no consonant elements exist, Equation 1 is reduced to the following equation:

$$d = D^{\theta_2} \times K^{\theta_3}. \qquad (2)$$

Equation 2 shows that the magnitude of dissonance can vary when all relations are dissonant. Equation 2 also indicates that Equation 1 includes the definition of the magnitude of dissonance when two elements are dissonant with one another. The magnitude of the dissonance is given by Equation 2, the reduced form of Equation 1, on the assumption that one element is K, another element is D_1, and no remaining Ds are present in Figure 1.

Equation 1 has clear advantages over the verbal definitions of Festinger (1957). The mathematical formulation represents all the essential features of his verbal definitions in one simple function. It eliminates the ambiguities of the verbal definitions and opens a new way to calculate the magnitude of dissonance associated with any key element.

The predictions that were not explicit in Festinger (1957) are derivable from Equation 1. The D-aimed modes are more effective than the C-aimed modes in dissonance reduction. As long as the dissonant elements are not extremely resistant to change, the C-aimed modes will be used less than the D-aimed modes. The K-aimed mode is a hidden but viable mode of dissonance reduction. If the value of $[D/(D + C)]$ is greater than .50, the reversal of the key element is a most reasonable way to reduce dissonance.

Difficulties in the Alternative Definitions of the Magnitude of Dissonance

The ratio definition of the total magnitude of dissonance is typically presented as "D divided by D plus C" (Festinger & Carlsmith, 1959, p. 204), where "D" and "C" denote the sum of the weighted dissonant relations and the sum of the weighted consonant relations associated with some particular cognition, respectively. Each relevant relation is weighted according to the importance of the elements involved in that relation. However, this ratio definition has two difficulties.

First, dissonance cannot vary within and between situations in which the values of the ratios are the same. For example, imagine one situation: Ms. B has just made a public statement counter to her private opinion about abortion. Suppose that "D" = 35 and "C" = 40, associated with this public statement as the key element. Then the magnitude of dissonance = $[35/(35 + 40)]$ = .47. However, imagine another situation: Ms. B has just chosen pizza and rejected hamburger as her lunch. Suppose that "D" = 7 and "C" = 8, associated with the choice as the key element. Then the magnitude of dissonance = $[7/(7 + 8)]$ = .47. Imagine one more situation: Ms. B has just decided to be a scientist rather than an artist. Suppose that "D" = 63 and "C" = 72, associated with this decision as the key element. Then the magnitude of dissonance = $[63/(63 + 72)]$ = .47. Thus, the amount of dissonance for Ms. B is the same in all these situations. Note that this equal-ratio problem can be solved by the second part and third part of the right side of Equation 1 (see also Footnote 2).

Second, the ratio definition cannot deal with situations in which no consonant relations are present ("C" = 0). Assume two situations in which "D_1" = 10 and "D_2" = 30. Then the ratio definition indicates that the magnitude of dissonance in both situations = $[10/(10 + 0)]$ =

$[30/(30 + 0)] = 1$. Dissonance always becomes unity, independent of the number and importance of dissonant relations (except "D" = 0).

Some researchers may suspect that it is impossible to have situations in which no consonant element exists around the key element. Imagine, however, a situation such as the extermination camps of the Nazis: A person who is going to be put to death says in a low voice, "I am completely innocent," "There is no reason for me to be killed," and "I do not want to die." In this situation, the key element should be "I am going to be put to death." Although the person can come to believe in life after death to reduce dissonance, the dissonance will disappear if the person is set free by a liberator just before being put to death.

Wyer (1974) supported the ratio definition with one exception: He postulated a new concept, *dissonance threshold.* According to Wyer, participants actually do not reduce dissonance to zero but rather reduce it to below the dissonance threshold that they can tolerate. Differential attitude change is neither predictable nor interpretable from differential magnitude of dissonance without this concept. If dissonance must be reduced to zero, the amount of dissonance-mediated attitude change must be the same with any magnitude of dissonance. However, assume that the greater the dissonance, the greater the likelihood of overcoming resistance to change of the target cognitions. Then the differential attitude change is predictable and interpretable without the threshold concept.[4]

Viewed from the MPF model, whether Wyer's (1974) dissonance threshold notion can solve the problems in the ratio definition may be of interest. Suppose, in Ms. B's example, that her dissonance threshold is .20. She may reduce the value of "D" from 35 to 10 after her public statement about abortion and from 7 to 2 after her choice for lunch, respectively. Then, the remaining dissonance = $[10/(10 + 40)] = [2/(2 + 8)] = .20$, which she can tolerate. The amount of attitude change is 25 and 5, respectively. However, why does the same magnitude of dis-

---

[4]Festinger (1957) did not assume that dissonance must always be reduced to zero. He discussed the situation in which a prophecy was successively disconfirmed, "where the dissonance can no longer be reduced to *a point where it is tolerable*" [italics added] (p. 251), although he did not use the term *dissonance threshold.*

sonance (.47) produce such differential attitude change (25 vs. 5)? Wyer's postulate may hold true if the value of $[35/(35 + 40)]$ is greater than the value of $[7/(7 + 8)]$.

Wyer's (1974) dissonance threshold notion is of little logical importance for distinguishing between the D-aimed and C-aimed modes in dissonance reduction and merely requires the amount of dissonance to reach the threshold, whether through the D-aimed or the C-aimed modes. It is evident that even if the threshold concept is introduced into the ratio definition, dissonance cannot vary when all relations are dissonant.

Shultz and Lepper (1996) also presented a formal mathematical definition of the magnitude of dissonance (see chap. 10, this volume). In their neural network model (the *consonance* model), the networks correspond to a participant's representation of the situations in the classic dissonance research. Each cognition consists of a pair of units. One unit represents a positive direction of the cognition, and another unit represents a negative direction. Thus, if a network consists of three cognitions (e.g., cognitions about counterattitudinal behavior, external justification, and internal evaluation), it constitutes a six-unit network. In these networks, activations of various units represent the direction and strength of the individual's beliefs and attitudes. *Connection weights* between cognitions represent psychological implications among the person's beliefs and attitudes. The connections between any two units can be either positive or negative, or the two units can be irrelevant to one another.

In this consonance model, any pair of units i and j are in a consonant relation if the value of the triple product of w_{ij}, a_i, and a_j is greater than zero. Here w_{ij} denotes the connection weight ($-1 \leq w_{ij} \leq 1$) between units i and j, and a_i and a_j denote the activations of units i and j, respectively. The amount of consonance is defined as the value of the triple product. *Total dissonance* in a network is defined as the negative of total consonance divided by the number of nonzero intercognition relations in the network. Shultz and Lepper (1996) have claimed that their definition "goes beyond the ratio definition of Festinger (1957), because it is formalized, assesses the amount of dissonance in each intercognition relation, includes within-cognition ambivalence, includes 'consonant' relations with positive triple products, and can vary when all relations are dissonant (i.e., all triple products are negative) or all relations are consonant (i.e., all triple products are positive)" (p. 223).

It is doubtful, however, that the amount of consonance can be defined as the value of the triple product, (w_{ij}) (a_i) (a_j). The value of the connection weight and the values of the activations of units i and j are located in two different categorical dimensions. Therefore, the product of these values has no exact quantitative meaning. It may be possible to check with the sign of the triple product to see whether the relation is consonant or dissonant; however, it is almost impossible to tell which amount of consonance is greater, .1 (.8) (.8) or .8 (.2) (.4), where the values represent w_{ij}, a_i, and a_j, respectively.[5]

Also, the total dissonance (d) in their definition cannot vary when all relations are dissonant if the activations of all units have the same values: for example, in a four-unit network with one dissonant intercognition relation, $d = -2[-.5 \ (.5) \ (.5)]/1 = 0.25$, and in a six-unit network with two dissonant intercognition relations, $d = -2[-.5 \ (.5) \ (.5) + (-.5) \ (.5) \ (.5)]/2 = 0.25$. Further, in a six-unit network or an eight-unit network with three dissonant intercognition relations, $d = -2[-.5 \ (.5) \ (.5) + (-.5) \ (.5) \ (.5) + (-.5) \ (.5) \ (.5)]/3 = 0.25$. Why should the dissonance be the same, 0.25, in all these networks? It seems necessary to exclude the number of nonzero intercognition relations from Shultz and Lepper's (1996) definition of *total* dissonance of a network. Finally, although this is not a major problem, dissonance varies even when all relations are consonant. The magnitude of dissonance should be equal to zero in no-dissonance situations.

---

[5]Shultz and Lepper (1996) made an additional assumption in the application. That is, the values of w_{ij} are invariably equal to 0.5 for excitatory relations and -0.5 for inhibitory relations. This means that the magnitude of consonance or dissonance between two units is defined as a multiplicative function of the a_i and a_j, with a constant (0.5 or -0.5) that represents the relation between the two units. Thus, the consonance model is similar to the present MPF model, though the consonance model includes neither the power parameters nor the key element.

IMPLICATIONS OF THE MPF MODEL

The present MPF model always requires the identification of what the key cognitive element is in the first place. The attempt to identify the key element in each of the other versions of dissonance should clarify the conceptual implications of the MPF model. The attempt to provide alternative bases for the new quantitative prediction derived from the consonance model may clarify the quantitative implications in the MPF model.

The Key Cognition in the Other Versions of Dissonance

It was found that dissonance has clear motivational and emotional properties (e.g., Elkin & Leippe, 1986; Elliot & Devine, 1994). It was also confirmed that the degree of dissonance arousal can be affected by factors (e.g., amphetamine) other than the relevant cognitive elements (e.g., Cooper, Zanna, & Taves, 1978; Steele, Southwick, & Critchlow, 1981; Zanna & Cooper, 1974). These findings are very interesting and important. However, such qualities of dissonance should extend beyond the particular situations. Thus, little significance can be given to the attempt to identify a single key cognitive element in this type of research.

Cognition about one's action or behavior has been regarded as the most important key element in most research and views on dissonance theory. This cognition is accompanied with commitment, certainty, and salience, which are expected to increase the resistance to change of the key element (cf. Beauvois & Joule, 1996; Brehm, 1992; Brehm & Cohen, 1962; Festinger, 1964; Joule, 1986; Mills & Ross, 1964). Brehm and Cohen (1962) stated that "dissonance theory, we have seen, is in part a theory of *postdecision* behavior" (p. 230; see the independent but identical statement in Wicklund & Brehm, 1976, p. 257). The MPF model does accept that cognition about one's action or behavior is one of the most important key elements. Nevertheless, the crucial principle is that the key element must not be restricted to one's action or behavior.

The *generative* cognition in Beauvois and Joule's (1996) radical dissonance theory is almost identical to the key element in the MPF model.

Using the *double* forced-compliance paradigm they showed that there were no empirical advantages to considering the relations among the dissonant and consonant cognitions without reference to the generative cognition. Beauvois and Joule's findings support the radial cognitive structure, with one key element, in the MPF model. However, generative cognition as a key element consists of a highly committing counterattitudinal action, so that act rationalization seems the only evidence of dissonance reduction in their theory.

Aronson (1968) made a drastic demarcation to Festinger's (1957) theory. His postulate is that dissonance at the center of the theory is created between one's self-concept and cognitions about a behavior that violates the self-concept. *Dissonance reduction* is a process by which the violated self-concept is restored. Viewed from the MPF model, *self-concept* is beliefs about oneself. Thus, Aronson (1968) regarded this particular belief as the most important key element. Aronson (1992) extended his model: Past behavior as well as present behavior can violate one's self-concept about being consistent, competent, and morally good. In this three-part self-concept model, a retrospective or framed feeling of hypocrisy threatens the self-concept. This feeling creates dissonance and hence produces behavioral bolstering and justification (e.g., Aronson, Fried, & Stone, 1991; Stone, Wiegand, Cooper, & Aronson, 1997).

Now assume that the following are true: (a) Dissonance is a motivation for self-protective behavior, and (b) this motivation is created mainly by the violation of one's self-concept. Then the syllogistically sound (but tautological) conclusion is as follows: Dissonance is created mainly by violation of the self-concept. I infer that what Aronson (1968, 1992) implied in his self-concept model was the very first premise: Dissonance theory is a theory of motivation for self-protective behavior. If researchers accept this statement, they may be willing to accept that dissonance theory has evolved into the theory of self (as noted by Greenwald & Ronis, 1978). They also may be willing to regard attitudinal and behavioral justification as the only evidence of dissonance reduction. However, it is not certain whether they will further accept the self-concept as the key element (cf. Cooper, 1992).

The present MPF model accepts that the self-concept is a probable key element. However, the model does not assume that it is necessary for dissonance theory to be a theory of motivation for self-protective behavior. The MPF model does not regard self-justification as the only evidence of dissonance reduction. Frey and Stahlberg (1986) found that participants who received reliable negative feedback about their intelligence test scores not only looked for more test-disparaging information but also evaluated being highly intelligent as less important than did the participants who received possibly unreliable negative feedback. Using the same intelligence-test paradigm, Götz-Marchand, Götz, and Irle (1974) also found that participants lowered the evaluation of their own intelligence after the negative feedback when this was offered as a first mode of dissonance reduction and the following modes were unknown. These findings suggest that reducing the importance of being intelligent is a viable way to reduce dissonance. This kind of dissonance reduction includes little self-justification.

Wicklund and Brehm (1976) concluded in their review of the forced-compliance literature that behavior and its consequence are two irrelevant cognitions without the perceived causal connection between oneself and the potentially dissonance-arousing event. They accepted that personal responsibility is a determinant of the nature of relation between cognitions. In contrast to Aronson (1968), however, they regarded cognition about one's behavior as the key element in principle. Viewed from the MPF model, it may be interesting to ask whether cognition about a behavior is dissonant with the cognition about its negative consequences when the person feels personally responsible for the consequences.

Consider the next two cognitions: $P = $ "I told a naive participant waiting for an experiment that I had just finished the experiment and the task was very interesting," and $Q = $ "The participant believed what I had said and strongly expected that the task would be very interesting." Considering these two alone, the cognition Q follows from the cognition P. Thus, these cognitions should be consonant with one another. To resolve this problem, it seems necessary for Wicklund and Brehm (1976) to further regard the behavior and its consequences to be a single key element. That is, when a person feels personally responsible for both his or her counterattitudinal behavior and its negative consequences, the cognition about the behavior and its consequences as a whole may be dissonant with his or her private attitude.

Cooper and Fazio's (1984) new look model (see chap. 7, this volume) introduced another kind of drastic change to dissonance theory. In this model, dissonance is brought about not simply by inconsistency among cognitions but rather by an aversive event. They proposed that the concept of dissonance must be differentiated into the concepts of *dissonance arousal* and *dissonance motivation.* An aversive and undesired event leads to dissonance arousal if and only if this event occurs because of something for which the actor is responsible. Dissonance motivation and attitude change are most likely to occur when the actors attribute the dissonance arousal to their own behavior. The actors change their private attitudes related to that behavior, to reduce the aversiveness of its consequences. Scher and Cooper (1989) found that even a proattitudinal behavior produces dissonance-mediated attitude change when the behavior brings about negative consequences for which the actor is responsible. They suggested that dissonance theory is a theory about the consequences of being responsible for negative events.[6]

Indeed, Cooper and Fazio's (1984) new look model is most straightforward in the specification of the conditions for dissonance arousal and in the explanation of attitude change. Viewed from the MPF model, however, it is not immediately clear what the key cognitive element is in the new look model. If the cognition about aversive and undesired consequences were the key element, what then would be another cognition that was dissonant with this cognition? Would it be one's belief in being efficacious, desire to avoid aversiveness, wish for some good end, action (behavior) counter to the norm of a given situation, or

---

[6]However, Harmon-Jones, Brehm, Greenberg, Simon, and Nelson (1996) found that a counterattitudinal action without any negative consequences produces physiological arousal and dissonance-mediated attitude change in a just barely sufficient justification situation. These findings support Festinger's (1957) initial view that attitude-discrepant behavior itself is sufficient to create dissonance. Harmon-Jones et al. suggested that the aversive state due to cognitive inconsistency is to be distinguished from the aversiveness of the behavioral consequences.

none of these? If the answer were "none of these," the new look model might not be able to claim the concept of dissonance.

Alternative Bases for the New Quantitative Prediction Derived From the Consonance Model

Shultz and Lepper's (1996) consonance model includes no single key cognition around which dissonance is calculated. Viewed from the MPF model, their success in the computer simulations of the classic dissonance experiments is likely due to their two critical assumptions (i.e., not only the invariant values of the connection weights but also the high resistance to change of the behavior and justification and the low resistance to change of the evaluation).

They claimed that although dissonance theory merely predicts a separation of the alternatives in a free-choice situation, the consonance model generates a new prediction. That is, the rise in evaluation of the chosen alternative between undesirable alternatives is greater than the fall in evaluation of the rejected alternative between desirable alternatives. Actual as well as simulated results in Shultz and Lepper (1996) seem to support this prediction. They regarded it as very important evidence for the consonance model.

Note, however, that the choice between undesirable alternatives would not have been made without external pressure that constituted a consonant element and that this was not considered in Shultz and Lepper's (1996) calculation of consonance. The present MPF model will provide alternative bases for their prediction and results. In a free-choice situation, each of the choice alternatives is dividable into positive and negative aspects.

For example, suppose that immediately after the choice between undesirable alternatives, evaluations of the positive and negative aspects of the chosen alternative are 0 and -4 and evaluations of the positive and negative aspects of the rejected alternative are 0 and -5, respectively. Then the negative aspect of the chosen alternative and the negative aspect of the rejected alternative are dissonant and consonant with the choice, respectively. As previously stated, it is predicted in the MPF model that the D-aimed modes are more effective than the C-aimed modes in dissonance reduction. Thus, the amount of change will be greater in evaluation of the negative aspect of the chosen alternative (e.g., from -4 to -1) than in evaluation of the negative aspect of the rejected alternative (e.g., from -5 to -6). In this example, then, evaluation change in the chosen alternative $= -1 - (-4) = 3$. Evaluation change in the rejected alternative $= -6 - (-5) = -1$.

This pattern of evaluation change is what Shultz and Lepper (1996) predicted and obtained in the choice between undesirable alternatives. In the same way, the pattern of evaluation change in the choice between desirable alternatives is predictable and interpretable from the MPF model. More important, the MPF model implies that the rise in evaluation of the chosen alternative between undesirable alternatives will be greater than the fall in evaluation of the rejected alternative between desirable alternatives, only if the resistance to change of the positive aspect of the rejected alternative between desirable alternatives is greater than the resistance to change of the negative aspect of the chosen alternative between undesirable alternatives.

PRELIMINARY FINDINGS IN SUPPORT OF THE MPF MODEL

Not Only Actors but Also Perceivers May Experience Dissonance: The Illusion of Control Over and Responsibility for One's Misfortune

Sakai and Andow (1980) hypothesized that when participants met with misfortune, they would be able to make use of the mechanisms of dissonance reduction to ameliorate it if they had the illusion of control over and responsibility for the misfortune. We used Wortman's (1975) method to create the illusion of control over and responsibility for an aversive event brought about by chance. In Wortman's study, one third of the participants were told which marble stood for which prize, and then they picked a marble to determine their prize. Another third were told which marble stood for which prize beforehand, but the experimenter picked a marble. The remaining participants picked a marble, but they had not been told which marble stood for which prize. Wortman found that participants perceived more control over the outcome and more responsibility for the outcome in the participant-caused–foreknowledge condition than in the experimenter-caused–foreknowledge and the participant-caused–no-foreknowledge conditions, although the outcomes were obviously determined by chance.

Eighty students at the University of Tokyo participated in a 2 × 2 × 2 factorial experiment. The three factors were (a) strong versus weak electric shock, (b) long versus short duration of the anticipated task with shocks, and (c) the person who threw a dice to determine the level of shock: the participant versus the experimenter. Participants were first told that the purpose of the experiment was to examine effects of tension state on performance of the Stroop (1935) Color–word test and that electric shocks would be used to manipulate the tension state. Next they were told that the level of shock was determined by oddness or evenness of the spots of a dice. Finally, they were told which spots stood for which level of the shock. Then the participant or the experimenter threw the dice. According to the spots of the dice, participants were given a strong or a weak shock as a sample during the experiment. The dependent variables were measured after the sample shock.

Most important for the present discussion, there was a significant main effect of the person who threw the dice. The participants who threw a dice estimated that their heart rate increased less as a result of the shock than did the participants for whom the experimenter threw a dice. Actual heart rate did not differ significantly between the two conditions. In addition, the participants who threw a dice evaluated the experimenter as more intelligent and more favorable than did the participants for whom the experimenter threw a dice.

Note that the participants who threw a dice were the perceivers rather than the actors. Indeed, they performed a behavior, but they were not actually responsible for their behavior. The findings suggest that the illusion of control over and responsibility for an aversive event creates dissonance and that the illusion not only reduces the aversiveness of the event but also produces attitude change to alleviate the whole situation. One's misfortune may be greatly ameliorated by actively having the illusion of control over and responsibility for it. The findings extend the notion that "dissonance is aroused by freely bringing about aversive consequences that are foreseeable" (Cooper & Fazio, 1984, p. 240).

Not Only Actors but Also Observers May Experience Dissonance: Shared Responsibility for the Other Person's Advocacy and Its Negative Consequences

Sakai (1997) tested the hypothesis that the notion of personal responsibility for negative consequences (Calder, Ross, & Insko, 1973; Collins & Hoyt, 1972; Cooper, 1971; Cooper & Fazio, 1984; Wicklund & Brehm, 1976) was extendable to shared responsibility for the other person's advocacy and its negative consequences. In this experiment, two unit-forming factors (proximity and common fate; discussed by Heider, 1958) were used to manipulate shared responsibility. Up to the time of introducing the manipulation of shared responsibility, the procedure was similar to that of Festinger and Carlsmith (1959). After performing a boring task, participants were induced to have either unit or no-unit relation to their coparticipant (a confederate). Then the experimenter asked the coparticipant to tell the next participant (in fact, a second confederate) that the task had been very interesting. The second confederate pretended to be persuaded.

In the unit condition, the experimenter requested that one of the two participants perform the behavior of telling the next participant that the task was interesting. Then the confederate proposed to the naive participant that they should go together and added that he or she (the confederate) would deliver the counterattitudinal message to the next participant. Further, the confederate asked whether it was okay with the participant. In the no-unit condition, the experimenter told the confederate to do the work, and the confederate said nothing more to the naive participant. During the advocacy, participants in the unit condition sat next to their partner, face-to-face with the next participant. Participants in the no-unit condition stood alone, distant from their partner and the second confederate. The results indicated that participants in the unit condition expressed more familiarity toward their partner than did participants in the no-unit condition. Participants in the unit condition also felt more joint responsibility for the negative consequences and evaluated the boring task as more interesting than did participants in the no-unit condition.

These findings suggest that the person put in the unit relationship with the other person by proximity and common fate felt jointly responsible for the other person's advocacy and its negative consequences, experienced dissonance, and manifested self-justificatory attitude change, even if the person himself or herself did not make any counterattitudinal advocacy. What then was the key element in this experimental situation? On the basis of the results about familiarity, Sakai (1997) suggested that the key element would be *we concept*, that is, the extended self. However, it is also likely that the key element was the participant's own action to agree and go along with the other's decision.[7]

Are the Dissonance Phenomena Limited to Western Cultures?

It seems evident that Japanese people can feel cognitive dissonance. However, using the free-choice paradigm, Heine and Lehman (1997) found no dissonance effects in Japanese participants. In their experiment, Canadian and Japanese participants, who were in Vancouver, chose one of two attractive CDs of Western music as reward for their participation in the study on music preferences and personality. After

---

[7]As mentioned, shared responsibility was manipulated by both proximity and common fate in Sakai's (1997) study. To introduce and increase the feeling of common fate, the partner made the proposal to a participant in the unit condition that they should go together, added that the partner would make the counterattitudinal advocacy alone, and asked whether it was okay with the participant. Neither the proposal nor the question was put to the participant in the no-unit condition. It seems certain from the data on the familiarity toward the partner that participants in the unit condition felt more common fate and developed more the sense of we with their partner than did participants in the no-unit condition. However, when the feeling of common fate was manipulated, it is likely that participants in the unit condition agreed to allow their partner lie to the next participant and went along with their partner's decision, whereas participants in the no-unit condition did not act. This alternative explanation of the effects of Sakai (1997) renders it difficult to draw a clear conclusion about what the key element is and whether one's own action is necessary to create dissonance in this kind of situation. Future research is needed to clarify the key element and the cause of the very interesting effect.

the choice, they were given positive, negative, or no feedback about their personality test scores. The no-feedback control group showed the typical separation of the alternatives (i.e., the *spreading-apart* effects), the negative-feedback group showed more enhanced spreading-apart effects, and the positive-feedback group showed no spreading-apart effects, but only among Canadian participants. Japanese participants showed no separation of the alternatives in any feedback conditions. On the basis of these results, they suggested that the Japanese do not rationalize their decisions, and dissonance effects are in general limited to Western cultures.

Heine and Lehman's (1997) study is very interesting in terms of culture and dissonance. Their results, however, may be due to the effects of *cognitive overlap*. In a free-decision situation, "the greater the cognitive overlap between the two alternatives, that is, the less the qualitative distinction between them, the smaller the dissonance that exists after the choice has been made" (Festiginer, 1957, p. 41). Viewed from the words of songs, it is likely that cognitive overlap between the alternative CDs of Western rock and pop music, such as Janet Jackson, was much higher in the Japanese participants, who spoke English as a foreign language, than in the Canadian participants, who spoke it as a mother tongue.

Unfortunately, little research on the spreading-apart effects using the free-choice paradigm has been done by Japanese social psychologists. However, using the forced-compliance paradigm with a high-choice manipulation, Sakai (1981) found that Japanese male high school students who advocated abolishing the coeducational system of their school evaluated the abolition more favorably in the public advocacy conditions than in the anonymous advocacy and control conditions. The results of this study as well as those of Sakai and Andow (1980) and Sakai (1997) suggest that Japanese people do show dissonance and dissonance reduction.

CONCLUSION

The MPF model has been proposed to expand and refine dissonance theory. In this model, any cognitive element is qualified to be the key element around which dissonance exists. A cognitive element is redefined as a state of mind that is verbalizable as a sentence. This redefinition will facilitate the construction of a conceptual bridge between balance theories and dissonance theory. The importance of a cognitive element is defined as the importance of its corresponding sentence. The mathematical formulation of the magnitude of dissonance provides new quantitative perspectives on the process of dissonance generation and reduction. The identification of the key element in each of the other versions of dissonance has clarified the implications of the MPF model that the other revisions do not have. The MPF model is useful for specifying one cognition as the key element, calculating the magnitude of existing and remaining dissonance between and within situations, predicting the K-aimed, D-aimed, and C-aimed modes in dissonance reduction, and performing an empirical test of the quantitative as well as qualitative hypotheses about dissonance processes. The findings in Sakai (1997) and Sakai and Andow (1980) offer potentially interesting evidence in support of the principles in the MPF model and indicate that dissonance effects are not limited to Western cultures.

REFERENCES

Abelson, R. P. (1983). Whatever became of consistency theory? *Personality and Social Psychology Bulletin, 9*, 37–54.

Aronson, E. (1968). Dissonance theory: Progress and problems. In R. P. Abelson, E. Aronson, W. J. McGuire, T. M. Newcomb, M. J. Rosenberg, & P. H. Tannenbaum (Eds.), *Theories of cognitive consistency: A sourcebook* (pp. 5–27). Chicago: Rand McNally.

Aronson, E. (1992). The return of the repressed: Dissonance theory makes a comeback. *Psychological Inquiry, 3*, 303–311.

Aronson, E., Fried, C., & Stone, J. (1991). Overcoming denial and increasing the intention to use condoms through the induction of hypocrisy. *American Journal of Public Health, 81*, 1636–1638.

Beauvois, J.-L., & Joule, R.-V. (1996). *A radical dissonance theory*. London: Taylor & Francis.

Bem, D. J. (1972). Self-perception theory. In L. Berkowitz (Ed.), *Advances in experimental social psychology* (Vol. 6, pp. 1–62). New York: Academic Press.

Brehm, J. W. (1992). An unidentified theoretical object. *Psychological Inquiry, 3*, 314–315.

Brehm, J. W., & Cohen, A. R. (1962). *Explorations in cognitive dissonance.* New York: Wiley.

Calder, B. J., Ross, M., & Insko, C. A. (1973). Attitude change and attitude attribution: Effects of incentive, choice, and consequences. *Journal of Personality and Social Psychology, 25*, 84–99.

Collins, B. E., & Hoyt, M. F. (1972). Personal responsibility-for-consequences: An integration and extension of the "forced compliance" literature. *Journal of Experimental Social Psychology, 8*, 558–593.

Cooper, J. (1971). Personal responsibility and dissonance: The role of foreseen consequences. *Journal of Personality and Social Psychology, 18*, 354–363.

Cooper, J. (1992). Dissonance and the return of the self-concept. *Psychological Inquiry, 3*, 320–323.

Cooper, J., & Fazio, R. H. (1984). A new look at dissonance theory. In L. Berkowitz (Ed.), *Advances in experimental social psychology* (Vol. 17, pp. 229–266). New York: Academic Press.

Cooper, J., Zanna, M. P., & Taves, P. A. (1978). Arousal as a necessary condition for attitude change following induced compliance. *Journal of Personality and Social Psychology, 36*, 1101–1106.

Elkin, R. A., & Leippe, M. R. (1986). Physiological arousal, dissonance, and attitude change: Evidence for a dissonance–arousal link and a "don't remind me" effect. *Journal of Personality and Social Psychology, 51*, 55–65.

Elliot, A. J., & Devine, P. G. (1994). On the motivational nature of cognitive dissonance: Dissonance as psychological discomfort. *Journal of Personality and Social Psychology, 67*, 382–394.

Festinger, L. (1957). *A theory of cognitive dissonance.* Evanston, IL: Row, Peterson.

Festinger, L. (1964). *Conflict, decision, and dissonance.* Stanford, CA: Stanford University Press.

Festinger, L., & Carlsmith, J. M. (1959). Cognitive consequences of forced compliance. *Journal of Abnormal and Social Psychology, 58*, 203–210.

Frey, D. (1986). Recent research on selective exposure to information. In L.

Berkowitz (Ed.), *Advances in experimental social psychology* (Vol. 19, pp. 41–80). New York: Academic Press.

Frey, D., & Stahlberg, D. (1986). Selection of information after receiving more or less reliable self-threatening information. *Personality and Social Psychology Bulletin, 12,* 434–441.

Götz-Marchand, B., Götz, J., & Irle, M. (1974). Preference of dissonance reduction modes as a function of their order, familiarity and reversibility. *European Journal of Social Psychology, 4,* 201–228.

Greenwald, A. G., & Ronis, D. L. (1978). Twenty years of cognitive dissonance: Case study of the evolution of a theory. *Psychological Review, 85,* 53–57.

Harmon-Jones, E., Brehm, J. W., Greenberg, J., Simon, L., & Nelson, D. E. (1996). Evidence that the production of aversive consequences is not necessary to create cognitive dissonance. *Journal of Personality and Social Psychology, 70,* 5–16.

Harris, R. J. (1975). This is a science? Social psychologists' aversion to knowing what their theories say. *Personality and Social Psychology Bulletin, 1,* 1–3.

Harris, R. J. (1976). The uncertain connection between verbal theories and research hypotheses in social psychology. *Journal of Experimental Social Psychology, 12,* 210–219.

Heider, F. (1946). Attitudes and cognitive organization. *Journal of Psychology, 21,* 107–112.

Heider, F. (1958). *The psychology of interpersonal relations.* New York: Wiley.

Heine, S. J., & Lehman, D. R. (1997). Culture, dissonance, and self-affirmation. *Personality and Social Psychology Bulletin, 23,* 389–400.

Jones, E. E. (1985). Major developments in social psychology during the past five decades. In G. Lindzey & E. Aronson (Eds.), *Handbook of social psychology: Vol. 1. Theory and methods* (3rd ed., pp. 47–107). New York: Random House.

Joule, R.-V. (1986). Twenty five on: Yet another version of cognitive dissonance theory? *European Journal of Social Psychology, 16,* 65–78.

Korn, J. H. (1997). *Illusions of reality: A history of deception in social psychology.* Albany: State University of New York Press.

Mills, J., & Ross, A. (1964). Effects of commitment and certainty upon interest in supporting information. *Journal of Abnormal and Social Psychology, 68,* 552–555.

Rosenberg, M. J. (1968). Hedonism, inauthenticity, and other goads toward expansion of a consistency theory. In R. P. Abelson, E. Aronson, W. J. McGuire, T. M. Newcomb, M. J. Rosenberg, & P. H. Tannenbaum (Eds.), *Theories of cognitive consistency: A sourcebook* (pp. 73–111). Chicago: Rand McNally.

Sakai, H. (1980). On the magnitude of cognitive dissonance: A theoretical note. *The Japanese Journal of Experimental Social Psychology, 20*, 81–84.

Sakai, H. (1981). Induced compliance and opinion change. *Japanese Psychological Research, 23*, 1–8.

Sakai, H. (1997, March 1). *Does shared responsibility for negative consequences generate cognitive dissonance?* Paper presented at the Cognitive Dissonance Theory 40 Years Later Conference, Arlington, TX.

Sakai, H., & Andow, K. (1980). Attribution of personal responsibility and dissonance reduction. *Japanese Psychological Research, 22*, 32–41.

Scher, S. J., & Cooper, J. (1989). Motivational basis of dissonance: The singular role of behavioral consequences. *Journal of Personality and Social Psychology, 56*, 899–906.

Shultz, T. R., & Lepper, M. R. (1996). Cognitive dissonance reduction as constraint satisfaction. *Psychological Review, 103*, 219–240.

Simon, L., Greenberg, J., & Brehm, J. (1995). Trivialization: The forgotten mode of dissonance reduction. *Journal of Personality and Social Psychology, 68*, 247–260.

Steele, C. M. (1988). The psychology of self-affirmation: Sustaining the integrity of the self. In L. Berkowitz (Ed.), *Advances in experimental social psychology* (Vol. 21, pp. 261–302). San Diego, CA: Academic Press.

Steele, C. M., Southwick, L. L., & Critchlow, B. (1981). Dissonance and alcohol: Drinking your troubles away. *Journal of Personality and Social Psychology, 41*, 831–846.

Stevens, S. S. (1962). The surprising simplicity of sensory metrics. *American Psychologist, 17*, 29–39.

Stone, J., Wiegand, A. W., Cooper, J., & Aronson, E. (1997). When exemplification fails: Hypocrisy and the motive for self-integrity. *Journal of Personality and Social Psychology, 72*, 54–65.

Stroop, J. R. (1935). Studies of interference in serial verbal reactions. *Journal of Experimental Psychology, 18*, 643–661.

Takata, T., Shirai, Y., & Hayashi, H. (1983). Cognitive dissonance revisited: II. A critical look at the evolution of the theory. *The Japanese Journal of Experimental Social Psychology, 22,* 167–181.

Tedeschi, J. T., & Rosenfeld, P. (1981). Impression management theory and the forced compliance situation. In J. T. Tedeschi (Ed.), *Impression management theory and social psychological research* (pp. 147–177). New York: Academic Press.

Wicklund, R. A., & Brehm, J. W. (1976). *Perspectives on cognitive dissonance.* Hillsdale, NJ: Erlbaum.

Wortman, C. B. (1975). Some determinants of perceived control. *Journal of Personality and Social Psychology, 31,* 282–294.

Wyer, R. S., Jr. (1974). *Cognitive organization and change: An information processing approach.* Potomac, MD: Erlbaum.

Zajonc, R. B. (1990). Leon Festinger (1919–1989). *American Psychologist, 45,* 661–662.

Zanna, M. P., & Cooper, J. (1974). Dissonance and the pill: An attribution approach to studying the arousal properties of dissonance. *Journal of Personality and Social Psychology, 29,* 703–709.

APPENDIX

How can the values of the power parameters, θ_1, θ_2, and θ_3 be estimated in Equation 1? Let Y denote the total amount of manifestations of the dissonance associated with a key element in a given situation. Y may be expressed as a function of d as follows:

$$Y = A \times d \times U, \qquad (A1)$$

where A is a constant ($A > 0$), and U is a disturbance, whose expected value $E(U) = 1$ and whose variance $V(U) = \sigma_U^2$. The random variable U is introduced into Equation A1 to permit trait and state variations in the manifestations of the dissonance. When Equation 1 is substituted into Equation A1, the following function is obtained:

$$Y = A \times [D/(D + C)]^{\theta_1} \times D^{\theta_2} \times K^{\theta_3} \times U. \quad (A2)$$

Taking the logarithm of both expressions in Equation A2, the following linear function is obtained:

$$y = \theta_0 + \theta_1 x_1 + \theta_2 x_2 + \theta_3 x_3 + \varepsilon, \qquad \text{(A3)}$$

where $y = \log Y$, $\theta_0 = \log A$, $x_1 = \log [D/(D + C)]$, $x_2 = \log D$, $x_3 = \log K$, $\varepsilon = \log U$, $E(\varepsilon) = 0$, and $V(\varepsilon) = \sigma_\varepsilon^2$. As can be seen in Equation A3, given the values of x_1, x_2, x_3, and y, the values of the parameters, θ_1, θ_2, and θ_3, can be estimated by using the least-squares method.

To estimate the values of the parameters, one must obtain the values of Y, D, C, and K in the first place. It has been difficult to measure these variables simultaneously. Now that the MPF model provides an operational definition of the importance of each cognitive element, the values of these parameters will be available in the near future.

PART FOUR

Dissonance and Affect

12

Moving Beyond Attitude Change in the Study of Dissonance-Related Processes

Patricia G. Devine, John M. Tauer, Kenneth E. Barron, Andrew J. Elliot, and Kristen M. Vance

In 1957, Leon Festinger outlined a straightforward set of assumptions concerning the motivational underpinnings of cognitive dissonance. Festinger posited that (a) an inconsistency between cognitions created an uncomfortable psychological tension state, and (b) people would be motivated to reduce the tension by implementing some change that would restore consonance among the inconsistent elements. Festinger's theory is essentially a process model, as represented in Figure 1. In Festinger's model, inconsistency between cognitions (A) leads to dissonance (B), an uncomfortable psychological tension and arousal state that the person will be motivated to reduce. According to the model, the motivational properties of dissonance will lead to a dissonance-reduction strategy (C), which if effective will alleviate dissonance (D).

Much of the imaginative work of dissonance researchers over the last 40 years has been devoted to documenting the motivational properties of dissonance, and an enormous amount of evidence consistent with the predictions of dissonance theory has been obtained. For example, hundreds of studies have shown that when people engage in counterattitudinal behaviors (A), ostensibly effective dissonance-reduction strategies, such as attitude change, are implemented (C)

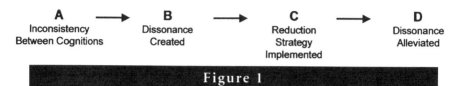

Figure 1

Schematic of Festinger's (1957) process model of dissonance.

(see Cooper & Fazio, 1984, for a review).[1] However, direct evidence regarding the arousal (B) and reduction (D) of dissonance has been more elusive. Given the extant evidence, the reasoning about dissonance arousal and its reduction has been necessarily indirect. The logic is as follows: Because dissonance-reduction strategies (e.g., attitude change) are implemented after a procedure designed to create inconsistencies between attitudes and behavior, it has been assumed that (a) dissonance was created, (b) dissonance motivated the use of the reduction strategy, and (c) the reduction strategy was successful in alleviating the dissonance. Although the well-established attitude-change findings are clearly consistent with theory-derived predictions, they do not provide direct tests of the process assumptions of dissonance theory. In short, the part of dissonance theory that has proven rather elusive has been the core assumption that the tension created is psychologically distressing and that this distress is alleviated after the implementation of a dissonance-reduction strategy.

In this chapter, we argue that outcome measures such as attitude change (or other ostensibly effective dissonance-reduction strategies, such as bolstering, self-affirmation, or trivialization) cannot provide this type of evidence because such measures are silent regarding underlying

---

[1]Throughout the chapter, we focus on induced-compliance paradigms that have traditionally used attitude change as the indicator of dissonance. We should be clear, however, that the induced-compliance paradigm is not the only one that suffers from an overreliance on the use of outcome measures as the indicator of dissonance. For example, the free-choice paradigm relies on the spreading of alternatives, and the selective-exposure paradigm relies on preference for attitude-consistent information. We suggest that these paradigms, with their emphasis on outcome measures to indicate dissonance arousal and reduction, are also limited in what they can reveal about the nature of the dissonance experience or the process of dissonance induction and reduction. The induced-compliance paradigm, however, has been the most frequently used paradigm in dissonance research. Therefore, we use this paradigm to illustrate our concerns regarding the overreliance on such outcome measures as indicators of both dissonance arousal and reduction.

processes. Thus, the methods most commonly used to test dissonance assumptions are limited in what they can reveal about the nature of the dissonance and whether dissonance-reduction strategies are effective in alleviating dissonance-related distress. Our position is that dissonance theorists have asked too much of attitude change (and other outcome measures). We suggest that more thorough and complete testing of dissonance theory may be possible if we expand our methodological tools in the assessment of dissonance. To this end, we offer one such tool and provide evidence supporting the efficacy of it as a measure that is sensitive to both dissonance induction (B) and reduction (D). Before introducing the measure, however, we review the historical approaches in which attitude change plays a central role.

ATTITUDE CHANGE AS THE INDICATOR OF DISSONANCE: THE GOOD, THE BAD, AND THE UGLY

Historically, the induced-compliance paradigm has been the most frequently used paradigm for studying dissonance hypotheses (see Cooper & Fazio, 1984). In this paradigm, participants are induced to freely choose to advocate a counterattitudinal position, which theoretically sets the stage for creating dissonance (commonly referred to as the *high-choice* condition). As a comparison condition, other participants are assigned to advocate a counterattitudinal position (commonly referred to as the *low-choice* condition); these participants theoretically do not experience dissonance, because they had no choice regarding the position they would advocate. After the counterattitudinal behavior, attitudes are assessed for participants in both choice conditions. In keeping with dissonance theory predictions, studies have repeatedly shown that high-choice participants show greater attitude change than their low-choice counterparts. Such findings have been interpreted to suggest that the dissonance experience is unpleasant and that it motivates attitude change that presumably alleviates dissonance-related distress. In addition, it has often been assumed that these attempts to reduce dissonance are successful. There are clearly some strengths to this empirical strategy.

The Good

Attitude change as the operational definition of dissonance reduction has served dissonance researchers well and yielded key insights regarding many aspects of cognitive dissonance. In the absence of any direct indicators of dissonance, testing outcomes that are consistent with the theory (e.g., attitude change among only high-choice participants after a counterattitudinal behavior) is a sensible and useful empirical strategy. Indeed, we are not suggesting that examining attitude change is in any way wrong or naive. Rather, we are suggesting that our overall understanding of the dynamics of dissonance processes may be improved by developing measures that can be used in conjunction with attitude change (and other outcome measures) to more fully reveal dissonance-related processes.

One of the primary goals early in the history of dissonance research was to demonstrate that the dominant theoretical paradigm in psychology at the time, reinforcement theory, could not account for the provocative findings generated in the tradition of dissonance experiments (see Aronson, 1992, for more detail). As such, the focus was on producing outcomes that were not readily interpretable from a reinforcement perspective. As an illustrative example, consider Festinger and Carlsmith's (1959) classic study in which participants who chose to convince an unsuspecting participant (actually a confederate) that a boring task was actually interesting came to like the task more if they were offered low ($1) compared with high ($20) compensation for their efforts. Thus, early on, the goal of the research was to produce outcomes that were consistent with dissonance theory and not easily handled by alternative theoretical accounts. It was assumed, rather than tested, that the processes outlined by Festinger (1957) were responsible for the outcomes.

As dissonance research moved forward, however, issues arose concerning whether the motivational assumptions outlined by Festinger (1957) were responsible for the observed outcomes (Bem, 1967; Chapanis & Chapanis, 1964; Tedeschi, Schlenker, & Bonoma, 1971) that highlighted the need for evidence beyond attitude change to support dissonance interpretations for these outcomes. In the absence of direct measures of dissonance, these issues were, to say the least, challenging for dissonance theorists. Such theoretical and empirical challenges, however, ultimately served to showcase the cleverness and ingenuity of a generation of dissonance researchers, who developed compelling ways to circumvent the fact that there were no good direct ways to measure dissonance. This was perhaps the most positive by-product of the need to rely on indirect assessment of dissonance. The creativity of these dissonance theorists served to inspire, and continues to inspire, subsequent generations of social psychologists both within and beyond dissonance research.

Consider, as just one of many possible examples, the creative solution to the problem of having no direct measure of dissonance evidenced in Zanna and Cooper's (1974) work on the arousal component of dissonance. Although they could not measure arousal directly, their theoretical resourcefulness led them to adopt a misattribution approach, which drew heavily on Schachter and Singer's (1962) two-factor theory of emotion in characterizing dissonance as an arousal state open to various cognitive labels. Zanna and Cooper reasoned that participants who freely chose to advocate a counterattitudinal position would not change their attitude if given the opportunity to misattribute their arousal.[2] In keeping with their predictions, high-choice participants given a placebo that would ostensibly make them feel tense changed their attitudes less than their high-choice counterparts, who had ingested a drug that supposedly would make them feel relaxed. Zanna and Cooper's study, along with a variety of conceptual replications (see

---

[2]It is of interest to note that Zanna and Cooper (1974) collected a measure of felt tension with a single item, ranging from *calm* (1) to *tense* (31). In general, participants who were expected to feel tension (e.g., standard high-choice condition and participants in the "drug"-creating-arousal conditions) reported higher levels of felt tension. Although these findings were reported, Zanna and Cooper's primary focus was to provide evidence that dissonance had arousal properties. Very few others have attempted to measure the felt discomfort created by dissonance tasks, and studies that did typically suffered from shortcomings that limited the informativeness of the measures (see Elliot & Devine, 1994, for a discussion).

review by Fazio & Cooper, 1983), makes a strong case for the position that dissonance has arousal properties. The key point to be emphasized here is that in the absence of any direct way to assess the arousal component of dissonance, Zanna and Cooper used their theoretical resourcefulness and empirical imaginativeness to circumvent the problem. However, there are also some limitations to the emphasis on arousal that have created interpretational difficulties, if not theory-damning concerns, for dissonance theorists through the years.

The Bad

Although the field got around the fact that there was not a direct indicator of dissonance (i.e., unpleasant tension and arousal) and progress was made, we argue that the field has asked too much of attitude change for informing the conceptual analysis of dissonance. That is, attitude change was the indicator that dissonance was induced *and* reduced. Thus, the fact that high-choice participants changed their attitudes more than low-choice participants was taken evidence that dissonance was experienced among the high-choice participants. Attitude change also served the function of telling researchers, by its absence, that dissonance was no longer present (although, as will become clear later, this may not always be a valid inference). For example, when people implement an ostensibly effective dissonance-reduction strategy, such as bolstering (Sherman & Gorkin, 1980), self-affirmation (Steele & Liu, 1983), or trivialization (Simon, Greenberg, & Brehm, 1995) and then attitudes do not change, it is assumed that dissonance motivation is no longer present. In short, attitude change has been the primary indicator that dissonance was created and that it was reduced.

We suggest that attitude change is at best an indirect indicator of whether dissonance has been induced or reduced. This observation is, of course, not novel. Overreliance on attitude change as an indicator of dissonance induction and reduction has created interpretational difficulties in many studies in which results did not conform with expected dissonance outcomes. For example, when attitude change is not observed in the induced-compliance paradigm, what can be concluded? Was dissonance not successfully created (e.g., perhaps one's procedure was flawed)? Did participants find alternative ways to alleviate their discomfort before attitudes were assessed? Was attitude change not a viable strategy for all participants? Did attitude change reduce dissonance for those who used this strategy? These are crucial questions and ones that attitude change cannot answer.

To illustrate the conceptual ambiguities associated with the use of attitude change as the sole indicator of dissonance, consider a classic study by Cooper and Worchel (1970). The goal of the study was to demonstrate that advocating a counterattitudinal position does not lead to the arousal of cognitive dissonance unless that advocacy results in undesirable consequences. In this study, participants were asked to perform an extremely dull task (cf. Festinger & Carlsmith, 1959) and were offered varying incentives for telling a waiting participant (actually a confederate) that the task was interesting and enjoyable. Before reporting their attitudes toward the task, half of the participants learned that they had successfully convinced the waiting participant that the task was interesting. The other half learned that the participant still believed that the task would be dull.

Cooper and Worchel's (1970) findings revealed that only those participants who believed that they had succeeded in convincing the waiting participant and complied for a small incentive came to believe the task was interesting (e.g., showed the classic dissonance-induced attitude shift). Cooper and Worchel suggested that those who were unsuccessful in convincing the participant (as well as those who received a sufficient incentive) did not change their attitudes because dissonance was not aroused in these participants. We would argue, however, that sole reliance on attitude change in this paradigm cannot reveal whether these participants experienced dissonance. It is at least conceptually possible that dissonance *was* created for the low-incentive participants who learned that their efforts to deceive the waiting participant failed but was reduced before participants' attitudes were assessed. Simply agreeing to the counterattitudinal behavior (i.e., to deceive the waiting participant) would be sufficient to induce dissonance (e.g., Elliot & Devine, 1994; Rabbie, Brehm, & Cohen, 1959). Indeed, learning that they had been unsuccessful in their deception efforts may have been sufficient to alleviate any dissonance-related distress that the deception caused them.

Similar ambiguities arise in other paradigms (with other theoretical agendas) as well. For example, Steele (1988; Steele & Liu, 1983) suggested that classic dissonance manipulations, such as the induced-compliance paradigm, serve to threaten people's global sense of self-integrity. He argued that to alleviate the discomfort, one need not make adjustments (e.g., attitude change) to the cognitions directly involved in the inconsistency but instead could engage in some activity that might restore (or reaffirm) one's global sense of self-integrity. To support this logic, Steele and Liu had participants write a counterattitudinal essay. Then, before reporting their attitudes, participants filled out a value-affirming scale on a dimension that was either important or unimportant to their self-identities. In keeping with Steele's theory, attitude change was observed only among participants for whom the self-affirmation opportunity was not important to their self-identities. However, Steele noted a couple of alternative explanations for the attitude data in Steele and Liu's studies, which suggest that attitude change may not be an adequate measure to demonstrate that dissonance was alleviated. He suggested that the important self-affirmations may have bolstered or frozen participants' initial attitudes, resulting in little attitude change. Thus, it appears that in the dissonance literature, the absence of a more direct measure of dissonance makes it difficult to make strong inferences about the presence or absence of dissonance.

Note that the studies reviewed in this section are not the only studies challenged by interpretational ambiguities that derive from having to reason indirectly about the arousal and reduction of dissonance. These studies were selected to illustrate the interpretational difficulties that arise under such circumstances. The ambiguities are clearly evident in other dissonance research as well. Consider, for example, the difficulties that could arise in a study if some participants' responses fit the classic dissonance attitude-change pattern, but other participants' responses did not. What is the researcher to make of such variability? Was dissonance successfully created for only some of the participants? Or is it possible that attitude change was not a dissonance-reduction option for some people (e.g., people who are highly committed to their attitudes; cf. Hardyck & Kardush, 1968)? Similarly, inconsistent findings (e.g., failure to reliably obtain preference for attitude-consistent information in the selective-exposure literature) proved difficult to resolve in the absence of some indicator that provided independent evidence that dissonance was successfully induced (Cialdini, Petty, & Cacioppo, 1981).

In short, although attitude change can be informative and has been useful in providing support for dissonance theory, it simply cannot rule out alternative explanations (i.e., dissonance was never created; dissonance was created, but not reduced; dissonance was reduced through some other strategy besides attitude change). And, finally, virtually no evidence exists to suggest that if attitude change occurred, participants felt better—that any discomfort that had been created by the dissonance-induction procedure was alleviated. This is perhaps the issue that has received the least empirical attention in the dissonance literature and one that, as illustrated below, raises some questions about the effectiveness of attitude change in explaining the mechanisms underlying the dissonance process.

The Ugly

According to dissonance theory, attitude change was the outcome of a presumed motivational state. The field generally, and dissonance researchers more specifically, was ultimately dissatisfied with having to rely exclusively on indirect evidence for the motivational state. In response to this set of circumstances, an exciting line of research ensued, the goal of which was to provide evidence that dissonance was at least arousing, if not directly psychologically unpleasant. Several studies attempted to show the arousal properties of dissonance by using indirect research techniques, such as incidental retention, response competition, and misattribution of arousal (e.g., Kiesler & Pallak, 1976; Pallak & Pittman, 1972; Zanna & Cooper, 1974).

Other investigators attempted to provide direct evidence regarding the arousal component of dissonance by measuring physiological changes that theoretically would accompany the dissonance. Although the early evidence was mixed, more recent studies provided evidence supporting the dissonance-as-physiological-arousal hypothesis (Elkin & Leippe, 1986; Harmon-Jones, Brehm, Greenberg, Simon, & Nelson, 1996; Losch & Cacioppo, 1990). In a set of induced-compliance experiments, Elkin and Leippe's (1986) participants displayed elevated galvanic skin responses (GSRs), as well as attitude change, after freely choosing to advocate a counterattitudinal position. Losch and Cacioppo (1990) obtained a similar pattern of results by means of a misattribution paradigm and frequency of nonspecific skin conductance responses (NS-SCRs) as the physiological indicator of dissonance arousal. Most recently, Harmon-Jones et al. (1996, Experiment 3) showed increased NS-SCRs in high- but not low-choice conditions. Taken together, these studies provide compelling evidence that there is a physiological component to the dissonance state.

With such strong evidence in hand for the arousal component of dissonance, Elkin and Leippe (1986; see also Harmon-Jones et al., 1996) also attempted to test the hypothesis that attitude change would lead to the reduction in the indicator of the presumed motivational state. Specifically, they tested the assumption that implementing a dissonance-reduction strategy, in this case attitude change, would lead to a reduction in dissonance. Elkin and Leippe argued that support for this assumption was critical to the contention that dissonance is a motivational state. Indeed, such studies provided the first opportunity to test the process assumptions suggested by Festinger's (1957) model. However, these efforts to directly support the hypothesis that dissonance reduction occurs after attitude change were foiled. That is, although Elkin and Leippe were able to show that GSR increased reliably when participants freely chose to advocate a counterattitudinal position (A → B) and that these participants changed their attitudes in the direction of the position they advocated (B → C), they failed to show dissonance reduction in the form of a significant decrease in GSRs in the post-attitude-change period (C did not lead to D).

Such findings were ultimately troublesome for the theory and led Elkin and Leippe (1986) to call into question the veracity of Festinger's (1957) assumptions regarding the motivational nature of dissonance arousal: "It is only though the arousal's subsequent reduction that motivation can be implied, and we found no evidence that explicit attitude change reduced arousal. ... Cognitive dissonance, then, may or may not be a motivational state" (p. 64). This type of statement was damning for the theory. Echoing these types of concerns, Wilder (1992) observed the following: "Questions of the reality of dissonance as a measurable tension or aversive state have always dogged the theory" (p. 352). In the wake of such disappointing findings regarding Festinger's dissonance-reduction postulate as well as the need to rely on indirect reasoning regarding dissonance-related processing, empirical progress regarding dissonance-related hypotheses was largely stalled. However, recent findings using an alternative measure of dissonance have paved the way to directly test Festinger's assumptions regarding dissonance arousal and reduction. This measure serves as a "dissonance thermometer" of sorts and is sensitive to both the induction and reduction of dissonance-related distress.[3] Used in conjunction with outcome measures such as attitude change, a measure of dissonance affect may yield insights concerning the dynamics of dissonance induction and reduction that would be impossible to obtain through outcome measures alone.

MEASURING DISSONANCE AS PSYCHOLOGICAL DISCOMFORT: A DISSONANCE THERMOMETER

Both indirect (e.g., attitude change) and direct (e.g., arousal) indicators of dissonance have created difficulties for testing core assumptions of dissonance theory. A close reading of Festinger's (1957) classic monograph, however, reveals that Festinger conceptualized dissonance in two distinguishable ways. He explicitly delineated psychological discomfort as a component of dissonance, and he alluded to dissonance as a bodily condition analogous to a tension or drive state like hunger (Croyle & Cooper, 1983). In Brehm and Cohen's (1962) restatement of dissonance

---

[3]We thank Mark Zanna for the suggestion of the label *dissonance thermometer*. We think this label is intuitive and captures the essence of the measure.

theory, they distinctly characterized dissonance as a state of arousal and focused extensively on its drivelike properties. As previously suggested, most research investigating the nature of dissonance, whether indirectly or directly, has primarily focused on Brehm and Cohen's derived arousal component of dissonance rather than the psychological discomfort component identified by Festinger. Indeed, the discomfort component of dissonance has most often been assumed rather than measured directly.

We believe the field has been too narrowly focused on arousal as the motivational component of dissonance. Recently, Elliot and Devine (1994) argued that for a variety of reasons psychological discomfort may be the preferred component of dissonance to consider when exploring the dissonance-reduction process. First, physiological measures are still in rather early stages of development, which may place limits on their use for tracking dissonance-reduction processes. Second, Cooper and Fazio (1984) suggested that arousal plays only a distal role in dissonance reduction. That is, although arousal is posited to instigate attributional interpretation, Cooper and Fazio argued that it is the phenomenological experience of discomfort created by the attributional judgment that is the proximal motivational force encouraging the implementation of a dissonance-reduction strategy. Third, even if both arousal and discomfort serve proximal functions in the dissonance process, the time course of dissonance reduction may be different for arousal and psychological discomfort. For example, the dissonance-reduction experience may be marked by immediate psychological relief after the implementation of a dissonance-reduction strategy, followed by more gradual reduction of dissonance-based arousal. Under these circumstances, it may be more feasible to empirically demonstrate the alleviation of the psychological discomfort component of dissonance than a reduction of the arousal component, which may require a time sequence of unknown length. Recent empirical work (Elliot & Devine, 1994) designed specifically to assess the psychological component of dissonance suggests that efforts to assess the psychological component of dissonance may be revealing regarding both the nature of the dissonance experience and the motivational properties of the dissonance state.

Elliot and Devine (1994) argued that to the extent that dissonance is experienced as psychological discomfort (cf. Festinger, 1957), it should be revealed as elevated feelings of discomfort (e.g., uncomfortable, uneasy, bothered) after a counterattitudinal advocacy (see also Devine, Monteith, Zuwerink, & Elliot, 1991). While acknowledging the potential limitations of self-report measures (cf. Nisbett & Wilson, 1977), Elliot and Devine argued that feelings of discomfort could be sensitively assessed with a self-report measure of affect. To the extent that this self-report measure of discomfort was successful, it could serve as a dissonance thermometer sensitive to increases and decreases in psychological discomfort. Elliot and Devine argued further that in the induced-compliance paradigm, if attitude change was truly motivated by an effort to alleviate dissonance, discomfort feelings would be alleviated after the implementation of this reduction strategy. Thus, in an attempt to directly measure psychological discomfort after a counterattitudinal advocacy and its presumed alleviation following attitude change, Elliot and Devine varied the order of the placement of measures of affect and attitude in two induced-compliance studies. To the extent that such a pattern could be shown, it would provide the first direct evidence to support Festinger's (1957) assertion that dissonance is fundamentally a motivational state. The minimum conditions needed to explore these issues are conditions that provide the opportunity to show that discomfort increases in the theoretically predicted circumstances (e.g., counterattitudinal advocacy), and that after an ostensibly effective dissonance-reduction strategy, the discomfort dissipates.

Initial Evidence for Dissonance as Psychological Discomfort

The utility of the affect measure for assessing dissonance is well illustrated in Elliot and Devine's (1994) second study. In this study, all participants wrote a counterattitudinal essay arguing for a 10% tuition increase. The study had three conditions. The low-choice control provided baseline affect and attitude scores. The two high-choice conditions differed only in the order in which participants reported affect and attitude. That is, after freely choosing to write and prepare the

Table 1

Mean Attitude Change and Discomfort Ratings as a Function of Experimental Condition

	Experimental condition		
Measure	High-choice affect–attitude	High-choice attitude–affect	Low choice
Attitude change	5.29_a	5.50_a	2.92_b
Discomfort	3.71_a	2.61_b	2.33_b

Note: Attitude-change values greater than 1 represent change in the direction favoring the proposed tuition increase. Discomfort values had a possible range of 1 to 7, with 7 representing the highest level of dissonance affect. Within each dependent measure, means with different subscripts differ significantly at $p < .01$ by the Fisher least significant difference test. Data from Elliot and Devine (1994, Study 2).

counterattitudinal essay, half of the high-choice participants immediately reported their attitude and then their affect. In the other high-choice condition, the affect measure preceded reports of attitude.[4]

Replicating the standard induced-compliance effect, participants in the high-choice conditions reported more attitude change than their counterparts in the low-choice condition (see Table 1). However, in keeping with Festinger's (1957) theorizing about dissonance induction and reduction, discomfort feelings were elevated only in the condition in which affect was reported before attitudes were assessed. These data suggest that preparing the counterattitudinal essay led to feelings of discomfort. Of critical importance for supporting Festinger's dissonance-reduction postulate, the level of discomfort feelings reported after participants were provided with an attitude-change opportunity dropped to baseline levels and did not differ from the affect reported by low-choice participants, who reported affect before preparing their counterattitudinal essays. Thus, it appears that feelings of discomfort

---

[4]In all of our studies reviewed, choice manipulation checks indicated the effectiveness of the choice manipulation.

dissipate after a dissonance-reduction strategy is implemented. Moreover, the affect findings are unique to discomfort feelings. The affect measure in Elliot and Devine's (1994) research included items that would tap other forms of psychological distress (e.g., guilt or depressed affect) as well as positive affect. None of these other affect measures were influenced by the experimental manipulations.

These findings are important in a number of respects. By focusing on and measuring the psychological discomfort component of dissonance, these data both clarify the nature of the dissonance experience and directly demonstrate the alleviation of dissonance on the implementation of an ostensibly effective dissonance-reduction strategy. Moreover, dissonance appears to be a distinct aversive feeling and not an undifferentiated arousal state. Perhaps most important, by demonstrating that attitude change was in the service of reducing the discomfort created by the counterattitudinal advocacy, Elliot and Devine (1994) obtained the first direct support for both dissonance induction and reduction.

Attitude Importance, Resistance to Change, and the Dissonance Thermometer

We have argued that in dissonance research, there has been an overreliance on attitude change as the key dissonance-reduction strategy (see also Simon et al., 1995; Steele, 1988). We believe that this strategy is, in part, responsible for a relative lack of attention to the study of dissonance-related processes involving important attitudes, which by definition may be more resistant to change than relatively unimportant attitudes (Boninger, Krosnick, Bernet, & Fabrigar, 1995; Zuwerink & Devine, 1996). In the induced-compliance literature, when participants freely choose to advocate a counterattitudinal position, the cognition about this behavior, partly because of its immediate salience, is highly resistant to change (hence attitudes are changed to restore consonance). When a counterattitudinal behavior conflicts with a personally important attitude, both the attitude and the cognition about one's behavior are likely to be resistant to change. When attitude change is not an option, other strategies for reducing dissonance-related distress would be required. A by-product of studying relatively unimportant attitudes is that there has been comparatively little focus on alternative dissonance-reduction strategies.

The issue of attitude importance did not escape the attention and theorizing of Festinger (1957) or the early dissonance researchers. Although it has long been assumed that attitude change may not be a viable dissonance-reduction strategy when the dissonance is associated with important attitudes, empirical attempts to explicate the role of attitude importance are scant. Both classic and more recent theorists have articulated some of the challenges associated with studying important attitudes within the dissonance framework (e.g., Cooper & Mackie, 1983; Hardyck & Kardush, 1968; Pilisuk, 1968; Sherman & Gorkin, 1980). As noted by Sherman and Gorkin (1980), "when the original attitude is an especially strong and central one, involving a large degree of relevance and prior commitment, attitude change is unlikely" (p. 389). In response, Sherman and Gorkin examined a form of attitude bolstering, arguing that neither attitude change nor denying the behavior was possible.

In our recent work, we have sought to document the role of attitude importance in the dissonance process. Specifically, we have begun to investigate how attitude importance influences the nature of the dissonance experience and the types of dissonance-reduction strategies that may prove effective (or ineffective) in alleviating distress. In one study, using a counterattitudinal advocacy paradigm with recycling as the issue, we replicated the essential design of Elliot and Devine (1994) but included participants who varied in the self-reported importance of their recycling attitudes (Devine, Froning, & Elliot, 1995). That is, some of the participants reported that their recycling attitudes were highly personally important, whereas others, although equally in favor of recycling, indicated that their attitudes were less personally important. Low- and high-importance participants were then randomly assigned to one of three conditions. Following Elliot and Devine (1994), this study included a low-choice condition, to establish baseline affect and attitude scores, and two high-choice conditions that differed only in the order in which participants reported their affect and their atti-

Table 2

Mean Attitude Change and Discomfort Ratings as a Function of Experimental Condition and Importance Level

	Experimental condition					
	High-choice affect–attitude		High-choice attitude–affect		Low choice	
Measure	Low imp	High imp	Low imp	High imp	Low imp	High imp
Attitude change	3.75$_a$	1.86$_c$	5.30$_b$	2.57$_c$	2.83$_c$	1.42$_c$
Discomfort	3.60$_a$	3.70$_a$	2.10$_c$	3.84$_a$	2.67$_b$	2.44$_{bc}$

Note: Imp = importance. Attitude-change values greater than 1 represent change in the direction favoring reduction of recycling efforts. Discomfort values had a possible range of 1 to 7, with 7 representing the highest level of dissonance affect. Within each dependent measure, means with different subscripts differ significantly at $p < .01$ by the Fisher least significant difference test.

tude. Under low choice, as can be seen in Table 2, both low- and high-importance participants reported little discomfort or attitude change.[5] Under high choice, the effects were moderated by attitude importance. For low-importance participants, both the attitude change and the discomfort data replicated the findings of Elliot and Devine. Specifically, attitude change for low-importance participants was elevated under both high-choice conditions; however, discomfort feelings were elevated only for low-importance–high-choice participants when affect was reported before attitudes were assessed. For high-importance participants, however, attitude change was not a viable dissonance-reduction strategy. In neither high-choice condition did high-importance participants

---

[5]In this study, all measures were taken after the essay was prepared. In Elliot and Devine (1994), low-choice participants reported affect before the essay task was introduced. Although this provided a nice baseline affect measure, it did not directly address whether the low-choice instructions were dissonance inducing. The data from the Devine et al. (1995) study suggests that the low-choice instructions did not lead to elevated levels of discomfort for high- or low-importance participants. Assessing affect after rather than before the essay task is, we think, generally a preferred strategy.

change their attitudes against campus recycling. Moreover, their discomfort was elevated whether they reported attitude or affect first.

When attitude change is not viable, are there strategies that can be effective for alleviating dissonance-related distress? Two recent lines of research suggest an affirmative answer to this question. One line of work follows directly from the Devine et al. (1995) study examining dissonance and attitude change in people of varying levels of attitude importance. Because high-importance people continue to experience discomfort after the attitude-change opportunity, they will still be motivated to reduce their distress. Thus, in a follow-up study, Tauer and Devine (1998) have replicated Devine et al.'s (1995) basic design, but they have provided all participants with a subsequent alternative dissonance-reduction opportunity, in this case, altering the perception of the strength of their essay (cf. Scheier & Carver, 1980; Simon et al., 1995). Theoretically, low-importance people, who are likely to change their attitudes and therefore be free from dissonance motivation, would not take advantage of this subsequent opportunity. High-importance people, however, would alter the perception of the strength of their essay because they continued to experience high levels of discomfort and thus dissonance motivation. To the extent that altering the perception of essay strength was an effective dissonance-reduction strategy for high-importance people, they would experience a reduction of discomfort. This line of work is important because it will help to shed light on the effectiveness of different strategies and the conditions under which alternative strategies are most optimal.

In another study, Tauer, Devine, and Elliot (1998) garnered evidence that self-affirmations are effective at reducing dissonance for people low and high in attitude importance. Once again using the recycling issue, half of their low- and high-importance participants completed a self-affirmation task before reporting their affect; for the other half of the participants, the order of these tasks was reversed. The self-affirmation task involved generating four examples of times when they had demonstrated their most cherished characteristics (see Vance, Devine, & Barron, 1997). When the affect measure preceded the self-affirmation task, feelings of discomfort were elevated for both high-

($M = 3.83$) and low- ($M = 2.94$) importance participants. When the affect measure followed the self-affirmation task, feelings of discomfort for both high- ($M = 3.09$) and low- ($M = 2.22$) importance participants were reduced, although discomfort was still somewhat elevated for high-importance participants. It is also of interest to note that there was no evidence of attitude change for either high- or low-importance participants in this study. In all conditions, attitudes were assessed after the affect and self-affirmation opportunities. High-importance participants, of course, were not expected to show evidence of attitude change (cf. Devine et al., 1995). Of particular interest, however, was that low-importance participants, after having completed a self-affirmation task, did not change their attitudes. The self-affirmation opportunity appeared to alleviate their discomfort and, thus, reduced the motivational force that produces attitude change (cf. Elliot & Devine, 1994; Festinger, 1957).

METHODOLOGICAL AND THEORETICAL BENEFITS OF USING THE DISSONANCE THERMOMETER

Several methodological and theoretical benefits accrue from having a measure that is both easy to implement and sensitive to dissonance induction as well as reduction. First, and most obviously, the measure can serve as a manipulation check for both dissonance induction and reduction. As noted previously, the absence of a manipulation check created interpretational difficulties for dissonance researchers when results did not conform to theoretical predictions. It was not possible to determine whether the experimental procedures had failed to evoke dissonance or whether the dissonance that had been created was reduced through the implementation of an alternative reduction strategy. Cialdini et al. (1981) suggested that research on selective exposure and dissonance was (temporarily) abandoned against a backdrop of seemingly inconsistent results. These inconsistencies proved difficult to interpret, in part due to the absence of an effective dissonance manipulation check. Use of the dissonance thermometer may facilitate progress in such areas.

Having an effective dissonance manipulation check may also provide efficient ways for validating new procedures for instilling dissonance, such as the hypocrisy procedure developed by Aronson and colleagues (see Aronson, 1992; Stone, Aronson, Crain, Winslow, & Fried, 1994). The goal of the hypocrisy manipulation is to show that dissonance can be created and can lead to dissonance-related cognitive and behavioral changes even when participants advocate a proattitudinal position (e.g., in favor of safe sex). In developing the technique, Stone et al. (1994), in the long tradition of dissonance research, relied on producing theory-consistent changes in behavior or attitudes to validate the hypocrisy procedure. We suggest that more efficient and potentially more informative progress can be made by using a measure like the dissonance thermometer during the validation process. For example, it would be immediately apparent if new procedures were effective if they led to increases in psychological discomfort.

In a similar fashion, the dissonance thermometer can be used to assess the efficacy of alternative dissonance-reduction strategies without relying exclusively on attitude change (see Tauer & Devine, 1998). The most often used strategy for validating the efficacy of alternative dissonance-reduction strategies (e.g., trivialization or self-affirmation) is to show that after implementing an ostensibly effective strategy, attitudes do not change (e.g., Simon et al., 1995; Steele & Liu, 1983, respectively). The dissonance thermometer can provide information on the efficacy of dissonance-reduction strategies much more directly (i.e., discomfort decreases) and may, as a result, enable new progress to be made in exploring alternative strategies for alleviating dissonance-related discomfort.

Finally, use of a dissonance manipulation check may ultimately permit the use of more efficient experimental designs. Historically, the dissonance literature has included low-choice conditions primarily to validate that little attitude change occurs when theoretically it should not. A direct measure of dissonance may obviate the need for such control conditions, at least in some circumstances.

Although the benefits of a dissonance manipulation check are considerable, some of the potentially more powerful benefits of a more direct dissonance measure may come in the form of improved theory testing and elaboration. As stated in the beginning of this chapter, Festinger (1957) proposed essentially a process model: A (inconsistency between cognitions) → B (dissonance) → C (some dissonance-reduction strategy) → D (alleviation of dissonance). However, empirical strategies to date have been largely limited to investigations in which A is created and C is observed. Although research investigating the arousal component of dissonance has attempted to explore the mediational processes suggested by the model, complications arise when arousal does not appear to dissipate after an ostensibly effective dissonance-reduction strategy is implemented (e.g., Elkin & Leippe, 1986). A measure of the psychological component of dissonance, which has been shown to be sensitive to dissonance induction and reduction, provides an additional tool for directly testing the process assumptions as they unfold over time. Specifically, a complete understanding of dissonance theory requires testing whether dissonance is created, whether a reduction opportunity is used, and whether dissonance reduction follows the implementation of an ostensibly effective dissonance-reduction strategy. Exploring these ideas calls for a mediational analysis that will allow researchers to directly test the process of dissonance induction and reduction.

Having a more direct measure of dissonance may ultimately help in addressing the long-standing debate concerning the necessary and sufficient conditions for dissonance arousal. Cooper and Fazio (1984) have maintained that taking responsibility for the production of aversive consequences is necessary for the arousal of dissonance. However, in using a discomfort measure of dissonance, Harmon-Jones (chap. 4, this volume) has shown that the production of aversive consequences is not necessary to create dissonance-related discomfort. That is, when participants advocated a counterattitudinal position for which there could be no aversive consequences (i.e., the evidence of their counterattitudinal behavior is literally thrown away), discomfort feelings were elevated. Moreover, discomfort feelings were associated with attitude change, supporting Festinger's (1957) dissonance-reduction postulate. Thus, although the production of aversive consequences may heighten the dissonance experience, Harmon-Jones's research suggests that aversive consequences are not necessary. As these findings suggest, when used in conjunction with other measures, the dissonance thermometer may enable more precise evaluation of the plausibility of the core assumptions of the various revisions of dissonance theory proposed over the years.

A final set of issues that may be fruitful to explore with the dissonance thermometer concerns the qualitative nature of the affect associated with different types of cognitive inconsistencies and the possibility that not all dissonances are created equal. Because the affect measure was designed to be sensitive to both global and more specific forms of affective distress, it may play a role in elucidating theory and enable the field to address issues that have long proved vexing for dissonance theorists. These include assessing the magnitude of dissonance experienced and how people resolve dissonance when inconsistencies involve important, central, or self-defining attitudes.

For example, following in the tradition of Aronson's (1968) reconceptualization of dissonance, Elliot and Devine (1994) suggested that the self may be implicated to varying degrees in the dissonance process. Specifically, the self-relevance of the threatened cognition may be critical in determining the qualitative nature of the affect experienced as a result of counterattitudinal behavior. Similarly, Aronson (1992) argued that dissonance-induction procedures, such as the hypocrisy manipulation, were likely to lead to feelings of guilt and not just global discomfort. The current strategies used to validate hypocrisy-induced dissonance reduction (e.g., cognitive or behavioral change) are silent on the qualitative nature of the affect created by the manipulation. To the extent that the quality of affect experienced is important in determining whether particular strategies are likely to be effective in reducing dissonance-related distress, it will be important to establish precisely what type of affect is evoked by alternative procedures (see Vance et al., 1997). Our measure, which was developed with the goal of assessing various qualities of affect elicited in response to cognitive inconsistencies, is well suited to these tasks (see Devine et al., 1991).

For example, our work on the affective consequences of prejudice-related discrepancies (i.e., actual responses revealing more prejudice than is permitted by one's nonprejudiced standards) has shown that violations of well-internalized, self-defining standards generate general negative affect (i.e., discomfort) and a more specific negative self-directed affect (i.e., guilt, see Devine et al., 1991). Violations of less internalized standards simply elicit more global negative affect. The dissonance thermometer was essential for detecting this difference in the experience of dissonance for attitudes that are more, compared with less, self-defining. Moreover, Vance and Devine (1997) recently used the dissonance thermometer after a hypocrisy manipulation relevant to nonprejudiced standards and behavior. Participants advocated the importance of treating Blacks in a nonprejudiced manner, then recalled times they had responded with prejudice. The combination of these experiences resulted in increased global discomfort, as well as elevated feelings of guilt and self-criticism. These findings support Aronson's (1992) general proposal about the consequences of hypocrisy but, perhaps more important, when combined with our previous findings, suggest that it may be prudent to think more completely about the specific qualities of affect associated with alternative dissonance manipulations. As emerging evidence suggests, it appears that not all dissonances are created or resolved equally. The use of a direct measure of affect makes it possible to more fully explore these issues.

CONCLUSION

Overreliance on attitude change has limited our ability to test core assumptions of dissonance theory. In response, we have offered an additional methodological tool and have reviewed evidence supporting its use. We have reviewed evidence from traditional dissonance paradigms that supports the efficacy of the dissonance thermometer and encourages dissonance researchers to revisit conceptual and theoretical issues that have been difficult to explore in the absence of a direct measure of dissonance. The use of an affect measure is not a panacea for the dissonance literature. Our purpose has been to illustrate how an affect measure can be used and may facilitate progress on central questions in the dissonance literature. Through its use, we have provided the first direct evidence to support the theoretical process outlined by Festinger (1957). Indeed, we expect that the most important developments afforded by the dissonance thermometer lie ahead and look forward to the next 40 years of dissonance-related theory and research.

REFERENCES

Aronson, E. (1968). Dissonance theory: Progress and problems. In R. Abelson, E. Aronson, W. McGuire, T. Newcomb, M. Rosenberg, & P. Tannenbaum (Eds.), *The cognitive consistency theories: A sourcebook* (pp. 5–27). Chicago: Rand McNally.

Aronson, E. (1992). The return of the repressed: Dissonance theory makes a comeback. *Psychological Inquiry, 3,* 303–311.

Bem, D. J. (1967). Self-perception: An alternative interpretation of cognitive dissonance phenomena. *Psychological Review, 74,* 183–200.

Boninger, D. S., Krosnick, J. A., Bernet, M. K., & Fabrigar, L. R. (1995). The causes and consequences of attitude importance. In R. E. Petty & J. A. Krosnick (Eds.), *Attitude strength: Antecedents and consequences* (pp. 159–189). Hillsdale, NJ: Erlbaum.

Brehm, J., & Cohen, A. (1962). *Explorations in cognitive dissonance.* New York: Wiley.

Chapanis, N. P., & Chapanis, A. (1964). Cognitive dissonance: Five years later. *Psychological Bulletin, 61,* 1–22.

Cialdini, R., Petty, R., & Cacioppo, J. (1981). Attitude and attitude change. *Annual Review of Psychology, 32,* 357–404.

Cooper, J., & Fazio, R. (1984). A new look at dissonance theory. In L. Berkowitz (Ed.), *Advances in experimental social psychology* (Vol. 17, pp. 229–266). San Diego, CA: Academic Press.

Cooper, J., & Mackie, D. (1983). Cognitive dissonance in an intergroup context. *Journal of Personality and Social Psychology, 44,* 536–544.

Cooper, J., & Worchel, S. (1970). Role of undesired consequences in arousing cognitive dissonance. *Journal of Personality and Social Psychology, 16,* 199–206.

Croyle, R., & Cooper, J. (1983). Dissonance arousal: Physiological evidence. *Journal of Personality and Social Psychology, 45,* 782–791.

Devine, P., Froning, D., & Elliot, A. (1995). [Attitude importance, dissonance, and resistance to attitude change]. Unpublished raw data.

Devine, P., Monteith, M., Zuwerink, J., & Elliot, A. (1991). Prejudice with and without compunction. *Journal of Personality and Social Psychology, 60,* 817–830.

Elkin, R. A., & Leippe, M. R. (1986). Physiological arousal, dissonance, and attitude change: Evidence for a dissonance-arousal link and a "don't remind me" effect. *Journal of Personality and Social Psychology, 51,* 55–65.

Elliot, A., & Devine, P. (1994). On the motivational significance of cognitive dissonance: Dissonance as psychological discomfort. *Journal of Personality and Social Psychology, 67,* 382–394.

Fazio, R. H., & Cooper, J. (1983). Arousal in the dissonance process. In J. Cacioppo & R. Petty (Eds.), *Social psychophysiology* (pp. 122–152). New York: Guilford Press.

Festinger, L. (1957). *A theory of cognitive dissonance.* Stanford, CA: Stanford University Press.

Festinger, L., & Carlsmith, J. (1959). Cognitive consequences of forced compliance. *Journal of Abnormal and Social Psychology, 58,* 203–210.

Hardyck, J., & Kardush, M. (1968). A modest modish model for dissonance reduction. In R. Abelson, E. Aronson, W. McGuire, T. Newcomb, M. Rosenberg, & P. Tannenbaum (Eds.), *Theories of cognitive consistency: A sourcebook* (pp. 684–692). Chicago: Rand McNally.

Harmon-Jones, E., Brehm, J., Greenberg, J., Simon, L., & Nelson, D. (1996). Evidence that the production of aversive consequences is not necessary to create cognitive dissonance. *Journal of Personality and Social Psychology, 70,* 5–16.

Kiesler, C., & Pallak, M. (1976). Arousal properties of dissonance manipulations. *Psychological Bulletin, 83,* 1014–1025.

Losch, M., & Cacioppo, J. (1990). Cognitive dissonance may enhance sympathetic tonus, but attitudes are changed to reduce negative affect rather than arousal. *Journal of Experimental Social Psychology, 26,* 289–304.

Nisbett, R., & Wilson, T. (1977). Telling more than we can know: Verbal reports on mental processes. *Psychological Review, 84,* 231–259.

Pallak, M., & Pittman, T. (1972). General motivation effects of dissonance arousal. *Journal of Personality and Social Psychology, 21,* 349–358.

Pilisuk, M. (1968). Depth, centrality, and tolerance in cognitive consistency. In R. Abelson, E. Aronson, W. McGuire, T. Newcomb, M. Rosenberg, & P. Tannenbaum (Eds.), *The cognitive consistency theories: A sourcebook* (pp. 693–699). Chicago: Rand McNally.

Rabbie, J., Brehm, J., & Cohen, A. (1959). Verbalization and reactions to cognitive dissonance. *Journal of Personality, 27,* 407–417.

Schachter, S., & Singer, J. E. (1962). Cognitive, social, and psychological determinants of emotional state. *Psychological Review, 69,* 379–399.

Scheier, M., & Carver, C. (1980). Private and public self-attention, resistance to change, and dissonance reduction. *Journal of Personality and Social Psychology, 39,* 390–405.

Sherman, S., & Gorkin, L. (1980). Attitude bolstering when behavior is inconsistent with central attitudes. *Journal of Experimental Social Psychology, 16,* 388–403.

Simon, L., Greenberg, J., & Brehm, J. (1995). Trivialization: The forgotten mode of dissonance reduction. *Journal of Personality and Social Psychology, 68,* 247–260.

Steele, C. M. (1988). The psychology of self-affirmation: Sustaining the integrity of the self. In L. Berkowitz (Ed.), *Advances in experimental social psychology* (Vol. 21, pp. 261–301). New York: Academic Press.

Steele, C. M., & Liu, T. J. (1983). Dissonance processes as self-affirmation. *Journal of Personality and Social Psychology, 45,* 5–19.

Stone, J., Aronson, E., Crain, A., Winslow, M., & Fried, C. (1994). Inducing hypocrisy as a means of encouraging young adults to use condoms. *Personality and Social Psychology Bulletin, 20,* 116–128.

Tauer, J., Devine, P., & Elliot, A. (1998, May). *Attitude importance, dissonance, and resistance to attitude change reduction.* Paper presented at the 7th annual meeting of the Midwestern Psychological Association, Chicago.

Tauer, J., & Devine, P. (1998). [Attitude importance and the efficacy of alternative dissonance reduction strategies]. Unpublished raw data.

Tedeschi, J. T., Schlenker, B. R., & Bonoma, T. V. (1971). Cognitive dissonance: Private ratiocination or public spectacle? *American Psychologist, 26,* 685–695.

Vance, K., & Devine, P. (1997). [How self-affirmations influence the motivation and behaviors associated with prejudice reduction]. Unpublished raw data.

Vance, K., Devine, P., & Barron, K. (1997, May). *The effects of self-affirmation on the prejudice reduction process.* Paper presented at the Midwestern Psychological Association Meeting, Chicago.

Wilder, D. (1992). Yes, Elliot, there is dissonance. *Psychological Inquiry, 3,* 351–352.

Zanna, M., & Cooper, J. (1974). Dissonance and the pill: An attribution approach to studying the arousal properties of dissonance. *Journal of Personality and Social Psychology, 29,* 703–709.

Zuwerink, J., & Devine, P. (1996). Attitude importance and resistance to persuasion: It's not just the thought that counts. *Journal of Personality and Social Psychology, 70,* 931–944.

13

"Remembering" Dissonance: Simultaneous Accessibility of Inconsistent Cognitive Elements Moderates Epistemic Discomfort

Ian McGregor, Ian R. Newby-Clark, and
Mark P. Zanna

The evolution of cognitive dissonance theory has been shaped by its research methods. Indirect, behaviorally based methods provided compelling demonstration of the theory's bold predictions but involved elaborate social interactions as well as the presumed epistemic dynamics. As such, they opened the door for revisions that moved the theory away from Festinger's (1957) core proposition that cognitive inconsistency, in itself, is aversive and motivates interesting cognitive and behavioral reactions. We submit that the *ambivalence* construct (Jamieson, 1993) is consistent with Festinger's original conception of dissonance and that ambivalence research, in conjunction with Bassili's (1994) notion of simultaneous accessibility, provides a fresh perspective that organizes and extends dissonance theory. Ambivalence research reasserts that cognitive inconsistency, in itself, is psychologically uncom-

Preparation of this chapter was supported in part by a Social Sciences and Humanities Research Council of Canada (SSHRC) Doctoral Fellowship, an Ontario Graduate Scholarship, and an SSHRC research grant. We gratefully acknowledge the assistance of Steve Bauer and Jill Dickinson in the data collection, Clay Boutilier in the computer programming, and John Bassili, Joel Cooper, Peter Gaskovski, Eddie Harmon-Jones, Judson Mills, Mike Ross, Steve Spencer, and Jeff Stone for their comments on drafts of this chapter.

fortable. We review older dissonance research and present our recent ambivalence research, which indicates that epistemic discomfort is moderated by the *simultaneous accessibility* of inconsistent cognitions. We propose that simultaneous accessibility can account for revisions to dissonance theory and some newer applications. We conclude by presenting recent research demonstrating a compensatory epistemic defense against accessible identity-related dissonance. When identity-related inconsistencies are made accessible, individuals compensate by hardening their attitudes about more circumscribed topics. Just as the discovery of this new dissonance defense derived from a new paradigm that incorporates the simultaneous accessibility concept, we propose that other burgeoning areas of social psychology may be informed and integrated by the concept. This chapter expands the purview of cognitive dissonance theory by returning to Festinger's core premise with a perspective that highlights the role of simultaneous accessibility in determining the effects of cognitive inconsistency.

COGNITIVE DISSONANCE THEORY
AND REVISIONS

The arrival of cognitive dissonance theory excited social psychologists for at least two reasons. First, it challenged the relatively bland version of reinforcement theory that was popular at the time (Aronson, 1992, p. 303). Second, it lent scientific support to the notion of motivated cognition, which had been percolating in other disciplines for many years. In philosophy, Schopenhauer (1818/1883) claimed that desire "is the strong blind man who carries on his shoulders the lame man (reason) who can see" (p. 421). In psychoanalytic psychology, rationalization was presented as a prevalent defense mechanism. The outcomes of the first high-impact dissonance studies lent vivid empirical support to the hypothesis that people sometimes act first and justify later.

Early high-impact studies cleverly demonstrated participants' tendency to justify their counterattitudinal behaviors, but in most experiments, inconsistent cognitions were assumed to follow from behaviors that implied an inconsistent position, and psychological discomfort was inferred from attitude change. Festinger's core proposition, that inconsistent cognitions cause psychological discomfort, was not directly tested. Reliance on behavioral induction and indirect assessment of dissonance opened the door for several challenges to the epistemic basis of the theory.

The first major challenge came from Bem's (1967) self-perception theory. Bem argued that attributional processes could explain attitude change in conventional dissonance paradigms and that no aversive motivational state need exist. According to Bem, participants noticed themselves behaving in a particular way, and because no external reason for their behavior was apparent, they inferred that their behavior must have arisen from internal factors (i.e., attitudes consistent with the behavior). The cognitive dissonance interpretation was eventually rescued from the self-perception challenge by the finding that if participants have an opportunity to misattribute dissonance arousal to another source, such as a pill (Zanna & Cooper, 1974) or an unpleasant environment (Fazio, Zanna, & Cooper, 1977), attitude change will not occur. Eventually both theories found their appropriate domain of applicability. Dissonance processes are operative when counterattitudinal behaviors are outside participants' latitude of acceptance; self-perception processes are operative when counterattitudinal behaviors are within participants' latitude of acceptance (Fazio et al., 1977).

Self-perception theory challenged dissonance theory at the back end of the counterattitudinal behavior paradigm, that is, it questioned Festinger's contention that psychological discomfort mediates the attitude change following counterattitudinal behavior. A second set of challenges to the original conception of cognitive dissonance theory came at the front end of the paradigm. Most notably, self-consistency (E. Aronson, 1968; see also chap. 5, this volume), self-affirmation (Steele, 1988; see also chap. 6, this volume), and the new look (Cooper & Fazio, 1984; see also chap. 7, this volume) perspectives questioned whether inconsistent cognitions were sufficient or even necessary to produce discomfort and attitude change. E. Aronson proposed that inconsistent cognitions are only uncomfortable when they implicate the self-concept.

For example, most people believe that they are competent and good. Thus, when they are tricked by a dissonance researcher into doing something stupid or bad, they experience discomfort. According to E. Aronson, discomfort arises, not because, for example, a counterattitudinal essay is inconsistent with a prior attitude, but because the negative behavior of writing in support of the wrong cause is inconsistent with a positive self-concept. Two subsequent revisions took E. Aronson's focus on stupid or bad actions even further and contended that inconsistency is not even a necessary condition for dissonance to be experienced. Cooper and Fazio (1984) proposed a new look for dissonance theory, arguing that psychological discomfort in dissonance experiments occurs because people feel personally responsible for the production of aversive consequences. Similarly, Steele's (1988) self-affirmation revision posited that it is not inconsistency but threat to global self-integrity that causes the discomfort in dissonance experiments. According to new look and self-affirmation perspectives, people rationalize behaviors that imply their incompetence or immorality.

As evidence that cognitive dissonance theory has drifted from its epistemic roots, introductory social psychology texts now typically allocate more space to the revisions than to the original theory. Indeed, textbooks now routinely echo Abelson (1983) and conclude that dissonance reduction is primarily a social strategy for saving face following experimentally engineered embarrassment. From this perspective, the term *cognitive dissonance* is a misnomer. Discomfort in dissonance paradigms arises from social, not epistemic, factors.

AMBIVALENCE RESEARCH: RETURNING TO THE EPISTEMIC ROOTS OF DISSONANCE THEORY

Conventional dissonance paradigms made a huge contribution to the field's understanding of social behavior and motivated cognition but invited revisions that deemphasized the theory's initial focus on epistemic motivation. Recent research on ambivalence complements findings from conventional paradigms by investigating implications of *native* inconsistencies (i.e., naturally occurring inconsistencies that are not behaviorally induced by a researcher). A direct technology for assessing inconsistency, developed by Scott (1968) and later by Kaplan (1972), separately measures both the positive and negative aspects of a given attitude (holding aspects of the opposite valence constant) and provides the means for direct assessment of native discrepancies within attitudes. Using this technique, Thompson, Zanna, and Griffin (1995) found that intra-attitudinal discrepancies were associated ($r = .40$) with the experience of ambivalence—or feeling "torn and conflicted," as measured by Jamieson's (1993) Simultaneous Ambivalence Scale (SIMAS).[1] Thus, although devoid of the provocative outcomes and high-impact appeal associated with the original dissonance tradition, ambivalence research quietly reaffirmed the epistemic core of Festinger's proposition that had been deemphasized by the new look and self-affirmation revisions. Inconsistent cognitions are experienced as uncomfortable. Indeed, recent research using a conventional dissonance research method also bolsters Festinger's original epistemic conception. Harmon-Jones, Brehm, Greenberg, Simon, and Nelson (1996) have found that dissonance (directly measured by skin conductance) is aroused and that attitude change occurs after "freely" chosen counterattitudinal expression, even when participants discard their counterattitudinal statements before anyone else can see them. This contradicts the new look revision's requirement that negative consequences be present. In another experiment, Elliot and Devine (1994) have found that counterattitudinal expression increases self-reported psycho-

---

[1]Two questions refer to experienced conflict between cognitive elements (e.g., "I'm not at all confused about abortion because I have strong thoughts about it and have easily made up my mind in one way"), two to conflict between affective elements (e.g., "I do not find myself feeling torn between the two sides of the issue of abortion; my feelings go in one direction only"), and two to conflict across modalities (e.g., "my head and my heart seem to be in disagreement on the issue of abortion"). One question in each pair refers to the absence of ambivalence and is reverse scored, and the six items are averaged to form a Felt Ambivalence score. We see ambivalence as a measure of targeted dissonance. In dissonance research, discomfort is usually assessed on a global level, that is, "how uncomfortable do you feel right now?" Felt ambivalence as a dependent variable is measured by having participants report on how uncomfortable they feel about a particular issue, thereby focusing participants on a relevant subset of their feelings and away from irrelevant influences.

logical discomfort and that the discomfort is alleviated by attitude change.[2]

How can the reassertion of the original conception of dissonance theory be reconciled with the various revisions? We think that the revisions may have capitalized on factors that influence the simultaneous accessibility (Bassili, 1994) of inconsistent cognitions. If inconsistent cognitions are not accessible at the same time, dissonance discomfort will be minimized. On the other hand, if inconsistent cognitions are simultaneously accessible, dissonance discomfort will be maximized. Indeed, according to Festinger, Riecken, and Schachter (1956), one way to reduce dissonance is to "forget or reduce the importance of those cognitions that are in dissonant relationship" (p. 26).

A SIMULTANEOUS-ACCESSIBILITY ACCOUNT OF THE REVISIONS

E. Aronson's (1968) original claim that dissonance will occur only when the dissonant cognitions are self-relevant can easily be understood in terms of accessibility. According to the *self-reference effect*, information related to the self is recalled more easily than non-self-related information (Rogers, Kuiper, & Kirker, 1977). Dissonance may be heightened when self-related cognitions are involved because the two cognitions may be more likely to remain simultaneously accessible and less likely to drift out of awareness.

Cooper and Fazio's (1984) new look revision can similarly be explained in terms of accessibility. The perception that one has just done harm to an audience that does not deserve it is likely a relatively novel and unexpected realization for most participants. The increase in attributional activity (Pyszczynski & Greenberg, 1981; Wong & Weiner, 1981) that accompanies such experientially bizarre behavior may very

---

[2]The affective response to dissonance, assessed by Elliot and Devine's (1994) "dissonance thermometer," is different from that measured by typical mood scales. This may be why it has eluded reliable assessment in the past. Dissonance causes feelings of tension, irritation, and discomfort, as opposed to the affective states more typically measured, such as sadness, depression, or anger. See also McGregor and Little (1998) for a distinction between unhappiness and dissonance-related discomfort.

well render the behavior, and the inconsistent cognition the behavior implies, hyperaccessible. In addition, guilt associated with a bad behavior might motivate an attempt to suppress awareness of it, which could cause rebound hyperaccessibility (Wegner, 1994). Note also that in the Harmon-Jones et al. (1996) research in which dissonance ensued without the presence of aversive consequences, the "recall task" cover story may have inadvertently ensured that the original attitude and the counterattitudinal expression remained simultaneously accessible.

The self-affirmation revision of dissonance theory is also amenable to an accessibility interpretation. As mentioned above, "stupid" or "bad" behaviors are more likely to remain accessible because of self-reference and heightened attributional activity. Moreover, Steele and Liu (1983) have demonstrated that affirmation can alleviate dissonance but have not demonstrated that dissonance discomfort arises from threatened self-worth. We propose that affirmation ameliorates dissonance because it offers an attractive distraction from the inconsistent behavior just performed. In keeping with this interpretation, J. Aronson, Blanton, and Cooper (1995) have found that participants prefer to affirm themselves in domains unrelated to the dissonant elements (see also Blanton, Cooper, Skurnik, & Aronson, 1997).

Steele and Liu (1983) have attempted to rule out a distraction account of their results by demonstrating in a counterattitudinal essay paradigm that affirmation still reduces attitude change (and therefore dissonance) even when participants are reminded of their dissonant essay after the affirmation and before the attitude measure. We are not convinced that their reminder was effective, however. The reminder procedure simply required participants to write down three key words from their earlier essay. As we discuss later in the context of some earlier dissonance research and recent research on hypocrisy, individuals seem to have a remarkable capacity for avoiding awareness of inconsistencies unless their noses are quite vigorously rubbed in them. It is unclear whether simply reminding participants of three words from their essays was sufficient to remind them that they had advocated tuition increases of their own free will. Instead, they may have been motivated to continue to forget about the free-choice aspect (cf. Kunda, 1990). A more convincing rebuttal of the distraction account would require a reminder more difficult for participants to wiggle out of.

SIMULTANEOUS ACCESSIBILITY AND EARLY DISSONANCE RESEARCH

The importance of accessibility as a moderator of cognitive dissonance was supported by experimental results from the early days of cognitive dissonance research. Several studies demonstrated that dissonance reduction through attitude change depends on whether participants are distracted from or have their "noses rubbed" in the dissonant cognitions—conditions that presumably render the dissonant cognitions less or more accessible. In one of the first accessibility experiments, Brock (1962) found that after being induced to "freely" write an essay about why they would like to become Catholic, non-Catholics' attitudes became more favorable toward Catholicism if they focused on essay convincingness as opposed to grammatical structure in the interval between the essay writing and attitude assessment. Thus, extra attention to inconsistent elements apparently increased dissonance. In contrast, one of the first distraction experiments (Allen, 1965) found that when participants engaged in an absorbing technical task between a free-choice behavior and the assessment of attitudes, the dissonance-reducing spread of alternatives was eliminated (see also Zanna & Aziza, 1976).

In these early experiments, all avenues of dissonance reduction were closed off except attitude change, and the inconsistent cognitions were extremely salient (unless a distraction was introduced). This state of affairs maximized the likelihood of finding self-justificatory attitude change but obscured investigation of distraction as a natural route of dissonance reduction. According to Rosenberg and Abelson (1960), people follow a principle of least effort when attempting to restore cognitive consistency. Because changing one's attitude presumably takes some cognitive work, Hardyck and Kardush (1968) proposed that stopping thinking, a form of self-distraction, might be the preferred strategy for coping with dissonance. A research technique was needed that would incorporate the spontaneous distraction that presumably occurs in real life.

The forbidden-toy paradigm (E. Aronson & Carlsmith, 1963) is unique in that during the "temptation period," in which children are forbidden to play with a well-liked toy, they can easily take their minds off their cognitive dilemma by playing with toys that are not forbidden. Thus, in contrast to other kinds of dissonance procedures in which participants are left to simmer in their counterattitudinal behavior, participants are free to immerse themselves in other engaging activities. This provides a relatively naturalistic setting for the dissonance-reduction strategy that Pallak, Brock, and Kiesler (1967) referred to as throwing oneself into one's work. Carlsmith et al. (1969) augmented the built-in distraction feature of the forbidden-toy paradigm with two manipulations of forced attention. In one experiment, a "janitor" made the forbidden toy salient by walking into the room during the temptation period and incidentally asking the children why they were not playing with it. In the other experiment, the forbidden toy was made salient by a "defective" lamp, which flashed on and off above it. The general procedure and results were as follows.

Each child was brought into a room, shown how to use six attractive toys, and asked to rank the attractiveness of the toys. The experimenter then explained that he had to run an errand and that while he was gone, the child was forbidden to play with the second-ranked toy (which was placed on a different table). In the mild-threat condition, the experimenter said, "If you play with the [second-ranked toy], I will be a little bit annoyed with you." In the severe-threat condition, he said instead, "If you play with the [second-ranked toy], I will be very upset and very angry with you, and I'll have to do something about it." The experimenter then left the room for a 6-min temptation period, during which the forced-attention manipulations occurred for those in the experimental conditions. After the temptation period, the experimenter asked the children to rerank the toys. Thus, both experiments had a simple 2 (mild threat vs. severe threat) × 2 (forced attention vs. control) format.

In both experiments, two main effects resulted. There was more derogation of the second-ranked toy in the mild-threat conditions than in the severe-threat conditions, and there was more derogation in the forced-attention conditions than the control conditions. Carlsmith et al. (1969) had expected that attention would increase derogation, but only when dissonance existed in the first place, that is, in the mild-threat condition. Zanna, Lepper, and Abelson (1973) conducted a follow-up experiment, to see whether the expected interaction (forced attention increasing derogation only under mild threat) might result if forced attention was directed simultaneously toward both of the inconsistent cognitions ("I'm not playing with the desirable toy" and "there's no strong reason not to") instead of just the one ("I'm not playing with the desirable toy"). They reasoned that the absence of an interaction in the first two experiments might be due to the fact that although the blinking light or janitor's comment focused the children's attention on the fact that they were not playing with a valued toy, it did not simultaneously remind them of the initial justification for that compliant behavior. For dissonance to occur, both cognitions would have to be simultaneously accessible.

To accomplish forced attention to both cognitions, the janitor experiment was modified in two ways. First, after the threat manipulation, the experimenter placed a sticker marked with an X on the side of the forbidden toy. Children were told that this sticker was being put on the toy as a reminder that the experimenter would either be a little annoyed or very angry and upset (depending on the threat condition) if they played with the forbidden toy. Second, in the high-accessibility condition, when the janitor entered the room in the middle of the temptation period, instead of simply calling attention to the forbidden toy, he said, "What's this toy doing over here on the table?" and "How come this toy has a sticker on it?" These two modifications apparently succeeded in simultaneously focusing children's attention on both of the dissonant cognitions. The expected interaction between potential dissonance (severe vs. mild threat) and simultaneous accessibility (control vs. reminder) resulted, with the greatest amount of dissonance reduction (toy derogation) in the high-reminder–mild-threat condition, suggesting that the experience of dissonance does seem to be moderated by the simultaneous accessibility of the potentially dissonant cognitions (see Figure 1). These studies underscore how easily inconsistent elements can become inaccessible when distraction opportunities are present.

SIMULTANEOUS ACCESSIBILITY
AND AMBIVALENCE

The early experiments suggest that simultaneous accessibility can play an important role in dissonance processes, but like most dissonance research in the counterattitudinal behavior paradigm, interpretation is vulnerable to the revisionist critiques mentioned above. Further, the early experiments manipulated salience. Although it is likely that salient elements will also be highly accessible, it would still be desirable to measure accessibility directly. Fortunately, the rise of social cognition in the 1980s brought new techniques for manipulating and measuring accessibility of knowledge structures (e.g., Bassili & Fletcher, 1991; Fazio, Sanbonmatsu, Powell, & Kardes, 1986). We have used some of this technology to measure simultaneous accessibility in our research on ambivalence, in a relatively high-tech attempt to corroborate the accessibility results from the early high-impact experiments. In two studies, we have used Bassili's (1996) technique for measuring simultaneous accessibility of attitude components, to see whether psychological discomfort may be influenced not just by the existence of discrepant cognitions but also by the simultaneous accessibility of those cognitions (Newby-Clark, McGregor, & Zanna, 1997). These studies are described below.

Recall that Thompson et al. (1995) found that intra-attitudinal inconsistency was correlated at .40 with Jamieson's (1993) measure of felt ambivalence (i.e., how torn people felt about that attitude issue). This finding is consistent with the core of Festinger's (1957) original thesis, that the existence of nonfitting cognitions leads to psychological discomfort (see Footnote 1). In the following two studies, we were interested in whether simultaneous accessibility of inconsistent cognitions would moderate the relation between the existence of inconsistent cognitions (what we call *potential* ambivalence), as measured by the Kaplan

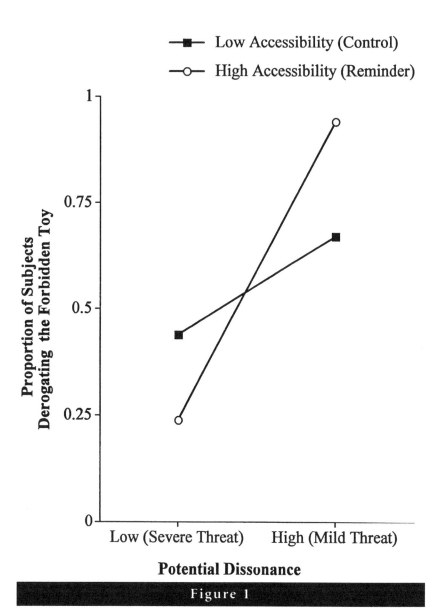

Figure 1

Toy derogation as a function of potential dissonance and simultaneous accessibility in the forbidden-toy paradigm.

(1972) technique,[3] and *felt* ambivalence, as measured by Jamieson's (1993) SIMAS (see Footnote 1). We hypothesized that felt ambivalence would be highest when inconsistent cognitions not only existed, but were available to awareness at the same time. We recorded how long it took participants to answer the Kaplan questions about the positives and negatives of each issue and used these latencies to calculate an index of simultaneous accessibility.[4] Our contention is that potential ambivalence is experienced as felt ambivalence when contradictory cognitions are highly and equally accessible.

In the first study, we telephoned 187 undergraduates and asked them questions about two issues: abortion and capital punishment. As expected, there was a significant positive relation between felt ambivalence and potential ambivalence for both attitude issues. Further, the interaction between potential ambivalence and simultaneous accessibility was significantly associated with felt ambivalence for abortion and marginally associated with felt ambivalence for capital punishment. These results supported our hypothesis that the relation between potential and felt ambivalence would be moderated by the simultaneous

---

[3] To assess potential ambivalence, we asked participants to separately rate the positive and negative aspects of each attitude issue (Kaplan, 1972). For each issue, one pair of ratings referred to overall evaluation (i.e., favorable and unfavorable), a second to affect (i.e., positive and negative), and a third to cognitive responses (i.e., beneficial and harmful) toward the issues under consideration. Response options ranged from 1 (*not at all*) to 4 (*extremely*). Responses to each pair of questions were used to calculate a partial potential ambivalence score according to the following procedure. The partial potential ambivalence score was calculated from the two overall evaluation ratings. One rating referred to how unfavorably one viewed the unfavorable aspects of the issue (ignoring the favorable), and the other rating referred to how favorably one viewed the favorable aspects of the issue (ignoring the unfavorable). For each person, a partial potential ambivalence score for overall evaluation was calculated by means of a formula developed by Jamieson (personal communication, June 23, 1991) based on Scott (1968): The lower of the two ratings (in this example either favorability or unfavorability) was squared and divided by the higher rating. Thus, as the positive and negative components became increasingly and equally extreme, potential ambivalence scores increased. We averaged the three partial potential ambivalence scores to form one potential ambivalence score for each issue.

[4] We performed a reciprocal transformation on the latency data, to normalize the positive skew and translate latency scores to speed scores. Speed scores for the three pairs of potential ambivalence questions were then used to calculate simultaneous accessibility, by means of the formula devised by Bassili (1996). Within each attitude issue, for each of the three pairs of speed scores, we squared the slower response time and divided it by the faster. Thus, as the two response speeds within each pair became increasingly and equally extreme, simultaneous-accessibility scores increased. We averaged the three partial simultaneous-accessibility scores within each issue, to create overall indices of simultaneous accessibility for each attitude issue.

accessibility of the relevant cognitions (see the results of the meta-analysis below, for the pattern of the interaction).

In a computerized replication, 69 undergraduates responded to the same questions as in Study 1, but the questions were presented on a computer screen, and response latencies were more automatically recorded. Results were almost identical. Again, potential ambivalence and felt ambivalence were significantly correlated, and again, the interaction between simultaneous accessibility and potential ambivalence was significantly associated with felt ambivalence for abortion and marginally for capital punishment. Meta-analyses across the two studies yielded significant interactions for both attitude issues. For descriptive purposes, we also combined participants from the upper and lower quartiles of simultaneous accessibility from both studies and (a) calculated the correlation between potential and felt ambivalence and (b) regressed felt ambivalence on potential ambivalence.[5] For participants high in simultaneous accessibility, the correlation between potential and felt ambivalence about abortion was .73; for those low in simultaneous accessibility, the correlation was only .32. Finally, as shown in Figure 2, the slope of felt ambivalence (standardized) about abortion regressed on potential ambivalence (low = -2 SD, high = 2 SD) was clearly steeper for those in the upper (as compared with the lower) quartile of simultaneous accessibility.

In keeping with Bassili's (1994) conception of ambivalence, the results from these two ambivalence studies demonstrate that felt ambivalence arising from the existence of inconsistent cognitions is moderated by the extent to which both cognitions are readily and equally accessible. Taken in conjunction with distraction–attention findings from conventional dissonance paradigms, our results demonstrate that the simultaneous accessibility of inconsistent cognitive elements is an important factor in determining how much epistemic discomfort will be experienced. We see simultaneous accessibility as an essential and underemphasized aspect of dissonance theory that helps explain revi-

---

[5]We computed upper and lower quartiles separately within each sample. All measures were standardized within each sample because of different metrics. For economy, aggregated results are presented only for the abortion issue. Results for the capital punishment issue were comparable.

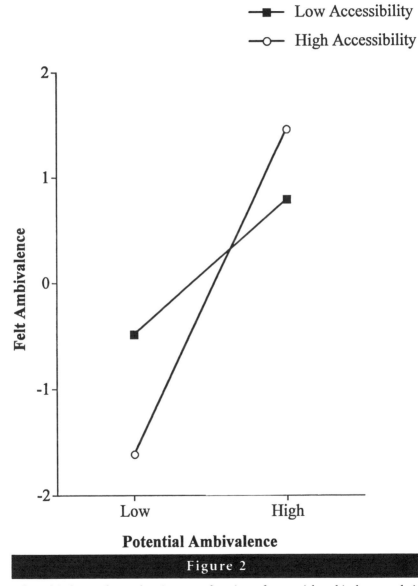

Figure 2

Felt ambivalence about abortion as a function of potential ambivalence and simultaneous accessibility.

sions and recent applications of the theory to dissonance-reducing mechanisms other than behavioral justification. We now turn to some of these newer applications.

A SIMULTANEOUS-ACCESSIBILITY ACCOUNT OF RECENT DISSONANCE RESEARCH

Recently, there has been increasing attention to modes of dissonance reduction, other than attitude change, that may occur in everyday life. Simon, Greenberg, and Brehm (1995) have demonstrated that under certain circumstances, participants will resolve dissonance by trivializing counterattitudinal behavior. Steele has demonstrated that one can indirectly cope with dissonance by affirming oneself in a different domain (Steele, 1988) or by reducing the breadth of one's thoughts by consuming alcohol (Steele, Southwick, & Critchlow, 1981). Hypocrisy researchers have demonstrated that after being made mindful of their hypocrisy, individuals reduce dissonance by changing their future behaviors and intentions (e.g., Stone, Wiegand, Cooper, & Aronson 1997). Accessibility interpretations of these phenomena are provided below.

Trivialization

Imagine that you are a participant in a trivialization experiment. You have just completed a counterattitudinal essay and are experiencing dissonance discomfort as a result. Four questions are now provided by the researcher that essentially ask whether it is really so important in the grand scheme of things that you wrote a counterattitudinal essay. Would you not gladly agree with this suggestion and use it as an excuse to become less preoccupied with the counterattitudinal behavior? In essence, the four questions suggest not to worry about it, it doesn't really matter all that much. It seems plausible that trivialization works because it gives participants permission to forget about their inconsistent behavior. Trivialization may relieve dissonance by decreasing the simultaneous accessibility of the inconsistent cognitions, that is, less important cognitions may wander from awareness more easily.

Affirmation and Alcohol

As discussed previously, affirmation may reduce dissonance by providing a powerful distraction from inconsistent elements (rendering them less accessible). The relation between alcohol and accessibility is more direct. According to Steele and Joseph's (1990), when intoxicated, individuals are able to focus only on the most salient cue in the environment. Steele et al. (1981) have found evidence that alcohol relieves discomfort from internal inconsistencies as well, presumably because alcohol permits awareness of only one element of the inconsistency. Although no direct evidence indicates that people spontaneously use alcohol to quell dissonance, it seems probable, given the ubiquitous appeal of alcohol and the effectiveness of alcohol and distraction for reducing dissonance.

Hypocrisy

Hypocrisy research capitalizes on individuals' considerable effectiveness at keeping discrepant cognitions out of focal awareness even when they are sober. In the typical hypocrisy experiment, after participants publicly advocate a prosocial attitude (e.g., condom use, water conservation, recycling), they are reminded of their past failures to practice what they have just preached. Participants caught in this dilemma, of high simultaneous accessibility of an advocated attitude and awareness of past behavioral shortcomings, resolve the predicament by acting and intending to act in a manner consistent with the advocated attitude. But it is only when participants are reminded of their past behavior that they experience dissonance. Remarkably, even when asked to think about behaviors of friends or roommates (that are inconsistent with the advocated attitude), intentions and behaviors do not change, indicating that participants' own contradictory past behavior somehow eludes awareness. The hypocrisy paradigm highlights a seemingly impressive capacity to limit awareness of personal inconsistencies under normal circumstances.

ACCESSIBLE IDENTITY INCONSISTENCIES AND COMPENSATORY HARDENING OF THE ATTITUDES

For the remainder of this chapter, we focus on new research akin to hypocrisy research, in which participants are confronted with native inconsistencies that normally elude awareness. This departure from the conventional dissonance paradigm (in which inconsistent cognitions are experimentally implanted by means of a counterattitudinal behavior) enables investigation of inconsistencies that are fundamental to self-definition.[6] We propose that induced awareness of such inconsistencies will motivate a generalized and compensatory attitudinal rigidity response, that is, when the foundation of identity is shaken by dissonance, people will seek epistemic solace in more circumscribed certainties by hardening their attitudes. This section presents theoretical and empirical evidence that attitudinal extremism may be a defensive response to identity dissonance.

Mindset and Hardening of the Attitudes

Taylor and Gollwitzer (1995) have recently developed "mindset" manipulations, which we think are essentially manipulations of the simultaneous accessibility of inconsistent alternative selves. They have found that when participants are induced to ruminate about both sides of a personal dilemma (deliberative mindset), mood, self-esteem, and positive illusions become depressed. In contrast, when participants are immersed in the particulars of one course of action that has already been decided on (implemental mindset), mood, self-esteem, and illusions are elevated. Taylor and Gollwitzer have suggested that individuals usually keep themselves somewhat implemental because the tunnel vision associated with implemental mindset provides required motivation for sustained effort on challenging tasks. In addition to this functional

---

[6]Such inconsistencies may arise from mismatches between and among the implications of a diverse array of self-elements (e.g., defining memories, future possible selves, personal values, and priorities). These are referred to interchangeably as *inconsistent self-elements, self-relevant inconsistencies,* and *alternative selves* in the remainder of this chapter.

motive, we suggest that an epistemic motive might also be present. Perhaps individuals try to avoid deliberation and keep themselves implemental as a means of escaping the self (Baumeister, 1991; Vallacher & Wegner, 1985), that is, to shield against the dissonance discomfort associated with simultaneous awareness of inconsistent priorities and possible selves. Whereas deliberative mindset instructions increase participants' awareness of inconsistent alternative futures and associated benefits and drawbacks, implemental mindset may protect individuals from dissonance the same way that alcohol does: limiting simultaneous awareness of inconsistencies by myopic focus on one alternative (in this case, successful completion of the project in question).

On the basis of this interpretation of the mindset manipulations, McGregor (1998, Experiment 4) conducted an experiment to ascertain whether deliberative mindset would cause epistemic discomfort and arouse defensive hardening of the attitudes, as measured by increased conviction, decreased felt ambivalence, and increased consensus estimates about one's attitudes.[7] In the baseline condition, epistemic discomfort was assessed after a control manipulation that involved deliberating about someone else's dilemma. In the deliberation-only condition, epistemic discomfort was assessed after the deliberative-mindset manipulation. In the deliberation/hardening-opportunity condition, participants completed the deliberative-mindset materials; answered 10 questions on their conviction, ambivalence, and consensus estimates about their attitudes toward capital punishment and abortion (this provided the opportunity for them to harden their attitudes); and then completed the measure of epistemic discomfort.

As expected, in the deliberation-only condition, epistemic discomfort was significantly higher than in the baseline condition. Most important for our hypothesis, however, in the deliberation/hardening-opportunity condition, there was an apparently compensatory

---

[7]The 19 epistemic-discomfort items were gleaned from literature on dissonance (e.g., Elliot & Devine, 1994), ambivalence (e.g., Jamieson, 1993), and contradictory self-guides (e.g., VanHook & Higgins, 1988). The items were mixed, uneasy, torn, bothered, preoccupied, confused, unsure of self or goals, contradictory, distractible, unclear, of two minds, muddled, restless, confused about identity, jumbled, uncomfortable, conflicted, indecisive, and chaotic. The scale was unifactorial and had a Cronbach alpha of .91.

hardening of attitudes about capital punishment and abortion, and epistemic discomfort was reduced to baseline levels. Moreover, attitude hardening succeeded in reducing the epistemic discomfort. A within-cell correlation revealed a significant negative relation between attitude hardening and epistemic discomfort in the deliberation/hardening-opportunity condition. These results indicate that compensatory hardening of attitudes can ameliorate the identity dissonance associated with the simultaneous accessibility of inconsistent alternative selves.[8]

Mindset and Terror-Management Theory

The nature of the dependent and independent variables in the experiment just reported suggest a new perspective on terror-management (TM) research, which has found that people become more rigid about their attitudes and values after being reminded of their own mortality (see Greenberg, Solomon, & Pyszczynski, 1997, for a review of the past 10 years of TM theory and research).[9] On the dependent variable side, the attitude and value rigidity in TM research resemble hardening of the attitudes. On the independent variable side, mortality salience and the deliberative mindset both can be seen as initiating the simultaneous accessibility of identity inconsistencies.

According to TM theory, adhering to consensual attitudes and values links one to one's culture (which transcends death) and thereby provides a measure of symbolic immortality that serves as an anxiety buffer against death terror. The explanation for the results in TM experiments that we prefer, however, is that consensual values simply provide epistemic solace in the face of the identity dissonance made accessible by mortality salience. Theoretical support of this interpretation comes from Yalom's (1980) review of existentialist literature. Yalom

---

[8] Negative affect and state self-esteem also were assessed at the same time as epistemic discomfort, and neither was significantly affected by the experimental manipulations. This may be because the cell size ($N = 17$) was about half that used in the Taylor and Gollwitzer (1995) experiments. Indeed, having less power in the present experiment may have made it possible to detect the discriminant validity of the epistemic-discomfort scale.

[9] The typical result in TM research is that evaluations of attitudinally similar and attitudinally dissimilar others become more polarized. Other kinds of psychological distress—such as concerns about dental pain, giving a speech, or unemployment—do not cause polarization.

highlights three kinds of experiences that can effectively underscore responsibility for authorship of one's identity and render the multiple possibilities associated with the "who am I" question simultaneously accessible: *important decision making, mortality salience,* and *awareness of the self across time.* Important decision making explicitly underscores the alternative possible selves and values associated with the alternative courses of action. Mortality salience provides an urgent reminder about responsibility for making choices in life to avoid existential guilt—regret about not having lived well. Similarly, awareness of the self across time accentuates the reality of personal becoming and thereby draws simultaneous attention to choices one has and different selves one has been. Thus, all three phenomena can be seen as confronting individuals with increased simultaneous accessibility of inconsistent identity alternatives. The experiments that follow provide further support for our contention that all three phenomena can cause compensatory epistemic rigidity. When identity inconsistencies are made accessible, we propose that individuals will attempt to cope with the identity dissonance by claiming compensatory conviction about their attitudes in more circumscribed domains.

One of the first markers of attitude rigidity used in TM research was the monetary punishment assigned to a prostitute. Mortality salience causes harsher punishment recommendations. Empirical support for our proposed relation between mindset and TM research comes from McGregor (1996), who investigated the effects of mindset on monetary punishment recommendations for a prostitute. Mirroring past mortality salience results, he found that deliberative mindset caused harsher punishment recommendations toward prostitutes than implemental mindset did.

The results of the two experiments just discussed provide support for a new perspective on TM theory. If typical TM outcomes can be induced using epistemic threat as well as mortality salience, perhaps the TM outcomes are ultimately mediated by aversion to dissonance associated with the "who am I" question rather than by abject fear of creaturely annihilation, as argued by TM theorists. From this perspective, mortality salience could be considered one kind of existential prime that makes alternative selves simultaneously accessible. We contend that mortality salience exposes participants to a potent strain of dissonance in the identity domain and that TM outcomes exemplify compensatory hardening of the attitudes.

Mortality Salience, Time Salience, and Attitude Hardening

To provide more empirical support for this interpretation of TM theory and our hypothesis that simultaneous accessibility of inconsistent self-elements causes compensatory hardening of attitudes, McGregor (1998, Experiment 3) investigated whether mortality salience and awareness of the self across time (the third existential prime suggested by Yalom, 1980) would cause the same kind of attitude hardening as deliberative mindset did in the previous two experiments. For a manipulation of mortality salience, participants responded to two short questions asking them what would happen to their physical bodies once they died and how they felt about their own death (Greenberg et al., 1997). As a manipulation of awareness of the passage of time, participants were asked to briefly comment on what it would be like to revisit the physical scene of an important childhood memory in the year 2035. The dependent variable was the difference between participants' evaluations of glowingly positive and very negative essays about the University of Waterloo.[10]

Results indicated that relative to controls, participants in both the time-salient and mortality-salient conditions reported a greater preference for the positive essay over the negative one. With the results from the previous two experiments, this supports the hypothesis that all three existential primes can motivate generalized epistemic rigidity as a response to dissonance associated with simultaneous accessibility

---

[10] TM research indicates that mortality salience causes more liking for individuals who share one's values. Data were collected from University of Waterloo 1st-year students in October. Presumably, most of our participants valued a Waterloo education 1 month into their 1st term.

of identity inconsistencies.[11] Furthermore, both the mortality and time manipulations caused significant increases in self-reported dissonance discomfort, and the dissonance discomfort partially mediated the epistemic rigidity reaction.

The Mediating Role of Identity Dissonance

Results from these three experiments demonstrate that all three manipulations can cause attitude hardening. To further explore our theory-based contention that mortality- and time-salience effects are mediated by the identity inconsistencies they remind participants of, McGregor (1998, Experiment 5) conducted an additional experiment based on findings of McGregor and Little (1998). McGregor and Little had found that identity inconsistencies are associated with the aversive experience of meaninglessness in life. If identity inconsistencies are associated with aversive meaninglessness, then reminding participants of their identity inconsistencies should increase feelings of meaninglessness and increase the desire to find meaning.

In keeping with this logic, McGregor (1998, Experiment 5) found that in comparison with control materials, time-salience and mortality-salience materials caused higher scores on Crumbaugh and Maholick's (1964) Seeking of Meaning scale (e.g., items include "I think about the ultimate meaning in life" and "Over my lifetime I have felt a strong urge to find myself"). Furthermore, mortality- and time-salience materials also caused intentions to engage in more meaningful personal projects over the next few weeks (i.e., projects that were more personally

---

[11]It could be argued however, that time salience is simply a subtle way of reminding people about their death. After all, it is over time that people grow old and die. To assess this possibility, McGregor (1998, Experiment 3) attempted to replicate the findings that Greenberg, Pyszczynski, Solomon, Simon, and Breus (1994) used as support for their contention that TM outcomes are ultimately mediated by death awareness. Greenberg et al. (1994) found that mortality salience caused an increase in death-related word-stem completions. If time salience is simply a subtle manipulation of mortality salience, then death-related word-stem completions should be as common after time salience as after mortality salience. In the present experiment, however, no increase in death awareness after the time manipulation was found. Death word-stem completions were significantly higher in the mortality-salience condition than in control or time-salient conditions, however, suggesting that mortality salience is a sufficient but not necessary condition for TM outcomes.

important, value congruent, and self-prototypical). These findings indirectly support our contention that mortality salience and temporal extension make inconsistent self-elements simultaneously accessible.

In summary, the five experiments described in this section converge on the conclusion that simultaneously accessible identity inconsistencies can cause compensatory hardening of the attitudes. When important self-relevant inconsistencies are highlighted by deliberating about dilemmas, mortality salience, or awareness of the self across time, participants attempt to reestablish epistemic equilibrium by claiming conviction about attitudes in more circumscribed domains. Just as the simultaneous-accessibility notion provides an integrative perspective on past dissonance research, in conjunction with dissonance theory, it provides a powerful explanatory tool for integrating some other burgeoning directions in social psychology.

CONCLUSION

The main theme in this chapter is that for dissonance (or ambivalence) to be aroused, inconsistent cognitions must be simultaneously accessible. Simultaneous accessibility is an important variable that has considerable power for integrating disparate findings from a variety of dissonance paradigms (see also chap. 8, this volume) and from other research areas as well. In addition, recognition of the role of accessibility allows for a shift in focus from experimentally implanted inconsistency (through counterattitudinal behavior) to the investigation of native inconsistencies (see also Higgins, Shah, & Friedman, 1997). This shift holds promise for revealing the full power of cognitive dissonance. When exposed, important self-relevant inconsistencies that are normally defended against should have more motivational power than, for example, awareness that one has written an essay in favor of tuition increases. The identity-dissonance research reported in the final section suggests several new directions that might be fruitfully investigated. In particular, it suggests that extremism and zealotry may be motivated by the identity dissonance associated with simultaneously accessible alternative selves.

REFERENCES

Abelson, R. P. (1983). Whatever became of consistency theory? *Personality and Social Psychology Bulletin, 9,* 37–54.

Allen, V. L. (1965). Effect of extraneous cognitive activity on dissonance reduction. *Psychological Reports, 16,* 1145–1151.

Aronson, E. (1968). Dissonance theory: Progress and problems. In R. P. Abelson, E. Aronson, W. J. McGuire, T. M. Newcomb, M. J. Rosenberg, & P. H. Tannenbaum (Eds.), *Theories of cognitive consistency: A sourcebook* (pp. 5–27). Chicago, IL: Rand McNally.

Aronson, E. (1992). The return of the repressed: Dissonance theory makes a comeback. *Psychological Inquiry, 3,* 303–311.

Aronson, E., & Carlsmith, J. M. (1963). Effect of the severity of threat on the valuation of forbidden behavior. *Journal of Abnormal and Social Psychology, 66,* 584–588.

Aronson, J., Blanton, H., & Cooper, J. (1995). From dissonance to disidentification: Selectivity in the self-affirmation process. *Journal of Personality and Social Psychology, 68,* 986–996.

Bassili, J. N. (1994, November). *On the relationship between attitude ambivalence and attitude accessibility.* Paper presented at the University of Waterloo, Waterloo, Ontario, Canada.

Bassili, J. (1996). The "how" and "why" of response latency measurement in telephone surveys. In N. Schwarz & S. Sudman (Eds.), *Answering questions: Methodology for determining cognitive and communicative processes in survey research* (pp. 319–346). San Francisco: Jossey-Bass.

Bassili, J. N., & Fletcher, J. F. (1991). Response time measurement in survey research: A method for CATI and a new look at nonattitudes. *Public Opinion Quarterly, 55,* 331–346.

Baumeister, R. F. (1991). *Escaping the self.* New York: Basic Books.

Bem, D. J. (1967). Self-perception: An alternative interpretation of cognitive dissonance phenomena. *Psychological Review, 74,* 183–200.

Blanton, H., Cooper, J., Skurnik, I., & Aronson, J. (1997). When bad things happen to good feedback: Exacerbating the need for self-justification with self-affirmations. *Personality and Social Psychology Bulletin, 23,* 684–692.

Brock, T. C. (1962). Cognitive restructuring and attitude change. *Journal of Abnormal and Social Psychology, 64,* 264–271.

Carlsmith, J. M., Ebbesen, E. B., Lepper, M. R., Zanna, M. P., Joncas, A. J., & Abelson, R. P. (1969). Dissonance reduction following forced attention to the dissonance. *Proceedings of the 77th Annual Convention of the American Psychological Association, 4* (Pt.1), 321–322.

Cooper, J., & Fazio, R. H. (1984). A new look at dissonance theory. In L. Berkowitz (Ed.), *Advances in experimental social psychology* (Vol. 17, pp. 229–266). Orlando, FL: Academic Press.

Crumbaugh, J. C., & Maholick, L. T. (1964). An experimental study in existentialism: The psychometric approach to Frankl's concept of noogenic neurosis. *Journal of Clinical Psychology, 20,* 200–207.

Elliot, A. J., & Devine, P. (1994). On the motivational nature of cognitive dissonance: Dissonance as psychological discomfort. *Journal of Personality and Social Psychology, 67,* 382–394.

Fazio, R. H., Sanbonmatsu, D. M., Powell, M. C., & Kardes, F. R. (1986). On the automatic activation of attitudes. *Journal of Personality and Social Psychology, 50,* 229–238.

Fazio, R. H., Zanna, M. P., & Cooper, J. (1977). Dissonance and self-perception: An integrative view of each theory's proper domain of application. *Journal of Experimental Social Psychology, 13,* 464–479.

Festinger, L. (1957). A theory of cognitive dissonance. Evanston, IL: Row, Peterson.

Festinger, L., Riecken, H. W., & Schachter, S. (1956). *When prophecy fails.* Minneapolis: University of Minnesota Press.

Greenberg, J., Pyszczynski, T., Solomon, S., Simon, L., & Breus, M. (1994). Role of consciousness and accessibility of death-related thoughts in mortality salience effects. *Journal of Personality and Social Psychology, 67,* 627–637.

Greenberg, J., Solomon, S., & Pyszczynski, T. (1997). Terror management theory of self-esteem and cultural worldviews: Empirical assessments and conceptual refinements. In M. P. Zanna (Ed.), *Advances in experimental social psychology* (Vol. 29, pp. 66–139). San Diego, CA: Academic Press.

Hardyck, J. A., & Kardush, M. (1968). A modest modish model for dissonance reduction. In R. P. Abelson, E. Aronson, W. J. McGuire, T. M. Newcomb, M. J. Rosenberg, & P. H. Tannenbaum (Eds.), *Theories of cognitive consistency: A sourcebook* (pp. 684–692). Chicago: Rand McNally.

Harmon-Jones, E., Brehm, J. W., Greenberg, J., Simon, L., & Nelson, D. E.

(1996). Evidence that the production of aversive consequences is not necessary to create cognitive dissonance. *Journal of Personality and Social Psychology, 70,* 5–16.

Higgins, E. T., Shah, J., & Friedman, R. (1997). Emotional responses to goal attainment: Strength of regulatory focus as moderator. *Journal of Personality and Social Psychology, 72,* 515–525.

Jamieson, D. W. (1993, August). *The attitude ambivalence construct: Validity, utility, and measurement.* Paper presented at the 101st Annual Convention of the American Psychological Association, Toronto, Ontario, Canada.

Kaplan, K. J. (1972). On the ambivalence–indifference problem in attitude theory and measurement: A suggested modification of the semantic differential technique. *Psychological Bulletin, 77,* 361–372.

Kunda, Z. (1990). The case for motivated reasoning. *Psychological Bulletin, 108,* 480–498.

McGregor, I. (1996). [Effects of mindset manipulations on a terror management theory outcome measure]. Unpublished raw data, University of Waterloo, Waterloo, Ontario, Canada.

McGregor, I. (1998). *An identity consolidation view of social phenomena: Rigid and integrative responses to identity confrontation.* Unpublished doctoral dissertation, University of Waterloo, Waterloo, Ontario, Canada.

McGregor, I., & Little, B. R. (1998). Personal projects, happiness and meaning: On doing well and being yourself. *Journal of Personality and Social Psychology, 74,* 494–512.

Myers, D. G. (1996). *Social psychology* (5th ed.). New York: McGraw Hill.

Newby-Clark, I. R., McGregor, I., & Zanna, M. P. (1997, August). *The relation between felt ambivalence and conflicting cognitions is moderated by the simultaneous accessibility of the conflicting cognitions.* Paper presented at the 105th Annual Convention of the American Psychological Association, Chicago.

Pallak, M. S., Brock, T. C., & Kiesler, C. A. (1967). Dissonance arousal and task performance in an incidental verbal learning paradigm. *Journal of Personality and Social Psychology, 7,* 11–21.

Pyszczynski, T. A., & Greenberg, J. (1981). Role of disconfirmed expectancies in the instigation of attributional processing. *Journal of Personality and Social Psychology, 40,* 31–38

Rogers, T. B., Kuiper, N. A., & Kirker, W. S. (1977). Self-reference and the encoding of personal information. *Journal of Personality and Social Psychology, 35,* 677–688.

Rosenberg, M. J., & Abelson, R. P. (1960). An analysis of cognitive balancing. In M. J. Rosenberg, C. I. Hovland, W. J. McGuire, R. P. Abelson, & J. W. Brehm (Eds.), *Attitude organization and change* (pp. 112–163). New Haven, CT: Yale University Press.

Schopenhauer, A. (1883). *The world as will and idea* (R. B. Haldane & J. Kemps, Trans.). London: Routledge & Kegan Paul. (Original work published 1818)

Scott, W. A. (1968). Measures of cognitive structure. *Multivariate Behavior Research, 1,* 391–395.

Simon, L., Greenberg, J., & Brehm, J. (1995). Trivialization: The forgotten mode of dissonance reduction. *Journal of Personality and Social Psychology, 68,* 247–260.

Steele, C. M. (1988). The psychology of self-affirmation: Sustaining the integrity of the self. In L. Berkowitz (Ed.), *Advances in experimental social psychology* (pp. 261–302). San Diego, CA: Academic Press.

Steele, C. M., & Josephs, R. A. (1990). Alcohol myopia: Its prized and dangerous effects. *American Psychologist, 45,* 921–933.

Steele, C. M., & Liu, T. J. (1983). Dissonance processes as self-affirmation. *Journal of Personality and Social Psychology, 45,* 5–19.

Steele, C. M., Southwick, L. L., & Critchlow, B. (1981). Dissonance and alcohol: Drinking your troubles away. *Journal of Personality and Social Psychology, 41,* 831–846.

Stone, J., Wiegand, A., Cooper, J., & Aronson, E. (1997). When exemplification fails: Hypocrisy and the motive for self-integrity. *Journal of Personality and Social Psychology, 72,* 54–65.

Taylor, S. E., & Gollwitzer, P. M. (1995). Effects of mindset on positive illusions. *Journal of Personality and Social Psychology, 69,* 213–226.

Thompson, M. M., Zanna, M. P., & Griffin, D. W. (1995). Let's not be indifferent about (attitudinal) ambivalence. In R. E. Petty & J. A. Krosnick (Eds.), *Attitude strength: Antecedents and consequences* (pp. 361–386). Hillsdale, NJ: Erlbaum.

VanHook, E., & Higgins, E. T. (1988). Self-related problems beyond the self-concept: Motivational consequences of discrepant self-guides. *Journal of Personality and Social Psychology, 55*, 625–633.

Wegner, D. M. (1994). Ironic processes of mental control. *Psychological Review, 101*, 34–52.

Wong, P. T., & Weiner, B. (1981). When people ask "why" questions, and the heuristic of attributional search. *Journal of Personality and Social Psychology, 40*, 650–663.

Yalom, I. D. (1980). *Existential psychotherapy.* New York: Basic Books.

Zanna, M. P., & Aziza, C. (1976). On the interaction of repression–sensitization and attention in resolving cognitive dissonance. *Journal of Personality, 44*, 577–593.

Zanna, M. P., & Cooper, J. (1974). Dissonance and the pill: An attribution approach to studying the arousal properties of dissonance. *Journal of Personality and Social Psychology, 29*, 703–709.

Zanna, M. P., Lepper, M. R., & Abelson, R. P. (1973). Attentional mechanisms in children's devaluation of a forbidden activity in a forced-compliance situation. *Journal of Personality and Social Psychology, 28*, 355–359.

Social Communication and Cognition: A Very Preliminary and Highly Tentative Draft

Leon Festinger

In order to understand and explain communication behavior in persons it is necessary to separate various kinds of communication since the whole area of communication is probably as all inclusive as human behavior. We shall here concern ourselves with one conceptually defined subarea under the rubric of communication which seems to be important. Specifically, we shall present a theory, together with some supporting data, to explain communication oriented toward acquiring or supporting one's cognition. We shall state the theory in a series of hypotheses along with derivations which can be made from them.

HYPOTHESES CONCERNING THE RELATION BETWEEN COMMUNICATION AND COGNITION

Here we will deal with the ways in which persons acquire cognition. Much of what we say under this heading may seem trivial and well known, but it is necessary to state these things as precisely as possible in order to develop our theory coherently.

Hypothesis 1. There are two major sources of cognition, namely, own experience and communication from others.

Acquiring cognition through one's own experience is, of course, the most direct way. We can think of the other source, that is, communication from others, as being an indirect way of acquiring cognition.

Frequently, cognition is acquired by a combination of both. Thus, for example, a child may learn from his mother that fire is dangerous and will hurt if touched. This cognition will undoubtedly be reinforced the first time the child gets burnt. One can raise the question of where, in this denotation of two sources of cognition, one would place such things as reading a newspaper, listening to a radio, hearing a political speech or seeing a sign along a road that says "15 miles to Peoria." These are all sources of cognition, none of them direct, but there seems to be a big difference among them. On logical grounds, according to our division, we would have to say that in each case the cognition that was acquired about the environment was acquired indirectly, through communication from others. Practically no one, however, will react to the traffic sign as anything other than fact while many will react to what the politician tells them as quite different from fact. (We will ignore here the cognition acquired about the politician himself from listening to him. This particular cognition is of course acquired directly through experience.) We see then, that in the case of acquiring cognition indirectly, there are factors which will affect the impact which the communication has on the cognition of the recipient. We will deal with this more in detail later.

Hypothesis 2. The impact of direct experience will exert pressure on the cognition to conform to the experience.

In other words, there will be forces acting on the person to have his cognition correspond to reality as he experiences it. The result of this will be that, in general, persons will have a correct picture of the world around them in which they live. This is, of course, not surprising since the organism would have a hard time surviving if this were not the case.

Hypothesis 3. The strength of the impact of indirect experience (communication) to make the cognition conform will vary with the relationship between the communicator and recipient.

To make this hypothesis specific enough to be useful we must specify something more about the dimensions of relationship between the communicator and recipient which are relevant and the direction of the effect on impact of the communication. We will do this by stating two subsidiary hypotheses.

Hypothesis 3.1. The greater the "trustworthiness" of the communicator, the greater will be the impact on the cognition.

Trustworthiness here means a complex of things which, in the future, might better be separated. We will, however, spell out some of the things which affect it. To the extent that the communicator is seen as in the same situation as the recipient and consequently likely to experience things from the same point of view he will be seen as trustworthy. Also, to the extent that the communicator is seen as performing an impartial service for the recipient he will be seen as trustworthy. A road sign, for example, is seen as a communication emanating from an impartial servant and is hence regarded as trustworthy. A union member will regard a statement of fact or of opinion or of interpretation as more trustworthy if it comes from another union member (a person in similar circumstances) than if it comes from an executive of the company.

Hypothesis 3.2. The stronger the attraction on the recipient toward association with the communicator, the greater will be the impact of the communication on cognition.

This hypothesis is related closely to others which will be stated later, and so no detailed explanation will be given at this point.

THE RELATION BETWEEN COGNITION AND BEHAVIOR

It has frequently been stated that cognition steers behavior. This is quite true and is important for an understanding of the directedness of behavior in an organism. For an understanding of cognition formation and the communication processes which determine and result from cognition formation it is also important to understand that behavior steers cognition. In the following hypotheses we will state our theory of how this takes place.

Hypothesis 4. There exists a tendency to make one's cognition and one's behavior consonant.

In order to explain this hypothesis, which is basic to the theory, we must spend some time in giving definitions of the terms we have used. First of all, although it may seem obvious, let us state more specifically the distinction between cognition and behavior. By cognition we wish to designate opinions, beliefs, values, knowledges and the like about one's environment, including oneself in this environment. By behavior we wish to designate actions of the person and reactions which he has. Actions would include driving a car, reading a book, being a man, residing in a certain place, and the like. Reactions would include things like being afraid, being hopeful, being anxious, and others.

It is also necessary to define consonance and the lack of consonance which we will call dissonance. There are three possible relations which can exist between items of behavior and items of cognition, namely, consonance, dissonance and irrelevance. (These same three relations may also exist among items of cognition or among items of behavior. To avoid confusion we shall not deal with these at this point but shall return to them later.) A relationship of irrelevance exists if a particular item of cognition has absolutely nothing to do with a particular item of behavior. Thus, for example, an irrelevant relation exists between having the opinion that elementary schools are overcrowded and the behavior of playing golf on a nice sunny Saturday morning. Such irrelevant relations produce no pressures on persons and we may, for the rest of the paper, ignore them.

A relationship of consonance exists between a particular item of cognition and some item of behavior if, holding the motivation the same, this behavior would follow upon this cognition in the absence of other cognitions and in the absence of restraints. Thus, for example, the knowledge that construction crews are working on a certain street would be consonant with the behavior of taking an alternate route in driving to work. The opinion that it is going to rain would be consonant with the behavior of carrying a raincoat. The belief that thieves are around would be consonant with feeling afraid when walking home alone on a dark night.

A relationship of dissonance exists between an item of cognition and an item of behavior if, under the same conditions described in the paragraph above, a different behavior would follow upon this cognition. Thus, for example, the belief that it is going to rain is dissonant with the behavior of going on a picnic. The opinion that some other person is a very excellent and very careful driver would be dissonant with having a fear reaction while driving with him in the ordinary course of events.

One may, of course, raise the question as to why dissonances ever arise. There are many circumstances in which dissonances are almost unavoidable, and it will help our discussion later to list now the various ways in which dissonances can occur.

1. A change occurs in the situation. A given behavior may have been consonant with cognition before a change occurred in the situation. This new set of circumstances impinges upon the person's cognition either directly or indirectly, and the new cognition is, at least momentarily, dissonant with the existing behavior.
2. Initial direct contact with a situation. A person's cognition may have been formed from communication with others. The first direct experience may impinge on the cognition so as to produce dissonance with the existing behavior at least temporarily.
3. New communication from others. This can function in the same way as the above two to introduce a new cognitive item which is dissonant with existing behavior.
4. Simultaneous existence of various cognitive elements. It is probably a usual state of affairs that there are several relevant cognitive items, some of which are consonant with a given behavior and others of which are dissonant with that same behavior. Under such circumstances it may not be possible for the person to find a behavior which eliminates all dissonances.

We can now return to an elaboration of Hypothesis 4. This hypothesis states then that if a state of consonance exists it is an equilibrium, that is, no forces to change the relation are acting. If a dissonance exists there will be forces set up to eliminate the dissonance and produce consonance. We will list the various ways in which these forces can act as subsidiary hypotheses.

Hypothesis 4.1. Given a dissonance between an item of cognition and an item of behavior there will be a tendency to change the behavior so as to make it consonant with the cognition.

When this tendency is strong enough to produce actual changes in behavior we will observe the kinds of things which have generally been treated as problems of learning or adaptation. For our present focus of interest we will not elaborate on these problem areas but will rather concern ourselves with those situations where the tendency to change one's behavior is not strong enough so that the existing behavior persists.

Hypothesis 4.2. Given a dissonance between an item of cognition and an item of behavior there will be a tendency to change the cognition so as to make it consonant with the behavior.

In general there are two ways in which the cognition can be changed, assuming we are dealing with persons who are in sufficient contact with reality so that Hypotheses 1, 2, and 3 hold. One of these is to actually act on the environment so as to produce a situation where the veridical cognition will be consonant with the behavior in question. Of course, such action would only be successful in producing consonance in circumstances where the person has control over the environment. We will leave this without further elaboration since, again, it is not our main focus of interest.

Probably the major way in which cognition is changed so as to make it consonant with behavior is by selective exposure to either direct or indirect impact from the environment and actively seeking communications which will change the cognition in the desired manner.

Thus, for example, a person who is afraid of riding in airplanes may avidly read and remember every account of an airplane disaster which he comes across and may avoid hearing about or reading about safety records and the like. Or let us imagine a person who has bought a new car just prior to the introduction of some new improvement. He may very actively try to persuade his friends that this new improvement is useless and will not work and adds unnecessarily to the expense of the car. If he succeeds in persuading them he will then have support for a cognition consonant with his possession of a car which does not have this new improvement.

Hypothesis 5. If a consonance exists there will be resistance to changes in behavior or cognition which would introduce dissonance.

Hypothesis 6. If a dissonance exists there will be resistance to changes in behavior or cognition which would increase the magnitude of the dissonance.

To summarize the statements involved in Hypotheses 4 through 6 we may say that tendencies operate to avoid increases and produce decreases of dissonance. These tendencies, when equilibrium does not exist, will manifest themselves either in changes of behavior or in changes of cognition. In order to make the theory more usable it is necessary to state some of the conditions which will determine whether the behavior or the cognition changes.

Hypothesis 7. Behavior or cognition will change in the presence of a dissonance if the strength of the dissonance is greater than the resistance to change of either the behavior or the cognition in question.

Hypothesis 8. Whether the behavior or the cognition changes will be determined by which has the weakest resistance to change.

The last two hypotheses will have meaning only to the extent that we can specify resistance to change and the determinants of the strength of resistance to change of both behavior and cognition. We shall consequently proceed to do this.

RESISTANCE TO CHANGE OF BEHAVIOR AND COGNITION

We will state two hypotheses which are in essence an attempt to state some of the sources of resistance to change.

Hypothesis 9. The resistance to changing behavior which is dissonant with cognition will be directly related to the strength of the motivation which this behavior satisfies, the amount of effort or pain or loss involved in changing the behavior and the number of cognitive elements which are consonant with the behavior.

Thus, for example, a person who has strong motivation toward having status and power might behave as if he had them even though his cognition was dissonant with this behavior. The stronger the motivation, the more resistant would the behavior be to change. Under these circumstances, provided the cognition is less resistant to change, the person will find ways to change his cognition rather than change his behavior.

An example of another source of resistance might be a person who has recently bought a new car and later knowledge tends to make his cognition dissonant with this behavior. Changing the behavior, that is, selling the car and getting another, might involve financial loss and might also involve admitting that he had been foolish to have made the original purchase. There will, consequently, be a certain resistance to changing the behavior.

The last factor mentioned in the hypothesis is, of course, clear. If the behavior in question is already consonant with many cognitive elements, it will be much more resistant to change than if there are no consonances between cognitive elements and this item of behavior.

Hypothesis 10. The resistance to changing an element of cognition which is dissonant with some behavior will vary directly with the number of behavior items with which this cognitive element is consonant, with the importance of those behavior items, and with the strength of the impact of the environment, directly or indirectly, which supports this cognition.

The last of the factors listed in the above hypothesis is relatively clear. If the paper on which I am writing this is white, and I continue to see it as white, it will be difficult to change this cognition. Or if someone believes that modern art is decadent and all his associates tell him that this opinion is correct, it will be rather resistant to change.

Also, if an element of cognition is consonant with many items of behavior in which the person engages, it will be more resistant to change than an element of cognition which is not consonant with any behavior. The more important a particular behavior, the more resistance will there be to changing an element of cognition which is consonant with it. Importance of the behavior would depend upon the strength of the motivation which the behavior satisfies.

At this point we would like to digress slightly to deal with a concept which has been used frequently by others but which we have not mentioned, namely, consistency among cognitive elements. Thus, for example, various persons have maintained, and it seems plausible, that new cognitions are absorbed by persons so that they are consistent with what already exists in the cognition. This has been maintained about opinions, attitudes, perceptions and the like. We have, however, not defined anything so far about relations among cognitive elements. Such definition is necessary, however. We will maintain here that any two or more cognitive elements which are consonant with the same behavior items and dissonant with the same behavior items are consonant with each other. Such a set of cognitive elements which are consonant with one another in this sense is a consistent cognitive system. The first part of Hypothesis 10, in light of this definition, could be stated as follows:

Corollary 10. The resistance to changing an element of cognition which is dissonant with some behavior will vary directly with the number and importance of the cognitive elements in the consistent system of which this particular element is a part.

THE RELATION OF COGNITION TO CHOICE

Thus far we have dealt only with the relation of cognition to behavior which already exists. There are many situations in which a person has decided or is forced to do something, but there are still alternatives which are available to him. We will here state a number of hypotheses dealing with the relationship between cognition and, at the moment, nonexistent behavior.

For the purposes of the following discussion let us distinguish three kinds of situations with respect to behavior in which a person might find himself.

1. A given realm of behavior may be entirely irrelevant for a person. This would mean that he does not engage in any of these behaviors nor is there a likelihood that he may. Thus, for example, the whole realm of behavior related to cars may be completely irrelevant to a poor farm worker in India. We will refer to this as an irrelevant realm of behavior.

2. A person may not engage in any number of possible specific behaviors, but there is the possibility, likelihood or even certainty that at some time in the future he will engage in at least one of them. Thus, for example, a person may have accepted a job in a different city from the one in which he now lives. This means that he is going to have to select a neighborhood in which to live, find a house to buy or an apartment to rent and the like. All of these behaviors are ones in which, at some future time, he will engage in. We will refer to this as relevant future behavior.

3. The person engages in some behavior or has committed himself to some specific course of action. This is the kind of situation which we have been discussing above, and we will not dwell on it again. It is clear that this situation, which we will call relevant present behavior, and the situation of relevant future behavior may exist simultaneously. The person in the example above is in both of these situations. His decision to accept the new job has committed him to a specific course of action and is, hence, present relevant behav-

ior. At the same time it has involved him in a situation of relevant future behavior.

Hypothesis 11. There will be no active seeking out or active avoidance of cognition related to an irrelevant realm of behavior.

A person in this situation may be a passive recipient of such cognition, but there will be no initiative on his part. Thus, for example, most persons do not exert effort to find out or to avoid finding out how far from the earth the moon is.

Hypotheses 12. In the situation of relevant future behavior there will be active seeking out of cognition relevant to each of the possible future behaviors.

If there are a variety of possible behavior items, one or more of which the person may engage in in the future, this person will actively seek cognition relevant to each of them. Thus, for example, if a person has decided to buy a new car, but has not yet decided what kind to buy, he will actively seek information about each of those which he regards as possible purchases. Of course, once a decision has been made, this type of cognition seeking stops. From then on the person will seek information consonant with his behavior and avoid information which is dissonant with it, as stated in Hypothesis 4. This partial reversal of information seeking behavior and the result of acquiring mainly consonant cognition after the decision results in what Lewin has called "freezing of decisions."

DERIVATIONS AND DATA

There is surprising little data extant in the literature which is relevant to the above set of hypotheses. The data which we have been able to find is not always such as to be completely trustworthy. We will present it for what it is worth along with the statement of the major derivations from the hypotheses.

Derivation A. If a person's action or reaction with respect to some event is dissonant with his cognition, he will communicate with others, the content of the communication being consonant with his action or reaction.

Derivation B. Such communications (the specific content) will be widespread if many persons have the same initial cognition and the same dissonant action or reaction.

There are data of a sort relevant to these derivations from two studies of rumors in India. Prasad (1950) systematically recorded rumors which were widely current immediately after the earthquake in the province of Bihar in India on January 15, 1934. The quake itself was a strong and prolonged one, felt over a wide geographical area. Actual damage was quite localized, and for a period of time communication with the damaged area was poor. We are, then, dealing with communication among persons who felt the shock of the quake but did not see any actual damage or destruction. While the study does not report anything about the specific reactions of these persons to the quake, it is probably plausible to assume that these persons, who knew nothing about earthquakes or their causes, had a very strong reaction of fear to the violent and prolonged quake which they felt. We will also assume that this reaction of being afraid persisted in them for some time after the shock was over. While the shock was going on, this fear reaction would be consonant with their cognition. But when the shock was over—the next day or even the day after that—when they could see no difference in anything around them, no destruction, no further threatening things, their cognition became dissonant with this reaction of fear which persisted. If this interpretation of the reactions of these persons is correct, then Derivation A would lead us to expect communication which would be consonant with fear reduction, namely communication, which would make it "appropriate" to be afraid. According to Derivation B we would expect these communications to be widespread since many of the persons would have had the same fear reaction.

Actually, the vast majority of the rumors which Prasad recorded were what one might call "fear provoking" rumors. The following are a fair sample of these rumors as illustrations.

> The water of the River Ganges disappeared at the time of the earthquake, and people bathing were imbedded in the sand.

> There will be a severe cyclone at Patna between 18 and 19 January. (The earthquake was on January 15.)

> There will be a severe earthquake on the lunar eclipse day.

> A flood was rushing from the Nepal borders to Madhubani.

> 23 January, 1934 will be a fatal day. Unforeseeable calamities will arise.

> There will be a *Pralaya* (total deluge and destruction) on 26 February, 1934.

It is clear that a goodly number of rumors arose which predicted that more disasters were shortly to come. This cognition is, of course, consonant with the reaction of being afraid. The data, interpreted in this way, tend to support our derivations. This support is, however, weak because so much has to be read into the situation to make an assumption about the reaction of persons and because there are many possible other explanations of why these particular kinds of rumors arose in such a situation. It is fortunate, however, that there is another study which can serve as sort of a control to compare with the one just discussed.

Sinha (1952) reports a careful collection of reports and rumors following a terrible disaster in Darjeeling, India. The author states, "There had been landslides before but nothing like this had ever happened. Loss of life and damage to property were heavy and extensive. . . . In the town itself houses collapsed and victims lay buried under the debris. . . . Over a hundred and fifty persons lost their lives in the district, about thirty of them in the town itself. Over a hundred were injured. More than 200 houses were damaged and over 2000 people were rendered homeless." In other words, it was a disaster easily comparable to that of an earthquake. The author states, "There was a feeling of instability and uncertainty similar to that which followed the Great Indian Earthquake of 1934," (p. 200).

We may then regard this aspect of the situation to be sufficiently comparable to allow us to compare the rumors which arose in this situation with those which arose following the 1934 earthquake. There is, however, one important difference which enables us to regard this study as a control. While the rumors following the earthquake were collected from persons who had no direct experience with the destruction, the rumors which Sinha reports were collected from persons in Darjeeling who did experience and see the destruction. In other words, we may again assume that the persons in this area had a strong fear reaction to the landslide all around them. However, there was evidence of the destruction, and consequently, their cognition was consonant with this fear reaction. In this situation then, we would *not* expect any rumors which predicted further disasters.

Actually there was a complete absence of rumors predicting further disasters. Some of the rumors represented slight exaggeration of the actual damage, and some rumors are even of the hopeful variety. The following is a selection of rumors to illustrate the general kind that existed.

> "Many houses have come down on the A-road." (p. 201) (Only one house had actually collapsed on this particular road.)
>
> Widespread belief that there had been a slight earthquake which had helped in producing the damage. (There had been no earthquake.)
>
> "It has been announced that the water supply will be restored in a week." (p. 203)
>
> "It will take months before the water supply is resumed." (p. 203)
>
> "There are extensive floods in the plains. . . . Many bridges have been washed away." (p. 204)

The remarkable thing about these rumors is the lack of serious exaggeration and even the presence of a few which are hopeful. The contrast with the rumors following the earthquake reported by Prasad is quite dramatic.

Since it seems that the two studies are comparable except for the fact that in one instance rumors were collected which circulated among persons not on the scene of destruction and in the other instance the rumors circulated among persons on the scene of destruction, this difference in the nature of the rumors tends to give further support to the derivation.

Derivation C. If cognition is consonant with behavior, and events occur which would tend to make the cognition dissonant with the behavior, there will be communication whose content reaffirms the consonant cognition and denies the dissonant cognition.

There are data relevant to this derivation from a study by Sady (1948) of rumors among the Japanese in the relocation centers during the second World War. The data are not ideal for our purposes since, just as in the case with the previous studies cited, there is relatively little information given as to the actions and reactions of the people in the various specific situations in which the rumors arose. The result is that, in order to interpret the data with reference to this derivation, we are forced to make various guesses about the reactions of the persons involved. These data are, however, the best that we have been able to discover.

Because of this problem of guessing the reaction of the residents of the relocation centers, we shall deal only with rumors that circulated near the beginning of the establishment of the camps or just prior to the closing of the camps. In both of these instances we can be reasonably sure about some of the reactions of the residents. When they were first sent to the camp they were very upset and anxious. They had been uprooted suddenly, and the major reaction, which persisted for some time, was fear and anxiety. Once in the camps, however, there was a tendency for cognition to become dissonant with the reaction of fear and anxiety. There were consequently many rumors which would tend to prevent this dissonance from arising. Rumors that many people were dying because of the heat and that their bodies were taken away secretly at night, or that the site for the relocation center had been deliberately chosen so that as many as possible of the evacuees would die, and many others of the same type were widely current. The following specific instance will illustrate the process.

During the first summer at the Poston Camp, temporary clinics operated before the regular hospital was ready. When the hospital was opened, these temporary clinics were closed, and a 24 hour home call service for emergencies was instituted. The change was, of course, an improvement in the medical services offered in the camp. This, according to our interpretation, would tend to introduce cognitions dissonant with the persisting reactions of fear and anxiety. In spite of (or perhaps to counteract) the fact of the introduction of the 24 hour home call service, the story circulated widely and was widely accepted that doctors would *not* make any more home calls. No matter how serious the case, the patient, they said, would have to go to the hospital before seeing a doctor. Thus, the change in medical services, through the rumor, was accepted into the cognition as a change for the worse and thus was consonant with their fear and anxiety.

Toward the end, when persons started to be resettled, the prevalent reactions, according to Sady, were again fear and anxiety, but this time about the problems of resettlement. There was apparently a considerable fear of how they would be treated by the communities on the outside. There were again quite a number of rumors which provided cognition consonant with this fear and which counteracted events which tended to produce dissonant cognitions. The following specific example will illustrate this.

The father and son of a family in one of the camps left to inspect their farm and to make arrangements for returning the entire family to their original home. A few hours after they left the rumor spread that they had been beaten up on the way and that one of them had been taken to the hospital. Administration personnel from the camp contacted the father and son and discovered the story was false, that they had been given an excellent reception. This was made public but the rumor persisted. The father and son then returned to camp, and the whole family left for their farm. Several letters were received from them telling about the good treatment they were receiving. Nevertheless, rumors continued to circulate, such as that they were having difficulty shopping and had become discouraged about staying on their farm. Again the rumors served to counteract dissonant cognition and preserve the consonance with their reactions of fear.

There is one other, rather dramatic, illustration of this process of avoiding dissonance from this same study. During the war some Nisei and some Issei requested repatriation to Japan, the Nisei renouncing their citizenship. While the majority of the Issei in the relocation centers believed and hoped that the war would end in a negotiated peace, most of those who had requested repatriation firmly believed that Japan would win the war and explained news of Japanese reverses as American propaganda. The renunciation of citizenship and the request for repatriation were rather irrevocable decisions, and at the time these decisions were made, the cognition of these persons was consonant with their decision. This group who had requested repatriation continued to believe that Japan had won the war even after the surrender. After having seen the newspapers and photographs attesting to the surrender of Japan, the great majority of the Japanese in the camps accepted the evidence. Those who had requested repatriation, however, held fast to their belief that Japan had won and continued to dismiss the evidence as American propaganda. This belief persisted all the way back to Japan on the boat. It was not until after landing in Japan that this belief was finally dispelled. The following Associated Press news story describes the situation.

Nippon Times, December 2, 1945

"Bitter Disappointment Marks Return Home of Nisei Who Wished They Had Stayed in U.S."

Why 95% of those who came back to Japan on the ship with me thought that Japan had won the war: They thought it just a bunch of American propaganda that Japan surrendered and they believed that they were being brought back to Japan because Japanese had won the war and were compelling the Americans to transport them.

We will now discuss some data relevant to Hypotheses 11 and 12. Baxter (1951) reports a study in which a number of persons were interviewed periodically during the election campaign of 1948. Particular attention was paid to the collection of data concerning discussions with others about the election. The panel of respondents was interviewed in June 1948 for the first time. Among other things, they were asked whether they were doing anything for their party in the present election, how interested they were in that election and whether or not they had talked politics with anyone that month. Table 1 presents the data based on these three questions.

An examination of the figures makes it clear that those who are doing something for their party talk more about politics than those who are not doing anything. If doing something for the party in the election campaign can be viewed as a behavioral commitment, then the interpretation would seem indicated that, having committed themselves behaviorally, there are pressures to talk politics and so make their cognition consonant with this behavior. Those who have not committed themselves behaviorally, with the election still so far in the future, show much lower incidence of seeking or giving opinions concerning politics. The possible interpretation that those who are doing something for the party are simply more interested in the election is ruled out by the fact that there are very similar proportions of interested and uninterested persons in both classifications.

Table 1
Percentage of Respondents Who Talked Politics in June

	% talked politics	Total #
Doing something for party		
High interest in election	65%	40
Low interest in election	68%	19
Doing nothing for party		
High interest in election	38%	487
Low interest in election	14%	217

This interpretation is supported more strongly if we examine this data more closely. To the extent that high interest in the election can be interpreted as indicating how important the person thinks the election is for himself, we would expect that the highly interested persons would talk politics more frequently than the less interested persons. This is indeed true for those who are not doing anything for the party, in other words, those not behaviorally committed. For those who are behaviorally committed, however, there is no difference at all in the frequency with which the highly and less interested persons discuss politics. In fact there is a slight difference in the opposite direction. It is possible that those who are behaviorally committed, and yet have low interest in the election, talk as much or even more than the others in order to make their cognition consonant with their behavior of working for the party.

Table 2 shows the percentage among those who did talk politics in June who talked frequently. It is clear that all the differences are in the same direction even to the reversal between the high and low interest groups who are committed to working for the party.

According to Hypotheses 11 and 12 we would, of course, explain the low percentages of persons talking politics in June among those highly interested but not working for the party by the fact that any decision (as to voting) was still a long way off. We would then expect

Table 2

Percents of Those Talking Politics in June Who Talked Often

	% talking often	#
Doing something for the party		
High interest	77%	26
Low interest	85%	13
Doing nothing for the party		
High interest	56%	183
Low interest	36%	31

that these percentages would increase enormously as the election drew near and the future implied behavior became salient. Table 3 shows the data for the percent in the various classifications who talked politics in October, just prior to the election.

Again, all of the differences are in the same direction as they were in the previous tabulations, including the reversal between the interest groups who were working for the party. The only difference now is that the two high interest groups talk almost as much. In other words, the immediacy of the election has had the anticipated effect.

In the preceding three tables which we have discussed, we cannot, because of the small numbers of cases in the group who are not very interested in the election and are working for the party, be very confident about the tendency for them to talk even more than those who are highly interested in the election. We can, however, be quite confident that among those committed to working for the party, the factor of interest in the election makes no difference in their tendency to talk politics.

Let us now turn our attention to the kind of data which is more usually obtained in studies of public opinion and mass media. The hypotheses and derivations which we have stated should be relevant to this type of material. Unfortunately, once more, we run up against the obstacle that there are practically no studies in which sufficient data

Table 3
Percents Talking Politics in October

	% talking often	#
Doing something for the party		
High interest	94%	46
Low interest	100%	6
Doing nothing for the party		
High interest	90%	418
Low interest	78%	152

were gathered to make a test of these hypotheses unequivocal. Typically, the elements of data which are missing are those concerning the behavior and reactions of the persons, the degree of commitment to the specific behavior or reaction which exists. We will discuss below a selection of material where plausible assumptions can be made regarding these missing items of data and see to what extent the results fit the theory we have presented.

There are many instances in the literature of reported relationships between information about or awareness of some item and some other variable which can usually be called "interest in the matter." Interest in something is, of course, a very vague term and does not usually refer to anything unambiguous. To the extent that interest is a measure of how important the problem is to the person, we would expect this relationship from our theory. That is, the more important an implied future behavior was, the stronger would be the tendency to acquire information relevant to it. Sometimes, however, the variable of "interest" seems to be interpretable as a reaction or behavior, and in such cases the data should conform to the predictions from the theory. We will give a few examples of such instances. It must be remembered that in most cases the data simply relate two variables with no indication of the direction of causality. That is, it is possible that a relationship between interest and amount of information could be found because once the person acquires the information, for whatever reason this may have occurred, it stimulates his interest in the problem. Probably this kind of thing always happens to some extent. In our interpretation, however, we will not dwell on this direction of causality but shall explore how the data can be interpreted from the other causal direction.

We will first examine a number of items of data from a report by the Survey Research Center (1948) of a survey concerning awareness of a recent Cancer Society campaign and attitudes toward cancer.

Respondents in this survey were asked which diseases they considered "most dangerous." Table 4 shows the relationship obtained between whether or not cancer was named as a "most dangerous disease" and the awareness of the cancer campaign.

Before interpreting this relationship let us speculate briefly about

Table 4

Relation of Awareness of Cancer Campaign to Choice of Cancer as a "Most Dangerous" Disease

Awareness	Cancer named	Cancer not named
Very high	11%	3%
High	34%	15%
Medium	37%	25%
Low	9%	28%
Very low	8%	27%
Not ascertained	1%	2%
	100%	100%

the meaning it has for a person to name cancer as one of the "most dangerous diseases." It will help in this speculation, of course, to know something about the reasons persons gave for feeling it was so dangerous. Actually, 74% of those who named cancer as one of the most dangerous diseases gave as a reason that it is incurable or that it is fatal. Let us imagine, then, that naming cancer as a most dangerous disease indicates some fear of cancer, or at least indicates the presence of an implied future behavior, namely, something must be done to avoid it. If this is true then the relationship obtained with awareness of the campaign would be consistent with our theory. A campaign by a cancer society may be expected to provide information about things to do to prevent cancer and may also be expected to provide cognition consonant with a "fear of cancer." We would then expect persons who are afraid of the disease or who have an implied future behavior to expose themselves to the campaign and hence be more highly aware of it than persons who are not afraid of it or have no implied future behavior. It can readily be seen that, interpreted in this way, such data support the theory. It can also readily be seen that an enormous amount of interpretation and conjecture is necessary in order to interpret the data at all. This, unfortunately, is true of almost all of the data in the literature.

Those data which we have had to infer or conjecture are precisely the ones that would have to be supplied to make a test of the theory rigorous. There is much material of this type which we could present and discuss, but there is little point in doing this since in all cases the same problems will obtain.

VOLUNTARY AUDIENCES

The theory which we have developed in the preceding pages has direct implications concerning who exposes himself to what. In other words, the theory predicts certain things about the composition of voluntary audiences. Specifically, it states the following things:

1. People with no present behavior or implied future behavior relevant to a given topic should not be found among purely voluntary audiences.
2. People who would expect to obtain cognition dissonant with present behavior should not be found in purely voluntary audiences.
3. Persons who expect to obtain cognition consonant with present behavior should be in voluntary audiences.
4. People with implied future behavior should expose themselves voluntarily irrespective of the bias of the communication.

Let us make clear, of course, that this does not refer to exposure for purposes of amusement or pleasure such as listening to a play or a dance band on the radio. That part of such a program that deals with propaganda, advertising or educational material is communicating to an involuntary audience, that is, an audience that was lured there for some other purpose. By a purely voluntary audience, we mean one which exposed itself voluntarily to the particular material in question.

One can find frequent remarks in the literature that tend to confirm these implications of the theory. It is often stated by persons writing on the subject that people listen to things they already agree with and do not expose themselves to things they disagree with. However, in going through the literature one begins to wonder where they reached this conclusion because there is almost a complete absence of data concerning it. For example, Klapper (1949) states, "this phenomenon of self-selection might well be called the most basic process thus far established by research on the effects of mass media. Operative in regard to intellectual or aesthetic level of material, its political tenor, or any of a dozen other aspects, the process of self-selection works toward two manifestations of the same end: every product of mass media (1) attracts an audience which already prefers that particular type of material, and (2) fails to attract any significant number of persons who are either of contrary inclination or who have been hitherto uninterested." He presents no data in support of this, however, except to quote Lazarsfeld (1942) as follows: "even so called educational programs are not free from this tendency. Some time ago there was a program on the air which showed in different installments how all the nationalities in this country have contributed to American culture. The purpose was to teach tolerance of other nationalities. The indications were, however, that the audience for each program consisted mainly of the national group which was currently being praised. There was little chance for the program to teach tolerance, because . . . self-selection . . . produced a body of listeners who heard only about the contributions of a country which they already approved."

Lazarsfeld, in turn, presents no data to support this impression. The one instance he mentions does, of course, support our derivations. Certainly being a member of a specific nationality group in America is an irrevocable behavior. Cognitions that this nationality group is important in American culture would be consonant with being a member of the group. Consequently they listen to a broadcast which provides this consonant cognition.[1]

REFERENCES

Baxter, D. (1951). *Interpersonal contact and exposure to mass media during a presidential campaign.* Unpublished doctoral dissertation, Columbia University, New York.

---

[1] Festinger reported the results of a study by Childs in the original version of this paper. Because the editors could not find the study to which he referred, the discussion of this study was eliminated from the present version.

Klapper, J. (1949, August). *Effects of the mass media* (A report to the director of the Public Library Inquiry). New York: Columbia University, Bureau of Applied Social Research.

Lazarsfeld, P. (1942). Effects of radio on public opinion. In D. Waples (Ed.), *Print, radio, and film in a democracy*. Chicago: University of Chicago Press.

Prasad, J. (1950). A comparative study of rumours and reports in earthquakes. *British Journal of Psychology, 41*, 129–144.

Sady, R. R. (1948). *The function of rumors in relocation centers*. Unpublished doctoral dissertation, University of Chicago.

Sinha, D. (1952). Behaviour in a catastrophic situation: A psychological study of reports and rumors. *British Journal of Psychology, 43*, 200–209.

Survey Research Center, University of Michigan. (1948, December). *The American public discuss cancer and the American Cancer Society campaign: A national survey*. Ann Arbor: Author.

Reflections on Cognitive Dissonance: 30 Years Later

Leon Festinger

This is a transcript of remarks Leon Festinger made as a discussant in the symposium Reflections on Cognitive Dissonance: 30 Years Later *at the 95th Annual Convention of the American Psychology Association. The other members of the symposium were Elliot Aronson, Jack Brehm, Joel Cooper, and Judson Mills.*

Let me try to touch a little on various things that have been mentioned, going back to history. I will try to be as amusing as I can be. Actually this isn't the 30th anniversary, it's perhaps the 31st or something like that. The manuscript of the book was finished in early 1956. I had signed a contract with Row, Peterson, who were very enthusiastic about publishing it. But by the time the manuscript was finished, the enthusiastic part of Row, Peterson had left that company, and Row, Peterson's enthusiasm diminished incredibly. After about eight months had gone by since they had the manuscript, I phoned them, expressed a bit of displeasure, and I was told in a very sympathetic terms that they had to put off production because a more important book had come in that they had to get out. Then the book appeared with a very flimsy cover and no slipcover at all, and when I complained about that, I was assured that was the new style in books. Then, after two years they let it go out of print, and there were no plans to reprint it. Fortunately, there was a captive press, that is, Stanford University Press. I was on the faculty committee, and they were persuaded to reprint it. So it came to life and continued living as a book.

I have never really thoroughly understood the early reactions to the theory of cognitive dissonance. The first thing I realized was the great wisdom of the decision of American Psychological Association to have a journal called *Contemporary Psychology*. Before *Contemporary Psychology* appeared, almost every APA journal carried reviews, and it is true that some books never got reviewed and some books got two or three reviews, but with the journal *Contemporary Psychology*, you were assured that there would be one and only one review of a book. The editors in their wisdom chose as their reviewer a gentleman called Solomon Asch, a great believer of human rationality, and he wrote a marvelous review. He approached the thing as a moral dilemma, and after considerable discussion he came out with the Scottish verdict not proven, implying that the alternatives were guilty or not guilty. But the reaction to it was more general than that. He was not alone. Others also went to great pains to try to demonstrate that the theory was incorrect. Which is OK. At least that was a more scientific approach. At that time at least, and I don't know whether it still exists today, there was a bit of an illness in social psychology, because people took more delight in countering rather than in exploring and questioning and conceivably supporting. I hope social psychology isn't that way any longer.

Other theories were also proposed, and there were a whole slew of inconsistency theories. For example, balance theory attempted a very, very elegant mathematical formulation of inconsistency at least among triads; you know, if A likes B and B likes C and A doesn't like C, that was imbalanced. I well remember several times protesting that it was demonstrably wrong because, for example, I like chicken, chickens like chicken food and I don't like chicken food. But everyone treated it as a joke, and nobody took it seriously. It's a rather serious criticism.

As I say, I never really understood the emotionality of the controversy. One result of that was that experiment after experiment on the part of the dissonance movement was oriented toward proving again and again and again that there is a process of dissonance reduction that occurs under certain conditions. They showed that it occurs here and it occurs there and perhaps, undoubtedly, it was very necessary at the time, but it was also a huge waste of effort of a lot of talented people who should have been devoting their efforts to clarifying the concepts, improving the definitions and changing it. No theory is going to be inviolate. Let me put it clearly. The only kind of theory that can be proposed and ever will be proposed that absolutely will remain inviolate for decades, certainly centuries, is a theory that is not testable. If a theory is at all testable, it will not remain unchanged. It has to change. All theories are wrong. One doesn't ask about theories, can I show that they are wrong or can I show that they are right, but rather one asks, how much of the empirical realm can it handle and how must it be modified and changed as it matures?

As a lot of people know, I ended up leaving social psychology, meaning dissonance theory, and I want to clarify that. Lack of activity is not the same as lack of interest. Lack of activity is not desertion. I left and stopped doing research on the theory of dissonance because I was in a total rut. The only thing I could think about was how correct the original statement had been. Let me give you an example. When Jack Brehm and Bob Cohen produced their excellent book, *Explorations in Cognitive Dissonance*, one of the things they highlighted was the necessity of choice. I've never said this to Jack before. If you're eavesdropping you'll hear it now. I said to myself, what kind of a contribution is this? It says in the original book that in order for dissonance to be large enough to exist there has to be minimal pressure on the person to do what the person does. If there is too much pressure, there is too much justification for having done it and it is all consonant with having done it, there is no dissonance. Doesn't that encompass the idea of choice? Isn't choice one part of that? I said to myself, these wonderful people whom I like and respect are taking one operation and elevating it to the status of a construct and it's terrible. I may have been right, I may have been wrong. But that is to illustrate to you how every word in that book was perfect. So to me, I did a good thing for cognitive dissonance by leaving it. I think if I had stayed in it, I might have retarded progress for cognitive dissonance for at least a decade.

It seems to me that all of that controversy is documented and today there is a much more normal course of events. I think the talk by Joel Cooper is a very fine illustration of what ought to be and what should have been going on for decades and decades. Trying to explicate, trying to pin down boundary conditions and not just in a way that says, well if this condition is fulfilled you get dissonance reduction and if this condition isn't fulfilled you don't get it, but to understand why and broaden the theory and elaborate it. In addition, the demonstration that there is some physiological evidence for arousal I think is an extremely important finding and needs more research done. Recent stuff that has started exploring alternative modes of dissonance reduction is perhaps some of the most encouraging work I think that is going on. The early experiments emphasizing predictions from the theory that were counterintuitive generally blocked off every conceivable avenue of dissonance reduction that we could block off, so that whatever effect there was would show itself in attitude change. But in the ordinary world and if the experimenter is not very careful, a little bit sloppy, there are lots and lots of avenues of dissonance reduction, and those have never been explored. I still think that one of the major avenues of dissonance reduction is to change your behavior. When I think of examples, I even go back to examples that are in the book. If somebody is in a room, wants to leave the room, and just walks straight into a wall where there is no door, I would think there was considerable dissonance. And the usual way in which that dissonance is reduced is the person looks around and says, O my God, the door is there, and he walks out the door. And that's not very remarkable. But there are also many other avenues of cognitive dissonance reduction aside from attitude change. There is intricate restructuring of whole kinds of networks and relations among cognitions. Somebody can remember what his grandmother told him when he was two years old which solves everything, et cetera. Exploration of that kind of thing is very, very important. I'm glad it's going on.

I am quite sure that there is enough validity to the theory, and as changes are made, emendations are made, there will be even more validity to the theory, that research on it will continue, and a lot will get clarified. One thing that I think has to be done is for more research to go on on dissonance producing situations and dissonance reduction processes as they occur in the "real world." I put it "real world" because Elliot is quite correct. In the good old days when you did laboratory experiments, we created a real world in the laboratory. I don't know how we would have gotten anything through ethics committees. One of the things about laboratory experiments is that you can only get out the stuff that you put into it and any good experimenter who is concerned in testing a part of the hypothesis is going to try to eliminate from that laboratory experiment all of the unwanted stuff that generally floats around, and dissonance arousing and dissonance reducing processes are not the only things that affect man, using man in the generic sense. I think we need to find out about how dissonance processes and dissonance reducing processes interact in the presence of other things that are powerful influences of human behavior and human cognition, and the only way to do that is to do studies in the real world. They're messy and difficult. You don't expect the precision out of those studies that you can get in the laboratory. But out of them will emerge more ideas which we can then bring into the laboratory to clarify and help to broaden and enrich the work.

Historical Note on Festinger's Tests of Dissonance Theory

Judson Mills

Leon Festinger is a famous figure in social psychology. Festinger was, according to Jones (1985), "the dominant figure in social psychology for a period roughly spanning the two decades from 1950 to 1970" (p. 68). His theory of cognitive dissonance "is generally recognized as Festinger's greatest creative contribution, and research related to dissonance dominated the journals of social psychology from the late 1950's to the early 1970's" (Jones, 1985, p. 69).

Stories of the foibles of famous figures hold a fascination, which leads them to be told and retold. When such a story about a famous figure in social psychology appears in the *Journal of Personality and Social Psychology*, which is considered to be archival, it takes on an appearance of authenticity and may be presumed accurate by scholars of the field. A statement in the *Journal of Personality and Social Psychology* about Festinger's tests of dissonance theory will be regarded as factual unless corrected.

In a recent article in the *Journal of Personality and Social Psychology*, Anderson and Anderson (1996) stated that "Festinger is reported to have tried a number of ways to experimentally test dissonance theory, with limited success. Finally, Festinger and Carlsmith (1959) succeeded in getting the various parameters set in the range necessary for replicable dissonance results to be obtained" (pp. 741–742). That statement cannot be commented on by Festinger, who is no longer living. However, I was in position to know about Festinger's tests of dissonance theory up to and including Festinger and Carlsmith (1959) and can attest, on the basis of personal knowledge, that the report in the *Journal of Personality and Social Psychology* about Festinger's tests of dissonance theory is inaccurate.

Festinger presented the first version of dissonance theory in January of 1954, in a graduate seminar at the University of Minnesota, which I attended, and I was Festinger's research assistant from the fall of 1954 through the spring of 1957. In September 1956 at Stanford, Festinger showed a written description of the procedure that was to be used in Festinger and Carlsmith (1959) to Leonard Hommel, who was then also a research assistant to Festinger, and me, and he asked us to find some boring tasks and to devise measures. At the start of that study in the fall of 1956, Hommel was the first experimenter and I was the second experimenter who collected the ratings of the boring tasks, a role later shared with Robert Terwilliger, who interviewed half the participants in the published study. J. Merrill Carlsmith replaced Hommel in January 1957.

Except for the change in the first experimenter, the only substantial change in the procedure in Festinger and Carlsmith (1959) from the original design given by Festinger to Hommel and myself was inclusion of the mention of being on call in the future in the $1 and $20 conditions (which I believe was done to reduce refusals to accept the money). Festinger did not, before devising the procedure in Festinger and Carlsmith, try a number of ways to experimentally test dissonance theory with limited success. The procedure of Festinger and Carlsmith was not developed by altering various parameters until finally succeeding in getting them set in the range necessary.

REFERENCES

Anderson, C. A., & Anderson, K. B. (1996). Violent crime rate studies in philosophical context: A destructive testing approach to heat and Southern culture of violence effects. *Journal of Personality and Social Psychology, 70,* 740–756.

Festinger, L., & Carlsmith, J. M. (1959). Cognitive consequences of forced compliance. *Journal of Abnormal and Social Psychology, 58,* 203–210.

Jones, E. E. (1985). Major developments in social psychology during the past five decades. In G. Lindzey & E. Aronson (Eds.), *Handbook of social psychology* (Vol. 1, 3rd ed., pp. 47–107). New York: Random House.

Author Index

Numbers that appear in italics indicate pages in a reference list.

Subject Index

Self-consistency theory (*continued*)
  self-cognition processes and, 194–195
  self-expectancies in, 177, 185
  standards for behavior, 185
  timing of self-focused attention in, 179–180
  vs. self-affirmation theory, 130
Self-esteem
  dispositional, 132–135
  in free-choice paradigm, 178
  high/low, 122–123, 155, 156, 178, 180–181, 182–183, 186, 190–191, 193–194
  interaction with self-focused attention, 181–185
  priming effects, 178, 184, 191
  production of aversive consequences and, 121–122
  rationalization of behavior and, 128–133
  resistance to immoral action and, 121–122
  in self-affirmation theory, 180
  in self-based theories of dissonance, 155
  in self-consistency theory, 186, 192
  in self-expectancy theory, 180–181
  self-standards interaction, 192–193
Self-evaluation maintenance, 177–178
Self-expectancies
  definition, 176
  in dissonance processes, 177, 192–194
  role of self-standards in, 185–187
  in self-consistency theory, 185
Self-focused attention
  function, 179–181, 194
  timing, 179, 181–185
Self-perception theory
  attitude change in, 327
  conceptual basis, 10–11, 327
  limitations, 12
  misattribution research, 11–12
Self-reference effect, 3300

Self-resources, 128–130, 132, 134, 177–178, 192–194
Self-standards, 185–187
  accessibility, 188–191
  self-esteem interactions, 193–194
Simultaneous accessibility of inconsistent cognitions, 326
  alcohol effects, 341
  ambivalence and, 335–340
  attitude hardening response to identity dissonance, 342–348
  dissonance theory revisions and, 330–331
  early dissonance research, 332–335
  hypocrisy paradigm, 341, 349
  principles, 348
  recent dissonance research, 340–341
  trivialization effects, 340–341
Skin conductance response, 81
Smoking, 4–5, 38, 67
Sociocultural factors
  dissonance as cultural phenomena, 287–288
  in self-accountability theory, 206–207
  terror-management theory, 344–345
Sociocultural standards, 185–186
Specific cognitions, 63–64
Spread of alternatives, 6, 31–32, 182
  consonance modeling, 262
  eliminating, 332
  in free-choice paradigm, 258
Stereotyping, 137–138, 139–141, 142

Temporal awareness, 345, 346–347
Terror-management theory, 344–346
Transcendence response, 89–90
Trivialization
  cognitive restructuring and, 207–213
  simultaneous accessibility account, 340–341
Truth-telling, 50–53

About the Editors

Eddie Harmon-Jones is an assistant professor of psychology at the University of Wisconsin—Madison. He received his doctorate at the University of Arizona in 1995. He has conducted research on the necessary and sufficient conditions for the arousal of cognitive dissonance and on the role of affect in the dissonance process. In addition to continuing these lines of research, he conducts research aimed at understanding the motivation underlying dissonance processes.

Judson Mills is a professor of psychology and director of the Graduate Program in Social Psychology at the University of Maryland, College Park. He studied with Leon Festinger at the University of Minnesota and at Stanford University, where he received his doctorate in psychology in 1958. He worked as Festinger's research assistant during the period 1954–1957, when Festinger was developing the theory of cognitive dissonance.

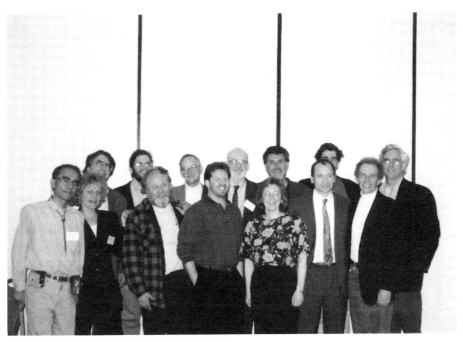

Top row, from left to right: Michael Leippe, Eddie Harmon-Jones, Jack Brehm, Judson Mills, Elliot Aronson, Joshua Aronson, and Mark Zanna.

Bottom row, from left to right: Haruki Sakai, Donna Eisenstadt, Jean-Léon Beauvois, Jeff Stone, Patricia Devine, Robert-Vincent Joule, and Joel Cooper.